Counseling Single Parents

Vera S. Maass, Ph.D., is a clinical psychologist, licensed in Indiana as Health Service Provider in Psychology and as a marriage and family therapist. She is a National Board Certified Counselor, a National Certified Addictions Counselor II, and a diplomate and clinical supervisor in the American Board of Sexology. She received her Ph.D. in 1978 from the University of Missouri-Kansas City and served a one-year clinical internship at the University of Kentucky Medical School in the Psychiatry Department, under the direction of Maxie C. Maultsby, Jr., M.D. During her training she had individual supervision by Albert Ellis, Ph.D.

Dr. Maass' professional memberships include American Psychological Association; American Counseling Association; American Association of Sex Educators, Counselors, and Therapists; The National Council on Family Relations; The National Association of Alcoholism and Drug Abuse Counselors; and the Indiana Psychological Association. Currently she serves on the board of the Indiana Council on Family Relations.

Dr. Maass combines influences from Dr. Maxie Maultsby, Jr., Dr. Albert Ellis, and others to create an internally consistent behavior change theory and a distinctive cognitive-behavioral therapy approach. She owns Living Skills Institute, Inc., a private practice agency in Indianapolis, and directs psychological services in a clinic that addresses sexual dysfunction issues. Dr. Maass is an active volunteer at the Indianapolis Museum of Art, and provides guest lectures at a local university.

Margery A. Neely, Ph.D., is a Kansas licensed psychologist (counseling), National Certified Counselor, and emeritus professor of counselor education at Kansas State University. She received her Ph.D. in 1971 from the University of Missouri-Columbia. She completed her internship at Southwest Missouri State University Counseling Center under Dr. Billy Rippee. She is a member of the American Psychological Association Divisions 17 (Counseling Psychology) and 51 (Society for the Psychological Study of Men and Masculinity); the American Counseling Association; Association for Counselor Education and Supervision; and, International Association of Marriage and Family Counselors.

Counseling Single Parents

A Cognitive-Behavioral Approach

Vera Sonja Maass
Margery A. Neely

 Springer Publishing Company

Copyright © 2000 by Springer Publishing Company, Inc.

All rights reserved

No part of this publication may be reproduced, stored in a retrieval system, or transmitted in any form or by any means, electronic, mechanical, photocopying, recording, or otherwise, without the prior permission of Springer Publishing Company, Inc.

Springer Publishing Company, Inc.
536 Broadway
New York, NY 10012-3955

Acquisitions Editor: Bill Tucker
Production Editor: Jeanne W. Libby
Cover design by James Scotto-Lavino

00 01 02 03 04 / 5 4 3 2 1

Library of Congress Cataloging-in-Publication Data

Maass, Vera Sonja.
   Counseling single parents : a cognitive-behavioral approach / Vera Sonja Maass and Margery A. Neely.
   p. cm.
   Includes bibliographical references and index.
   ISBN 0-8261-1313-3 (hc)
   1. Single parents—Counseling of. 2. Cognitive therapy.
3. Single-parent families. I. Neely, Margery A. II. Title.
HQ759.915.N43 2000
306.85'6—dc21
                                                           99-055582
                                                               CIP

Printed in the United States of America

Contents

Preface		*vii*
Acknowledgments		*ix*
List of Tables		*xi*
List of Figures		*xiii*
Chapter 1.	Background for Counseling and Therapy	1
Chapter 2.	Practical Theory-Building	27
Chapter 3.	Systematic Counseling Phases	49
Chapter 4.	Designating the Problem Area(s)	87
Chapter 5.	Identifying What Does Not Work	123
Chapter 6.	Introducing the Idea of Choices	163
Chapter 7.	Starting and Proceeding Along the Chosen Path	201
Chapter 8.	Reevaluating Progress	227
Chapter 9.	Generalizing Learning onto Other Situations	247
Chapter 10.	Reconceptualizing the Self	273
Chapter 11.	Coordinating and Balancing the Worlds We Live In	301
Chapter 12.	Where We Have Been—Where Are We Going?	329
References		*351*
Name Index		*365*
Subject Index		*369*

Preface

This book is written for advanced students in mental health professional training who have already learned the basic skills. It is also intended for professionals who desire additional information and stimulation for successfully counseling their single-parent clients. The phases of counseling/therapy are demonstrated through the use of composite cases. Our practice is based on cognitive theory, research, and clinical experience. The three assumptions behind the thrust of the chapters to assist professionals and advanced students are as follows:

1. The client has the responsibility and credit for any changes that occur.
2. The counselor can challenge defeating beliefs in a timely manner.
3. Successful changes may occur in small steps, but they reinforce new behavior and replace old self-defeating beliefs and behavior.

Acknowledgments

We appreciate the artwork prepared by Mary Hammel and the table prepared by Kathy Quigley and Julie Polson. Additional thanks to Alicia Neely for preparing the list of references.

List of Tables

Table 2.1. Single Parents' Beliefs
Table 2.2. Anxiety and Related Beliefs
Table 4.1. Cognitive Style
Table 5.1. Giving and Getting in Love Relations

List of Figures

Figure 3.1.   Susan's three worlds are depicted before and after therapy.
Figure 4.1.   Sample of the Interpersonal Growth Scale (IGS).
Figure 4.2.   Sample of the Intrapersonal Growth Scale (IGS).
Figure 4.3.   Ratings from Bill's Interpersonal Growth Scale (IGS).
Figure 6.1.   Ruth's list of activities.
Figure 6.2.   Becky's list of activities.
Figure 9.1.   Ratings from Bill's Intrapersonal Growth Scale (IGS).
Figure 11.1. Bill's three worlds—before and after therapy—reveal changes in his lifestyle.

1

Background for Counseling and Therapy

OBJECTIVES

1. To characterize the single-parent population.
2. To describe problems and potential strengths of single parents.
3. To sample research on attitudes and perceptions about single-parent families.
4. To introduce a therapeutic context.

BACKGROUND

Single parents face double difficulties and responsibilities. They handle twice the strain with half the resources found in two-parent families. In traditional families, both parents help manage children's health, education, behavior development, and emotional problems. Worries over job-related difficulties, finances, disappointments in friendships, and other setbacks can be shared. In single-parent families, all responsibilities fall upon one who is already stressed by emotional adjustment to the loss or absence of the other spouse. Single parents must combine several roles as they face financial and nurturing responsibilities that previously have been assumed by two parents. They may seek a counselor when they encounter problems without solutions, when friends and neighbors resort to, "You ought to find someone who can help." In her first session, Laura began to identify with other single parents. She said, "Yes, I'm a single parent—with double trouble!"

The purpose of this book is to demonstrate cognitive-behavioral counseling in action with examples of typical single-parent therapy sessions. All clients described in this book are composites of individuals in therapy. We provide information designed to shape realistic attitudes toward those who contribute major support for their children. We show some of the joy and travail that counselors experience when they choose to work with single parents.

SINGLE-PARENT POPULATION

Researchers consider single-parent families as significant components of our society, rather than atypical or pathological (Hetherington, Hagan, & Anderson, 1989). The so-called traditional family dates back to the 1940s (Women and work survey, 1998). Since 1970, there have been fewer than 20% of American families where father is synonymous with provider, mother means homemaker, and their two children are safely in school.

In context with the dramatic increase in the number of children living with a never-married parent—243,000 children in 1960, 3.7 million in 1983, and 6.3 million children in 1993—it has been predicted that out of 100 childbirths, 12 will be to unmarried mothers and that the parents of 40 children will divorce before the child reaches age 18. By the year 2000, it has been estimated that only 7% of the students attending public schools will be living in traditional two-parent nuclear families (Hodgkinson, 1985).

Incidence of Single-Parent Families in Various Parts of the World

Single-parent family formation incidence is increasing in other parts of the world as well. As they become urbanized, Hong Kong (Yeung, 1992), Singapore (Tan, 1992), and Thailand (Thailand Ministry of the Interior, 1988) report growth in single-parent families. As rural women in South Africa (Bester, 1995) and China (Li, 1994) are able to obtain divorce status, they establish single-parent families.

Background for Counseling and Therapy

In Europe, lone parents head almost one in five families in Great Britain, one in seven families in Denmark, and one in eight in Germany and France. Greece, Spain, and Italy maintain traditional families, about 19 to one, rather than join the single-parent-family incidence, according to an article about the family-value debate in Britain published in "The Economist" (1992). The divorce rates in the United States have led to a significant increase of single-parent households, demonstrated by a decline in the number of children younger than 18 years living with both their biological parents. In 1970 about 85% of children lived with both biological parents; in 1994 the percentage had dropped to 69 (Hines, 1997).

Characteristics of Single-Parent Households

Single parents become heads of household because they are widowed, divorced, never-married, or their spouses are absent for a significant period of time. U.S. Bureau of the Census (1997) statistics show that there were 50 million two-parent families in 1994, 12 million single-parent women heads of household, and 3 million men who were divorced, widowed, or never-married.

According to the Census report, almost 20 million children were living with a single parent. More than three-fourths of the children of divorce reportedly were living with their mothers (Hetherington, Bridges, & Insabella, 1998; U.S. Bureau of the Census, 1997). Mothers, who were divorced or living separately from spouses, were responsible for care of about half of these children; never-married mothers cared for more than 6 million of the children. Of the 3 million children living with a single father, about 2 million lived as children of divorce or separation. About 1 million children lived with never-married fathers. From 1995 to 1998 the number of single fathers in the United States has grown by 25%. Men represent one sixth of the nation's 11.9 million single parents. Although the number of single mothers is significantly higher, the increase in the number of single-father households seems to reflect changes in the attitudes of courts and society in general (Bart, 1999).

Traditionally, mothers were considered most capable in raising children and fathers were the main source for the family's financial resources. Many men leaving a marriage that was based on conventional sex roles initially have difficulty maintaining a household routine (Sprenkle & Cyrus, 1983). Single fathers are required to add homemaking and childrearing skills to their job skills. Single mothers, whose career orientation had not been strongly developed in the past, now may need to focus attention on acquiring job skills in addition to their homemaking tasks (Hogan, Buehler, & Robinson, 1983).

Problems and Potential Strengths in Single-Parent Households

Discussions about single-parent families have mainly focused on the difficulties experienced by these families. Several investigators have pointed out the negative aspects inherent in single-parent households (Garfinkel & McLanahan, 1986; McLanahan & Bumpass, 1988; McLanahan & Booth, 1989).

Single Fathers. Information concerning divorced fathers and their relationships with their children is scarce. Divorced fathers are less likely than mothers are to live with their children on a daily basis, although the number of fathers gaining custody for their children is increasing (Meyer & Garasky, 1993). Little is known about men's adjustment when they assume primary responsibility for the care of their children.

One recent study, using data from the National Survey of Families and Households, analyzed the impact of divorce on father-child relationships and fathers' psychological well-being (Shapiro & Lambert, 1999). The study was conducted over two time periods (Time 1: 1987 to 1988 and Time 2: 1992 to 1994). At Time 1, all 844 fathers were married and had at least one biological child below the age of 19 years on the full-time household roster. At Time 2, the majority (729) remained married, but 135 fathers had divorced or separated. Out of this group 33 fathers had the focal child living with them and 82 fathers' children lived elsewhere. Independent variables included marital status and child residence status, fathers' sociodemographic characteristics, characteristics of the focal child, time since separation, and relationship with former spouse.

The results, obtained at Time 2, supported the investigators' expectations that divorced fathers without their children in residence would report significantly poorer relationship quality than coresident fathers, regardless of marital status. An unexpected finding was that divorced fathers who had the focal child living with them reported significantly better relationship quality than continuously married coresident fathers. Regarding fathers' psychological well-being, regardless of child residence, divorced fathers had higher scores on depression than continuously married coresident fathers. Divorced nonresident fathers showed lower happiness levels than the continuously married fathers, but the lowest levels of happiness were obtained from the divorced coresident fathers. In summary, while divorced fathers who had their children living with them considered their father-child relationship to be of better quality than did any of the other groups of fathers, the levels of their own psychological well-being were the lowest.

The design of the study did not provide sufficient information to infer how much of the lack of happiness was due to the divorce and how much was due to the added stress of being the sole care providing parent. Apparently, information was obtained from the fathers only and, therefore, constitutes subjective descriptions. It might have been helpful to include the children as well as former spouses in the information-gathering process. As is, the conclusion can be reached that the stresses of single parenthood significantly impact the lives of both men and women. The case studies of Bill and Kent provide insight into the struggles experienced by fathers who combine the roles of provider and primary caregiver for their children. Bill had gained custody of his sons some time after the divorce due to his ex-wife's inability to provide adequate supervision. Kent became the sole responsible parent to his two children when his wife suddenly died as result of injuries sustained in an accident.

Single Mothers. Mother-only families have been regarded in the literature as a phenomenon that promises to change the social and economic context of family life for future generations (McLanahan & Booth, 1989). Single mothers are considered to be at greater risk for psychological problems and for ineffectual parenting practices than are married mothers. What are the factors accounting for the problems related to single-parent families? Compared to married parents, single parents likely experience economic hardship, reduced access to resources, and more stressful life events, while at the same time having less support from social networks (Kitson & Morgan, 1990; McLanahan & Booth, 1989). Another path of explanation focuses on traits or personality characteristics that places some people at risk for marital discord and other difficulties in functioning. The same characteristics that may have been instrumental in the marital problems leading to divorce may also impede the person's adjustment following the divorce (Kitson & Morgan, 1990).

Research about single mothers' mental health has mainly focused on symptoms of distress. Interviews with 518 single mothers and 502 married mothers in Ontario, Canada, revealed that single mothers were almost three times more likely than married mothers to have experienced a major depressive disorder. Additionally, single mothers were also found to have had a significantly greater number of adverse events during childhood and adolescence (Davies, Avison, & McAlpine, 1997). Analyzing the connections among adversities, depressive episodes, and family structure, the authors concluded that both depression and marital status are products of past experiences. Although there was a strong correlation between single parenthood and economic disadvantage, the authors did not believe that marital status and household income are collinear.

Effects on Children. Mother-only families have been described as reflecting economic insecurity and demonstrating negative intergenerational consequences. Children from mother-only families are considered more likely to be poor in adulthood and to become single parents themselves. The likelihood of adolescent antisocial behavior has been thought to be associated with mother-only households and conflict-ridden families (Demo & Acock, 1988). A study exploring the effects of single-mother families and nonresidential father's involvement on delinquency, drinking, and illicit drug use in Black and White adolescents found the highest rates of problem behavior among White male adolescents in single-mother families without the support of nonresident fathers (Thomas, Farrell, & Barnes, 1996). For Black male adolescents, fewer behavior problems were demonstrated in single-mother families without involvement of nonresidential fathers. Among Black families, the worst outcomes occurred when the nonresident father was involved with the adolescent male.

Some investigators expect the effects of socioeconomic disadvantage and certain maternal personality characteristics to be mediated to the children through the single mother's parenting practices (Bank, Forgatch, Patterson, & Fetrow, 1993). The authors focused on boys in elementary school and seemed to combine two studies. Subjects for one part were recruited through divorce application records and local advertising. They were divided into the "younger" group, consisting of 85 families with boys in K-2, and the "older" group, made up of 111 families with boys in grades 3 to 6. From another sample of boys recruited through the schools and thought to be at risk for delinquency, 56 single-mother head-of-household families were chosen. Measures used were structured interviews with the mother and child, laboratory parent/child problem-solving interactions, home observations, repeated telephone interviews, and questionnaires. The focus was on the three constructs of ineffective discipline, poor monitoring, and antisocial behavior problems.

The results supported the overall hypothesis that socioeconomic disadvantage and maternal antisocial qualities would have an impact on the sons' antisocial behavior problems and would be mediated through the mothers' family-management skills. Concerning the group of younger boys, neither ineffective discipline nor maternal antisocial behavior qualities were important predictor variables. With the older boys, mothers with antisocial behavior qualities—through their disrupted parenting practices—seemed to place their sons at risk for antisocial behavior problems. The authors concluded that it is not the divorce itself that causes antisocial behavior in boys, but that the demands and stresses of divorce and single parenting tend to reduce parent effectiveness and exacerbate the combined effects of negative contextual variables, such as socioeconomic disadvantage and maternal antisocial qualities. The study did not distinguish between boys who demonstrated adjustment problems before the divorce and those that developed problems after separation or divorce.

Larson and Gillman (1999) investigated the transmission of emotions in mother-only families. One hundred adolescents and their single mothers had been recruited through advertising. Participants carried alarm watches during their ordinary daily routines and reported their experiences at random times when signaled by the watches. Moderator variables focused on mother's characteristics, such as average anxiety and anger, mother's stress, social support, time spent in solitude, and parenting style. Time-sequence analyses of 651 contact occasions showed transmission of anxiety and anger from mother to adolescent but not from adolescent to mother. There were no significant differences for gender of the adolescents. The origins of mothers' transmitted anxiety and anger were indicated as being home- rather than job-related. Although transmission of anxiety was significantly correlated with high stress experienced by the mothers, the opposite was true for transmission of anger. It appeared that in families where mothers experienced high stress, their anger tended to produce anxiety, rather than anger, in their adolescent children. The amount of time a mother spent by herself moderated the transmission of both anxiety and anger.

The study did not involve single fathers and their children, nor did it look at transmission of emotions within two-parent families. Therefore, the findings need to be considered with caution.

Another study examining how tension is transmitted between the marital dyad and parent-child dyads showed that both mothers and fathers were more likely to have tense interactions with their children after experiencing marital stress. Fathers reported twice as much spillover of tension on days when experiencing work overloads or home demands than on stress-free days. Fathers also reported more spillover when wives were working full-time. Mothers reportedly experienced more stress spillover in families with adolescents in the house (Almeida, Wethington, & Chandler, 1999). Thus, the transmission of emotions does not appear to be limited to interactions between single mothers and their children. The observation of the beneficial effect of solitary time on the transmission of negative emotions reported by Larson and Gillman (1999) has valuable implications for counseling.

Marital conflict interferes with competent parenting, and children's externalized behavior, such as hostility directed toward other people or things, can be expected to occur (Mann & MacKenzie, 1996). To explore the effects of family environment on children's emotional and behavioral adjustment to parents' divorce predictor variables of parent-child relationships, marital conflict, and child temperament were used in a study involving a sample of 178 children. Greater marital conflict before divorce was found to be correlated with more problematic parent-child relationships after parental separation. In turn, poorer parent-child relationships are related to impaired emotional and behavioral adjustment in children after separation (Tschann, Johnston, Kline, & Wallerstein, 1989).

Judith Wallerstein's longitudinal study of 131 middle-class children and their divorcing parents seems to indicate that the impact of divorce increases over the first three decades of children's lives. Children of divorce continue to experience difficulties after high school and even after college (Wallerstein & Blakeslee, 1989). Hetherington and colleagues (1998) summarized research on children's adjustment after divorce, stating that 20 to 25% of children of divorce experienced adjustment problems, as compared with 10% of children in two-parent families. The authors concluded that children from disrupted families have a greater incidence of adjustment problems before as well as after divorce. The conclusion would be that marital conflict—rather than dissolution of the family system—is indicative of the children's adjustment problems.

Amato (1993) considered various perspectives that seem to influence children's adjustment to divorce, and offered several hypotheses. Frequency of contact with the noncustodial parent is important for children's well-being, but the presence of another adult to take over the role of the absent parent will have a positive effect on children's well-being. The literature provided inconsistent support for the assumption that frequency of noncustodial parent's contact was positively correlated with the level of children's well-being. The author's hypothesis that remarriage of the custodial parent will be more beneficial to the children's well-being than if the custodial parent remains single was not supported by the majority of studies reported in the literature. Also, due to the socialization effect, children were expected to fare better when they are older at the time of the parents' divorce, but conclusive support was not available in the literature. In conclusion, Amato suggested that a useful framework for further research should consider the total configuration of resources and stresses inherent in the whole divorce situation.

In response to Amato's proposal, Allen (1993) argued that considering the traditional family as the best environment for rearing children leads to a narrow focus on marital disruption as the most important factor in children's reduced well-being. In her opinion, the standard of the traditional nuclear family with the male head of household providing for his dependent wife and their children is a myth.

Recent exploration of parenting characteristics revealed that stability of the emotional connection between parent and child and predictability of the caretaking relationship are the most significant variables regarding children's adjustment (Silverstein & Auerbach, 1999). The authors considered these variables to be independent of the number of parents in the home or the sex of the parent.

Potential Strengths. Without doubt, the dissolution of a traditional family unit and the assumption of significantly increased responsibilities bring with them many difficulties for all members of these families—no matter what their specific circumstances. But as pointed out by Hetherington and Anderson (1987) while divorce and related family transitions constitute developmental vulnerabilities for some adolescents, they may promote growth opportunities for others. For some children of divorce, an increased sense of competence, creativity, and responsibility can be the result of family transitions. Such potential strengths within the new parent-child system need to be recognized and emphasized when working with this client population.

The case study of Susan, described in detail in Chapter 3, demonstrates how children's creativity and initiative can flourish in spite of the discomfort that accompanies the process of adjustment to the changed family system. In this particular case, the children's healthy adjustment to the transformation also assured a continuing relationship with their grandmother. The new interactions placed the relationship on a more meaningful basis for all concerned than had previously been the case.

As single parents assume exclusive or shared responsibility for the care of their children, an opportunity exists for reduced ambiguity and contradiction regarding behavioral rules within the family and consequences resulting from the violation of such rules (Maass, 1991). In two-parent families, children have chances to make use of the differences in discipline approaches between the two parents, and align themselves more closely with one or the other in attempts to emphasize the difference to their own advantage. Depending on the parenting style of the main care provider, the discipline systems can be established in simple and exact terms where rules are spelled out precisely and where consequences follow in a logical and predictable manner, leaving little room for unnecessary and destructive arguments. This did not work in the case study of Laura. After the divorce, her husband's more authoritarian approach no longer balanced her egalitarian parenting style. The relationship between her and her daughter evolved into an enmeshed family system where Laura's attempts at discipline became totally ineffective.

A different state of affairs is illustrated in the case of Betty, the widowed mother of three children. During her husband's lifetime, Betty's authority with her children was severely weakened. While still struggling with the emotions that accompany the loss of a spouse, Betty established herself firmly as head of her household and provided structure and limits for her children.

When too much month outlasts too little money (Neely, 1992b), parents' problems meet resources head on. Jon expects a quick trip to the sporting goods store when he says, "Mom, I have to have $135.00 for basketball shoes." In view of her limited resources, Jon's mother assumes the roles of financial manager, negotiator, and family CEO as she guides her son to a compromise, "Are you willing to help pay basketball team expenses by working a part-time weekend job?" By working together on decision making, parents help children understand how decisions can be mutually beneficial (Haines & Neely, 1989). Jon's affirmative response led to his gaining strength in the family. It also led to his mother's reaching a higher level of security in her single-parent role. Some problems resist parents' best efforts; some require rules and limitations, but many yield to patient negotiation.

Among the opportunities for growth that can evolve from reconstructions of family systems is an altered focus on the person's self-conception. Out of necessity the person may ask, "What are my strengths?" Concentration on self may be sharpened secondary to reduced distraction that comes from a shift from consideration about another person to consideration of the self. Again, the case of Susan is a good illustration. The combination of a perceived need for increased financial resources and the availability of mental and emotional energies that previously were used to focus on her husband's interests resulted in realistic appraisal of her abilities and careful planning of future actions. The process of exploring new directions and deciding which one to embark upon requires blocks of uninterrupted time. As wives and mothers, women are more accustomed than men are to respond immediately to interruptions. Their readiness to respond to interference leaves them ill-prepared to set aside significant periods of time to focus on themselves and concentrate on their ideas. When intense concentration on the well-being of family members is combined with lack of encouragement and derogatory remarks from significant others, focus on dreams of self-fulfillment and realistic appraisal of their feasibility become remote possibilities. The case study of Lynn depicts such a situation.

Additional case studies demonstrate how increased competencies and interests may develop out of new needs resulting from transformations of family systems. For single fathers, the required performance of household chores and food preparation may spark an interest in nutrition and increased community involvement, as can be seen in the case of Bill. From the initial reluctance to even consider the possibility of divorce, to the assumption of full custody for his sons, he faced many challenges. The successful resolution of those challenges expanded the range of stimulating interactions with others and the level of his personal satisfaction.

Just as male heads of households may have to learn skills that previously were the responsibility of their wives, suddenly-single female parents need additional preparation or training to improve their marketable job skills to achieve financial independence. Kahla, the young woman encountered in Chapters 9, 10, and 11, who was confronted with a long period of temporary single parenthood due to her husband's imprisonment, demonstrates the desperation a person would likely experience in such a situation as well as the strength and determination possible to gain control over her life.

Perhaps less frequent, but still probable, are problem situations involving parents or parents-in-law of the single heads of households. Grandparents may seize an opportunity to rejoin the family nucleus and may precipitate a struggle for head of household status (Jackson, 1995). Similarly, grandparents may attempt to remove the children from the custody of the single parent, with the rationalization that the grandparents are better equipped to care for the children than the single mother or father. Such attempts are more likely to occur when the father is the custodial parent. Kent, the widowed father of two children, encountered such demands from the parents of his deceased wife. His mother-in-law appeared quite adamant in her desire to take charge of her grandchildren. From the struggle over his children's care, Kent gained increased sensitivity and understanding about his own and others' feelings. His personal growth enabled him to successfully argue his case and to apply the lessons to other areas of his life as well. Similarly, Bill, who became primary caregiver to his sons, had to consider the likelihood that his former parents-in-law would attempt to gain custody over their grandsons.

Of course, dissolution of a marriage as a means to promote the development of individual potentials would not be recommended by anyone. But when family systems break down or disintegrate, adjustment to the new circumstances can be greatly helped by turning a situational loss into a learning experience that will eventually lead to other opportunities. The clinician's role is to facilitate the shift in emphasis from loss to opportunity. Strong attention to losses carries with it the risk that clients will see themselves as victims of some outside forces. Attitudes of victimology erode the notion of responsibility (Seligman, 1999). If people consider their difficulties to be caused by others, they tend to expect solutions to come from outside themselves. The therapist's role is to guide clients beyond the victim stance by encouraging them to recognize their strengths and stretch their abilities in the search for solutions.

ATTITUDES AND PERCEPTIONS ABOUT SINGLE-PARENT FAMILIES

Traditional families have set the family prototype, and any other structure is deemed inferior (Henderson, 1981). The messages that single parents present an immoral lifestyle model to their children, and that children must have male and female parents in order to grow up properly, are often delivered via school, religious institutions, and neighbors. As children from single-parent households are often expected by teachers, social workers, psychologists, and counselors to have more problems than children from intact families (Amato & Booth, 1991), these expectations may be expressed in the teachers' or counselors' behaviors toward the children. The overtly or covertly expressed expectations function as self-fulfilling prophecies, exacerbating or generating the anticipated difficulties (Amato, 1991).

Schools and public agencies have a job to do as they face the effect of family structure on community attitudes, social values, and achievement (Bogolup, 1995; Masten & Coatsworth, 1998). Some schools have initiated group counseling programs for children of divorce (Yauman, 1991) and guidance for children from non-traditional families (Crosbie-Burnett & Pulvino, 1990). It has been shown that role strain (Morrison, Page, Sehl, & Smith, 1986) can be reduced by supportive education in self-help techniques, communication skills, and conflict resolution (Neely, 1992a; Newhouse & Neely, 1993).

The facts of a dissolved marriage or an absent spouse do lend credence to single-parent family myths. Direct parental child care suffers when single parents work outside the home in order to pay the bills (Maass, 1992). When parents lack preparation for a family break-up, their bitterness leads to troubled children (Hetherington et al., 1998).

Because divorce is a common feature of single-parent families (Kelly, 1988), the assumption prevails that children of divorce will eventually end up divorced themselves. Testing the hypothesis that single-parent problems would be transmitted through generations, Prater (1991) reported a high pregnancy frequency among never-married women who were reared as children of never-married mothers. Another study focusing on never-married mothers (Coley & Chase-Lansdale, 1998) revealed that only about one third of the female children and 11% of the males became teen-age parents.

The significant number of nonmarital births in the United States, combined with the likelihood that these households will receive public assistance, has contributed to the unfavorable public opinion of single mothers being "welfare" mothers. Discussions of unmarried motherhood have generally focused on teenagers. More recently, though, it has become apparent that there is an increase of nonmarital births among women aged 20 years and over. In fact, women aged 20 years and older show a greater percentage of nonmarital births than women below age 20. Nonmarital birth rates since 1980 have increased 61% for teens, as compared to 69% for women aged 20 to 24 years, 67% for 25- to 29-year-olds, and 82% for women 30 to 34 years of age. Analysis of data from the Panel Study of Income Dynamics (PSID) describing a total of 2,613 births to 1,615 women between 1980 and 1990 revealed that the economic status of older, single mothers is closer to teenage mothers than to married childbearing women their age (Foster, Jones, & Hoffman, 1998). The total sample consisted of 23% unmarried and 77% married women. Among the older nonmarried childbearers, more than half (56%) were involved in the labor force to some degree in the year prior to the birth. After birth, involvement of older single mothers in the labor force dropped to 47%. Nearly three in five of them were using food stamps or AFDC after birth. The authors recommended that because postbirth rates of welfare use are nearly as high among nonteens (33%) as among teens (39%), further attention be given to the link between welfare and nonmarital childbearing at older ages.

The National Survey of Families and Households (NSFH) was conducted at two different time periods (1987 to 1988 and 1992 to 1994), involving a sample of 1,536 women who had a birth in the 5 years before the first interview (Driscoll et al., 1999). From the sample, 480 women were not married at the time of the birth and 285 of them were still unmarried at the time of the first interview period. At the time of the second interview period, women with nonmarital births at the first interview who were still unmarried had the poorest socioeconomic outcomes and were more likely to turn to welfare as a source of financial support. Women with nonmarital births at the first interview period who had married before having another birth were statistically indistinguishable from women who had only marital births.

Meyer and Cancian (1998) used data from the National Longitudinal Survey of Youth (NLSY) that were collected on over 5000 young women over a period of 14 years. They selected a sample of 594 women for whom detailed information regarding AFDC and non-AFDC income was available, in addition to data covering 5 years after leaving AFDC support. The investigators found great diversity in the economic status of young women after they left AFDC. In the third through fifth years after leaving welfare, more than one fifth of the women had incomes over twice the poverty line. One fifth of the sample did not receive any welfare payments during the entire 5-year period. The percentage of women not receiving welfare rose over the 5-year period from 40 to 55%, and the percentage of poor dropped from 56 to 41%. However, nearly four fifths of the women received a means-tested transfer at some time within the 5 years after exiting AFDC. Nearly one fifth of the women remained poor during the whole 5-year period.

Overall, women who were working and those who married at the time they exited AFDC, did better. Women with higher earnings potential demonstrated higher levels of success. More education, fewer children, or older children are contributing factors to higher earnings potential. The highest levels of economic well-being were found in women who worked and were married at the time they left welfare, but it is necessary to examine if the women's income alone would be enough to exceed the poverty line.

The studies mentioned above appear to support the dire prediction that the destiny of a significant portion of single-parent families headed by mothers is one of persisting poor socioeconomic and distress-ridden existence, unless the mother enters into another marriage.

Single mothers can refuse to succumb to the pessimistic outlook, and can seek counseling services to explore alternative solutions that will lead to increased independence and self-sufficiency. The concept of self-sufficiency should not include marriage as a long-term solution. If the woman remarries, subsequent marriages may be disrupted, as current statistics reflect, and she will find herself in the same problem situation as before. Thus, the woman's self-sufficient income is a more useful concept than a marriage-oriented definition of self-sufficiency. One path to increased self-sufficiency is work experience, but obtaining adequate child care is often difficult. Pursuing additional education or job-skills training present opportunities for future independence (Sandfort & Hill, 1996). Ruth, the young mother of two, was dependent on public assistance when she and her friend Becky came for conjoint therapy sessions to save money. Her case study is described in chapter 6 and serves as an illustration of how self-sufficiency can be achieved despite adverse conditions.

In-depth evaluation of the literature goes beyond the scope of this book, although it is important for therapists to keep informed about research relating to their areas of professional interest and to stay abreast with new developments. Even though reported results do not always conclusively point in one direction, they stimulate thoughts about the described dynamics and how the findings can be integrated into the therapist's particular theoretical approach.

THERAPEUTIC CONTEXT

"I've tried everything. Nothing works" is a common theme that clients bring to an initial therapy session. They urgently wish to reduce stressful feelings and remove roadblocks that seem to pop up in front of their goals. Therapists come prepared with an assortment of cognitive skills and behavioral techniques. They hope to set the process in motion with an effective interacting style.

Clients are often surprised when they recognize that counseling may be characterized as a confrontation between two complex belief systems. They may be taken aback when they face the notion that changing attitudes and thought processes lead to different emotions and behaviors.

Theoretical Orientation

Therapists seem to be achieving some convergence on theoretical orientation as well as agreement on optimum therapeutic approaches for different client groups. Warner (1991) reported surveys of American psychologists, Canadian psychologists, and Canadian counselors about theoretical orientation and influential theorists. All three groups preferred an eclectic orientation in first place. Cognitive-behavioral theory was chosen second by Canadian psychologists and third by Canadian counselors and American psychologists. Albert Ellis (rational-emotive behavior therapy) and Carl Rogers (person-centered therapy) were named among the top three as the most influential present-day therapists. Sigmund Freud (psychoanalytic therapy) was included in the top three by American psychologists, who also gave second place to psychoanalytic theory. The other two groups named Aaron Beck (cognitive therapy) as one of the top three influential therapists.

Another survey inquired about counseling approaches utilized in group therapy by certified alcohol and drug counselors and counselor trainees in the state of Arkansas. This revealed that most adhered to Reality Therapy. Behavior Therapy was second in preference, and Rational Emotive Therapy and Rogerian approaches tied for third place (Whisnant, Hammond, & Tilmon, 1999).

With the work of Ellis (1962, 1973) as foundation, this book incorporates ideas of Maultsby (1984) and other theorists to form an internally consistent theory of cognitive-behavioral therapy. The ancient question about what causes behavior remains intact for philosophical argument, social commentary, and chemical tinkering in the nervous system. A group of casino players may consist of lonely people who wish to be part of a crowd, some mathematics professors who are quite familiar with the theory of large numbers, and a few psychologists who see the others as candidates for Gamblers Anonymous. Here we prefer to describe behavioral choice as a continuous (Mahoney, 1991), purposeful process that has multiple influences.

Some theorists view thoughts as behavior determinants; some describe thoughts and beliefs similarly. We assume that environmental influences and thoughts about them trigger people's belief systems. We assume that people act as if their perceptions are accurate and their beliefs are true. Beliefs are major components of attitudes about situations and values that include goals, morals, and ethics.

Our mission as therapists is to help those who seem to be thwarted in their efforts to do well and feel good. We start therapy with the assumption that clients bring us their faulty beliefs and perceptions that are at odds with reality or are not in their best interests. We assume that clients who initiate treatment with us are stressed, in conflict, and have a history of doing some things poorly. But clients also have a record of achievements and talents that they can build on. New clients can be compared to athletes in a slump; they are looking for a coach.

Problem Identification

When John, a new client, comes to the office saying, "Everyone is on my back. My ex-wife, my kids—now the cops," it is obvious that he is hurting and is looking for help. John would do well to have a counselor and coach when he continues his complaints with, "Yeah, alcohol's the problem. But a drink or two makes me relax. It's good to relax, isn't it?" To the therapist, John signals urgent problems that form tentative treatment hypotheses. He is in conflict with himself, his primary relationships, and society when he reveals the connection of his difficulties to alcohol abuse. With the use of fractured logic, he came up with a belief, "Alcohol is good for me." The belief is false, life-threatening, and goal-blocking.

As phases of counseling follow one another, clients grow in natural and often predictable ways. From an initial painful situation, clients learn to challenge beliefs that are not worth having, and they obtain new coping skills. In time, clients acquire different views of themselves and their abilities. Finally they arrive at an improved set of life-building skills. Therapists have a role as teachers who help clients reach their goals. The therapy process consists of instruction, learning, and practicing goal-directed behavior. All three are required to change, to do better, and to feel better.

Relationship Dynamics

Therapists attempt to establish a collaborative relationship where clients feel safe, trusting, and free to explore historical and environmental influences that may lead to faulty or self-defeating decisions. Within this collaboration, clients acquire a new belief system and construct a behavior change model for future use.

"Tell me something about your decision to come in today" is an example of an ambiguous stimulus, a projective technique that one may adopt as a therapy opener. Clients' early responses may be equally vague and full of generalities. Their answers often take the form, "It's a mess. I can't stand the thought of going home from work." The example entails an opening for discovery of the client's cognitive style when the therapist asks, "At the end of work, what are some of the thoughts that come to mind when you think of home?" Therapists model elements of their therapeutic style when they attend to clients' responses, record exact quotations, and use clients' words to explain what happens in therapy or counseling.

Rapport. Emery (Beck, Emery, & Greenberg, 1985) points to the importance of good therapeutic relationships in effective time-limited cognitive therapy. He describes rapport in terms of sincerity and accurate mutual understanding between therapist and client. Albert Ellis (1995) teaches that people do well in relationships when they refuse to evaluate themselves or others, but instead freely appraise the behaviors and characteristics that bring them to therapy.

Ethical Structure. Therapists set the treatment pace and conditions that include payment terms, conditions of confidentiality, diagnosis, and their own competence limitations. Clients often want an answer to the question, "How long will this take?" Responsibility for duration of the counseling process can be transferred to the client with an answer such as, "The session schedule belongs to you. After the first session today, we hope that you will decide if you can benefit by further work. We will encourage you to evaluate your progress regularly and assess probability that this work will help you reach your goals."

Ivey and Ivey (1998) point to theoretical, diagnostic, and practice considerations that promote ethical decisions to accept or refer a client for treatment. They indicate the value of enhancing client strengths with the admonition, "If you can't find something positive in the client's behavior and history—refer!" The authors describe the *Diagnostic and Statistical Manual of Mental Disorders* (4th ed.) (DSM-IV) (American Psychiatric Association, 1994) as a classification system focused on labeling attitudes and behaviors, and instead propose a developmental approach. With reference to the concept of depression, they argue that labeling or naming the condition is a source of client victimization.

When the authors (Ivey & Ivey, 1998) describe developmental counseling on a path toward cultural awareness, they recognize the divergence between value systems in different cultures. It is important to recognize that some cultures regard interdependence and holism as family foundations, while others hold autonomy and independence as important developmental tasks. Therapists, who are in a developmental state, should realize that they face a multitude of variables when they attempt to locate all the issues in a client's life.

When clients come to therapy, the general expectation is that they have a goal in mind. A competent counselor will describe a therapy agenda that is goal-oriented and is based on a path that the client recognizes as a different way of going. In a recent description of his behavioral and emotional change theory, Albert Ellis (1996) stated that he attempts to help clients promote goals that are constructive and less hostile to themselves and others. He seeks to establish attitudes that are scientific, tolerant, and flexible.

Therapeutic Alliance. A working partnership between therapist and client develops over time. Each brings a complex belief system that evolves in its unique personal setting. It grows with different educational experiences, family influences, and cultural surroundings. Each partner comes to the session with a different set of skills and problems.

Clients and counselors face different tasks throughout the counseling process (Highlen & Hill, 1984). Orlinsky and Howard (1986) believe that collaborative effort can be measured by outcome success. They conclude that outcome depends on reciprocal role investment, empathic resonance, and mutual affirmation. With clients' goals in mind, therapists continually look for points of intervention, promote homework, and evaluate progress.

Process Variables. In a review that covered therapy process data from 1950, Orlinsky and Howard (1986, pp. 312–313) said that five conceptual elements are included as constituents of psychotherapeutic process:

> *Therapeutic contract* defines the purpose, format, terms, and limits of the enterprise.
>
> *Therapeutic interventions* comprise the "business" of helping carried on under the terms of the therapeutic contract.
>
> *Therapeutic bond* is an aspect of the relationship that develops between the participants as they perform their respective parts in therapeutic interventions.
>
> *Patient self-relatedness* refers to the patient's ability to absorb the impact of therapeutic interventions and the therapeutic bond.
>
> *Therapeutic realizations,* such as insight, catharsis, discriminant learning, and so on, occur within the session and presumably produce changes in the patient's life or personality. Measurable changes become the subject of outcome evaluations.

Cognitive Therapies. The stimulus effects of prior events and attractive goals have some influence, but cognitive therapy works on the notion that people make purposeful behavioral decisions from a wide range of choices. While therapy outcomes do not yield readily to rigorous scientific examination, clients do have an opportunity to learn a different way of feeling and behaving. They identify, challenge, and disconfirm old beliefs. Their new ways may be less than perfect, but they can free themselves from repeating the same behaviors and expecting different results.

John, the client who was dedicated to the use of alcohol, developed the belief that alcohol was good for him through a series of premises that seemed to withstand any challenge. Alcohol does lead to physical relaxation. Relaxation is good. In therapy, John learned that Aristotle worked on similar problems more than 2000 years ago when he proposed the form known as a practical syllogism. As therapists, we continue his teaching that when values become problems, it is a good idea to consider additional variables in the premises. John began to weigh the consequences of his drinking. He decided, with some reluctance, that abstinence would be a better choice than continued liver damage, ruptured relationships, and extensive jail time.

Dryden (1994) describes development of Albert Ellis' theory and practice of psychotherapy over 32 years. With added observations by psychologists who practice Rational Emotive Behavior Therapy (REBT), a huge library of reference to Ellis' contributions exists. As Ellis suggests, we resist the urge to imitate his style, and to some extent, we have changed his and other theorists' language to fit our approach.

We teach the notion that all of us fashion a complex belief system continuously. We form perceptual observations and judgments. In our purposeful search for fulfillment, joy, and happiness, we act as if our beliefs are true and our perceptions are accurate. On the other side of the coin, the conflicts we experience correlate with faulty beliefs and perceptual errors.

In consonance with many cognitive-behavioral practitioners, we disclaim most evaluative concepts that start with "self-". Clients usually open up entrenched belief systems brimful of anxiety, anger, and guilt when answering the question, "How would you know if you had self-confidence?" Their answers are likely to lead to one of REBT's well-established intervention targets, the belief that, "I must be a terrible, rotten, defective person." We minimize use of hypothetical variables. For example, we affirm that everyone is motivated to behave all the time. Therapy interventions point to ineffective behavioral choices and search for alternatives towards which clients are willing to work.

Phases

A therapist who understands clinical syndromes, has trained to become a good psychotherapist, and is well-versed in the conceptual framework is ready for supervised practice in cognitive therapy (Beck, Rush, Shaw, & Emery, 1979). Most therapists notice that clients follow a learning curve that has several stages.

1. Designating Problem Areas. Generalities often shroud reasons for initiating therapy. Client expressions may be limited to "I can't do anything right. There's no use trying." Clients begin to know that they can reconstruct their lives when they freely specify things they are willing to change.

2. Identifying What Does Not Work. We teach that thoughts trigger beliefs that lead to dysfunctional behavior and negative emotionality. Those beliefs are intervention targets. For practical, clinically based reasons, we declare thoughts as different from beliefs. We have yet to find a client who can successfully comply with a promise such as "Well, I'll just stop thinking about it." We identify what does not work because there are lessons that can be learned from less than perfect solutions.

3. Introducing the Idea of Choices. Our clients hear sage advice from Yogi Berra: "When you come to a fork in the road, take it." At important junctures, options include purposefully heading toward a goal that is potentially less than perfect, repeating old behaviors that have been shown to be ineffective, or exploring uncharted territory for new ways. The significance of this phase is to perceive and welcome additional options.

4. Starting and Proceeding along the Chosen Path. Clients often face and succumb to barriers such as "I might mess up. I might not like it." Such road-blocking thoughts summon beliefs that inspire capitulation. Techniques to strengthen goal-directed behaviors can be utilized. Imagery skills and behavior rehearsals are part of the preparation process that facilitates successful outcomes.

5. Reevaluating. Assuming responsibility for behavior and consequences allows for occasion to assess the quality of outcomes. Was the outcome worth the expenditure? There are also opportunities to challenge remaining destructive rituals, or to opt for a different course of action.

6. Generalizing Learning onto Other Life Situations. Each success provides a powerful analogy for future challenges. Repeated application of new behaviors serves to strengthen the new behaviors and increase the level of comfort that the individual experiences while performing on a new course of action.

7. *Reconceptualizing the Self.* Cognitive-behavioral theory and therapy techniques attend untiringly to individual responsibility. New behaviors and added competencies likely modify the concepts individuals have of themselves. Behavior changes do not occur in a vacuum, and realistic assessments include attention to reality and the influences of others in the environment (Bandura, 1977a).

8. *Coordinating and Balancing the Worlds We Live In.* Clients have but 24 hours each day to consider goals that they can pursue when they are alone, in solitude. They can work toward improving their relationships; they can act out aspirations in their competitive world of work. Therapists have the same tasks to accomplish each day, and they make room for social learning theory, existentialists' discoveries, and a reminder or two from Aristotle in their cognitive-behavioral way of thinking. Clients and therapists do well to achieve a healthy balance of activities in their day-to-day living.

The chapter that follows describes some of the contributions that lead to current practice. Chapter 3 recounts a clinical experience that contains elements of all eight phases. Chapters 4 through 11 are each dedicated to individual therapy process phases. Chapter 12 presents a brief historical reflection and contains a message of hope, along with a reality check for aspiring therapists.

Single parents see themselves alone on an emotional roller coaster. They learn to perceive intense feelings as part of their constantly changing family challenges. They gain confidence in the process when they agree to work toward moderating severe emotional responses. Their job in therapy is to recognize that normal family difficulties have minimal threat and danger; and that problems respond to competence, reason, and hard work.

SUMMARY

This chapter presents a description of various features of the single-parent population. Some of the problem areas that are characteristic for this population, as well as its potential strengths, are highlighted.

Equally important factors to consider are attitudes and perceptions about single parents and their families, because attitudes have an additional impact upon the way single parents regard themselves and their opportunities for sustained self-sufficiency.

Single-parent families are significant parts of most neighborhoods. They include characteristics as variable as those in traditional families, plus features usually associated with careers, time constraints, and relationships. Considering these families as making "normative lifestyle choices that are firmly established in society, rather than as social problems or pathological behaviors" (Coleman & Ganong, 1990, p. 930), would likely result in different attitudes. Emphasis would be placed on the inherent resiliency of these families, instead of subjecting them to an attitudinal system of victimology where society assumes responsibility for healing what is not broken. A family that undergoes transitions in the constellation of its members is not like a broken leg. Cognitive counseling offers a safe, neutral, accepting, and growth-stimulating atmosphere that encourages clients to focus on their strengths and abilities when learning new ways to cope, new ways to adjust, to their role as single parents.

The chapter concludes with a brief introduction and preview of the therapeutic context that is representative of the rest of the book.

EXERCISES

Write a short, one- or two-page description of your behavior change and emotional response theory. Compare your change theory with a classical theorist who tends to agree with you and with one who works on a different set of assumptions.

SUGGESTED READINGS

Bogolub, E. B. (1995). *Helping families through divorce: An eclectic approach.* New York: Springer Publishing Co.
   The author studied couples of different ages, their ethnicity, gender, and income levels in context of mental health professionals' roles.

Ellis, A. (1996). The humanism of Rational Emotive Behavior Therapy and other cognitive behavior therapies. *Journal of Humanistic Education and Development, 35*(2), 69–88.

The author presents a short description of his practice and application of the psychotherapy system that he has developed over the past 30 years.

Haines, J. M., & Neely, M. A. (1989). *Parents' work is never done.* Far Hills, NJ: New Horizon.

The authors offer suggestions for handling children ages 18 to 30 as the children face adult developmental tasks and crises.

2

Practical Theory-Building

OBJECTIVES

1. To describe preparatory theories of psychotherapy.
2. To introduce foundations for practical theory-building.
3. To choose theory applicable constructs and treatments.
4. To develop a practical psychotherapy.

THEORY-BUILDING

Individuals who seek psychotherapy make an appointment with a therapist, agree to a therapeutic contract, and take on the role of patient because they want to do better or feel better—or both. Those who pay the bills—employers, managed care companies, and prospective clients—confront a bewildering task when they approach treatment alternatives. New drugs and other procedures appear and disappear with regularity. Some are promising, and some just promise. The period from 1970 to 1980 may be remembered as the decade of proliferating psychotherapy theories, and third-party payers. In the 1990s there were hundreds of behavior-change theories, and a pronounced reduction in the number and willingness of payers. Raymond Corsini (Corsini & Wedding, 1995) recognized the trend toward eclecticism and suggested that counselors and psychotherapists would do well to develop their own theory and methodology.

In spite of a constantly changing treatment environment, therapists are continually responsible for coming to the appointment with an internally consistent behavior- and emotion-change theory that includes clinically tested treatment techniques.

In this chapter, we sample behavior and emotional change aspects of typical psychotherapy theories representing a range of conceptualizations that were available to us when we were students. The four preparatory theories present elements of clinical practice that we rejected or borrowed for our own. We trace the development of a practical cognitive-behavioral change theory that the senior author began in the 1970s. Albert Ellis (1962, 1973; Ellis & Harper, 1975) provided the foundation. Maxie C. Maultsby, Jr. (1971, 1975) provided the internship opportunity to work, learn, and continue the process of practical theory building. We respect and appreciate theorists who help us in our continuing search for effective therapeutic methods.

Preparatory Behavior Change Theories

As students, we were intimidated when we found that there were dozens of diverse psychotherapy theories and that the number multiplied each semester. In our attempt to wade through the theories, we grouped them according to the way that theorists conceptualize human behavior development. At least on one dimension, behavior modification and psychodynamic theories seem to be based on opposite suppositions. When B. F. Skinner (1972, p. 280) said that behavior modification is environment modification, he established a position that behavior development comes from outside the individual. Psychodynamic theories speak of drives, conflicting forces, and unconscious motivation; they emphasize that behavior development sources are within the person. Along the outside-inside continuum, social learning theories emphasize environmental influences, but include behavioral development by the individual. Cognitive theorists identify individuals as a primary source of affect and behavior, while they recognize influences in the environment.

Behavior Modification. We answered a psychology class challenge to use reading as a social reinforcer with a group of parents who had children in special education classes. Our assignment was, "If you develop an If-Then experiment and do the study this semester, you will get a grade for the course." One member of the experimental group, Ann, was separated from her husband; she had primary care responsibility for her 12-year-old son. The boy's father was short-tempered. He loved his son and wished to reunite the family. On visitation weekends, he requested that the family go to church together. The father was a talented barber and he was dedicated to Sunday football.

A devastating family ritual brought Ann to counseling. After church and lunch, the young boy went out to play while his parents discussed the possibility that they could work things out together again. Uneasiness dampened the atmosphere when Ann realized that it was time for her son's haircut. The parents had come to expect their son to fuss about coming indoors, knowing he would complain and squirm while the game was on. Ann knew the day was ruined when her husband looked at his watch, turned on the TV, and bellowed to the whole outdoors, "Get in here. You've got to have your hair cut."

For her part in the class experiment, Ann agreed to program church, lunch, and haircut followed by parental discussion while their son went out to play. Her directions to her son included, "If you follow the Sunday schedule, I will read a story to you before bedtime." Ann was supposed to record the story-reading times in a log. In a subsequent meeting of the mother's group, she reported that family Sundays had greatly improved. She said, "My son fell right into the new schedule. We haven't had a haircut temper tantrum since." When asked about story time and her reading log, she said, "Oh, I didn't have to do any of that. They both just fell into it."

While our response to the class assignment failed to reach the level of an experiment, we learned that family ritual development may be worthless, behaviors can change, and there are likely to be more variables in the process than those we measure. We also learned to have a high regard for Premack's principle: that people will perform some behavior that they dislike in order to do something they like (Neely, 1982). While Ann may have believed that her son and his father just fell into a new routine, behavior modifiers quickly observed that she held high-frequency behaviors, such as outdoor play and TV football, contingent upon completion of the haircut, a less enjoyable behavior for son and father.

Behavior therapy proceeds on the basis of behavior analysis that traces problem behaviors from their onset to the situations that currently control them. This includes a searching exploration of background conditions, family relations, and traumatic experiences. Human behavior is a result of what happened over the person's lifetime. An individual's behavior, its relevant situations, and consequences are interrelated. Together, they are called contingencies of reinforcement. Feelings and states of mind do not cause behavior; they are byproducts of behavioral contingencies.

Joseph Wolpe (1976) derived treatment procedures from behavior modification theory because "all of its techniques are based upon experimental findings" (p. 62). He asserts that successful therapy outcomes in modalities other than behavior modification are inadvertent, and that conditioning is the behavior change process. He refined his description of the change process when he said that behavioral and emotional response change treatment is conditioned inhibition based on reciprocal inhibition. Research on the autonomic nervous system parallels clinical experience. Anxiety and fear inhibit laughter, and laughter inhibits negative emotional responses. Counter-anxiety responses include relaxation, assertion, and sexual expression. After deep muscle relaxation, patients imagine anxiety-evoking situations from low to high disturbing capacity. As emotional responses diminish in the therapeutic imaging process, patients find that the real stimuli lose their power to evoke anxiety.

Social Learning Theory. In his development of Social Learning Theory, Albert Bandura (1977a) recognized that behavior is influenced by its consequences, that people learn new patterns of behavior by observing others, and that individuals participate in initiating and maintaining their behavior. Functional patterns develop by interaction between environmental events, individuals, and their behavior. He asserts that cognition has causal influence on behavior, but that most human behavior is learned through observation of successful behaviors modeled by others. On intake, Sue provided an account of her adoption of a new pattern of pervasively influential behaviors.

> Sue jammed on the brakes as her car hit an ice slick and began a sickening slide into a concrete post. She couldn't believe that her car was a total wreck. A few minutes before the accident Sue had finished her night shift work and left the company parking lot.

Sue responded to the accident immediately; she asked to be put on the day shift, and accepted a cut in pay in order to get the new position. She felt shaky and ill at ease when her son drove her to work. On the job, she complained that she couldn't focus, and she took temporary leave. In the next few months, Sue felt that she couldn't face the trip to work, and the job. She decided to quit work.

At first, Sue had a good support system. She lived next door to her parents and close to her son and his wife. She began to remove herself from social activities—one at a time. She did not drive; her son took on that responsibility. She felt sick to her stomach, dizzy, and nauseous in crowded places; her daughter-in-law took her shopping and agreed to accompany her at a weekly bingo evening. Sue spent most of her time inside her home. She reduced the frequency of her trips next door. Her parents increased their time with Sue in her home. Sue begged off shopping as often as she could. Her daughter-in-law began to pick up a shopping list and deliver the groceries to Sue at home. With each year, Sue drew a tighter circle around her diminishing activities.

Twenty-five years after Sue's slide on the icy street, her doctor moved to a new office on the fifth floor, and her daughter-in-law discontinued participation in the weekly outings. Sue found a new physician. Without friends, she could not find anyone who would take her to her favorite activity—bingo.

Sue presented none of the signs of intense emotionality. She seemed shy and retiring, but composed when she told her story of gradually diminishing well-established behaviors at work, driving an automobile, and encountering crowds in public places. She described her avoiding elevators and fear of leaving home alone. Tearfully, she told about leaving her family doctor and loss of her daughter-in-law's support.

When Maddux (1991) described acquisition of self-efficacy feelings, he drew the picture of Sue as she managed to create a 25-year-pattern of success at failure. She learned to dissemble a career in which she had progressed to shift supervisor. She surrounded herself with supporters who faced the crowds and operated complex machinery with her or on her behalf. She established a social environment peopled by those who would comfort her and cheer her on. Sue avoided adverse consequences of career loss when she qualified for disability benefits. She valued her son and other family members as she saw them take on the daily chores that she associated with fear, shakiness, and other odd feelings. In spite of hints from her supporters, Sue continued to restrict her behavioral repertoire over the years.

To promote durable and generalized behavioral and emotional changes, Bandura (1976) suggested that the best strategy is to model threatening activities repeatedly and to provide an environment in which the client can perform successfully. This restores formerly inhibited behavior and is followed by self-directed performance that extinguishes residual fears and reinforces personal efficacy. Sue expressed her goals in therapy as, "I want to find a way to get back to my regular doctor, and I want to play bingo again on Friday nights."

Force Theory. Lipson and Perkins (1990; see p. 209) developed a theory of human behavior that helps explain how people find themselves behaving contrary to their own best interests. Force Theory is a member of the group of theories that place behavioral and emotional development within the individual. They present the notion that external events—encounters in relationships and the environment—are processed as perceptions that form motivational forces. Force Theory incorporates ideas of individual differences. The theorists observe that Force Theory diminishes cultural and other group differences as behavioral determinants. Lipson and Perkins say that our daily behaviors proceed in response to the net effect of motivational forces. They recognize that we may find ourselves at the mercy of psychological forces that shape counterintentional behavior, and that our will power is often at a loss to cope with the combination of forces that lead us to respond. We chose Force Theory as an example of preparatory conceptualizations because the theorists present their ideas to us in everyday language, with a minimum of hypothetical variables, and limit their considerations to behavior that is counter to our intentions or best interests.

Psychological forces provide us with images of behavioral and emotional determinants that have power and direction. Peer pressure and moral imperatives direct and predict the way we act. Those who toe the mark and make an impact are known to be dependable and productive. Individuals who shilly-shally, hedge their bets, and beat around the bush can be counted upon to prolong negotiations and resist decision-making. People credit inner forces when they explain strategic successes with "I knew I had it in me." By their common names, motivational force attributions acquire characteristics of "good" and "bad" as well as "weak and strong."

Force Theory maintains that inner strength—will power—is a strong force among other strong forces, such as primary drives, the force of habits, and hidden forces that operate beyond our control or awareness. In combination with forces on the positive side of the good-bad continuum, will power contributes to desired behavior. Negative forces plus will power provide a framework when we attempt to explain violence and evil. Will power can be overcome by motive forces in combinations that result in behavior and emotionality that is contrary to our intentions and best interests.

Theorists believe that clients have a range of behavior change opportunities to augment inner strength in their quest for doing better and feeling better. They point to gaining insight as an aid, rather than a magical cure, for feelings that hurt and behavior that leaves a lot to be desired. In their development of Force-Field Analysis, Pfeiffer and Jones (1974) suggest a treatment technique that clients use to develop insight and decision-making resources. For the exercise, clients describe a problem behavior at the top of a piece of paper divided into two columns. One column is designated Restraining Forces; the other, Driving Forces. Restraining Forces are responsibilities or commitments to themselves, to others, or to outside factors. Driving Forces are alternative behavioral choices, help from others, or changes in the environment that help clear the way for goal achievement. The instructions are

1. List Restraining and Driving Forces.
2. Note forces in both columns that are outside of your control.
3. Renumber forces in each column, in order of importance; exclude those outside of your control.
4. Recognize Restraining Forces likely to yield to Driving Forces that you control.
5. Create a time-line for step-by-step action.

Cognitive Therapy. Cognitive therapists make the basic assumption that faulty thinking causes psychological problems. When they devise a treatment plan, treatment consists of identifying aberrations in thought processes, testing the validity of thoughts and beliefs, and modifying thoughts and attitudes that lead to unrealistic appraisals and misconceptions. Aaron Beck (1976) described cognitive therapy as a problem-solving exercise that includes active participation by his clients. Through learning and applying problem-solving techniques, clients generalize their skills to include new problems as they arise.

Beck, Emery, and Greenberg (1985) described anxiety as one of several mechanisms that people employ to cope with threat and danger. Anxiety is maintained by mistaken perceptions and distorted appraisals of life events. Excessive use of anxiety as a coping mechanism leads to the acquisition of involuntary, automatic thoughts and fantasies related to possible harm. Automatic thoughts are common points of intervention in cognitive therapy.

The theorists observe that an anxious person overreacts or reacts inappropriately in novel situations. Angry people respond to a startle by quickly assuming a combat-ready condition as their automatic thoughts promote verbal or physical display. Physical responses to startle and automatic thinking take form as recoil, stiffening, or flinching; voluntary muscle groups go into action automatically, involuntarily. Automatic thoughts exert continuous pressure on behavior, emotions, and physical feelings, even though an individual has evidence to show that the situation is neither threatening nor dangerous.

In his development of a cognitive therapy protocol, Gary Emery (Beck et al., 1985) described the cognitive change model in the initial session. He stated that patients often feel relief when they hear that their physical responses—sweating, increased heart rate and dizziness—are results of automatic thinking, rather than signs of impending death. His goals in the therapy process are to describe emotional problems in everyday language, relate emotion management to the patient's misconstructions, and lead patients to identify and correct their faulty thinking. Theorists find that patients who learn to develop options and use successful outcomes as analogies for future successes expand on these concepts and apply their therapy experiences in their daily lives.

Beck (1976) recognized that cognitive therapy and psychoanalysis are insight therapies in that both work with thoughts, feelings, and wishes that are reported by patients. Cognitive therapists rely on consciously derived meanings and inferences that are available to the patient for consideration and correction. They seek to understand the elements of how patients misinterpret reality, rather than find the answer to, "Why?"

Change Process Models. We included Behavior Modification, Social Learning Theory, Cognitive Therapy, and Force Theory because they present different answers to the question: "What are the sources of problems that people bring to a therapy appointment?" We chose models that place behavior development inside the person, and those that assume behavioral determinants are located in relationships, cultures, or other environmental factors. Therapists in training realize

Practical Theory-Building 35

that they have just begun to establish their theoretical framework when they find their place along the outside-inside continuum.

Practical Theory Foundation

Single parents come to therapy because they face stressful situations that refuse to yield to their best efforts. Statements by single parents (see Table 2.1) indicate a range of beliefs that they bring to the therapy session, provide a hint of their cognitive styles, and show that

TABLE 2.1 Single Parents' Beliefs

I'm responsible for peace and harmony in the family.

I'm the wife, homemaker, and mother, not the head of the household.

I won't ever grow up.

I know how a parent should behave.

I'm a gentle, loving woman who places others' needs above my own.

If I take care of things too well, people won't help me when I need it. In fact, people won't like me.

I am committed to honor a dying person's wish.

I have to be loyal to younger as well as older people in my family.

I value my individual independence.

I don't know what people think of me if I am stern with the children.

Good deeds will find their rewards.

It's a woman's duty to support her man.

What kind of a person am I to keep the children away from their friends?

What would people think if I . . . ?

Parents are responsible for their children's behavior.

Where there's a will, there's a way.

You can't lose by trying.

If at first I don't succeed, I try, try again.

there is usually a wide gap between events in their daily life and the experiences they are about to enlist. Few parents expect to confront a behavior-change theory when they decide to talk to a therapist.

In the absence of convincing philosophical assumptions or empirical evidence to support one among the hundreds of available theories, therapists choose training programs, treatment methods, and therapist-client interaction styles that are consistent with a personal philosophy and scientific approach. Because Albert Ellis' development of Rational Emotive Behavior Therapy (REBT) is ubiquitous in psychotherapist training programs, we present elements of Ellis (1994a) as a summary of our foundation theory. This serves as a behavior- and emotion-change model and as a specific treatment example related to a traumatic rape experience cited below.

Rational Emotive Behavior Therapy (REBT). Albert Ellis (1995) bases his theoretical work on the assumption that almost all human behavior, mood, and emotional response is attributable to a complex cognitive system that includes perceptions and beliefs. Ellis (1994a) described posttraumatic stress disorder (PTSD) in terms of REBT theory and stated that rape victims create PTSD by their dysfunctional beliefs. He recognized that response to severe trauma, such as exposure to rape and combat, may reach the threshold of PTSD diagnostic significance, or it may not. If the diagnostic level is reached, the rape victim may feel fearful and blame herself inappropriately. Some rape victims escalate their response to include recurrent nightmares, frantic avoidance measures, and panic.

As the victim's therapist, Dr. Ellis explained that her symptoms were real and painful, but normal and natural, in response to her appraisal of the attempted rape by an uncle and forced date rape by a man she trusted. Her appraisal included beliefs, such as the following:

> I must be weak, defective, rotten. I should have prevented it.
> All men are rotten. I can't trust anyone.
> I can't stand to live this way.
> I shouldn't have this panic. I shouldn't feel this way.

As she learned to identify and challenge her beliefs that were not true, in her best interests, or simply not good for her, she lessened her anxiety about anxiousness and panic. The intensity of her responses lessened. She recognized that while her physical feelings were uncomfortable, they were not intolerable or life-threatening.

The next step in therapy was to attend to the lifestyle consequences that the client had developed. She began to establish a belief that behaviors can be evaluated and changed if they are faulty. Ellis introduced several theoretical concepts and behavioral techniques that included the following:

1. Recording and reviewing therapy sessions.
2. Using REBT concepts in daily contexts with friends.
3. Considering and debating the usefulness of avoidance behavior.
4. Openly describing her part in the date rape that she considered a weakness.

As the client learned REBT theoretical constructs and put them into practice, she extended the time between sessions. She checked periodically for a review of her progress and new behavior acquisition.

Ellis (1994a) recounted constructions that people make to arrive at severe dysfunction. They include core beliefs, such as the following:

1. I must be approved by others. If not, I'm incompetent, defective.
2. Because I want others to approve of me, they are rotten, despicable if they don't.
3. Because I want to live comfortably, it's awful if I don't. I can't stand it.

Interaction with Clients. In his development of REBT, Ellis (1962, 1973, & 1994b) placed the client on center stage. Relationships, careers, and environmental conditions provide perceptions that exert influence on behavioral decisions and associated emotional responses. Misperceptions, faulty logic, and beliefs that are not worth having precipitate behavior that clients bring to the therapy session. Clients learn to change, to practice behavior- and emotion-change skills, and to assume responsibility for doing better and feeling better.

Theory-Applicable Constructs and Treatments

In his analysis of dysfunctional behavior, Albert Ellis put the human organism between the behaviorist's stimulus and response. He recognized that people construct a belief system over their lifetimes, and respond to their beliefs when they behave. Maxie C. Maultsby, Jr. (1975, 1984) developed criteria for beliefs that were subject to change because they were associated with dysfunctional behavior. We teach that it is a good idea to discard beliefs that are not true, not in our best interests, or not worth having. These criteria are at the base of a challenging process that leads to behavior and emotion change. A large part of our treatment session consists of identifying and challenging beliefs that our clients express as they tell us their stories and treatment goals.

The work of Ivey and Ivey (1998) that they named Developmental Counseling and Therapy (DCT) presents us with a dramatic example of theory and treatment implications that are different from our foundation. The authors note that external stress changes biological functioning, and build on that observation to say that atypical human behaviors are logical responses to environmental contingencies. They use war, rape, and natural disasters as obvious examples. DCT expands these stressful experiences to include migration, racism, and other external oppressions as sources of atypical behavior, defensive personality styles, and other PTSD symptoms. They conclude that implications of posttraumatic stress are basic components of therapy with severely distressed clients. Ivey and Ivey recognize that adoption of a culture-centered treatment approach would require changes in therapist training, educational systems, and political reorientation over several years.

Challenging Beliefs. We teach that perceptions and thoughts trigger beliefs. Beliefs that presume threat and danger lead to anxious feelings. The following table, Table 2.2, contains a selection of statements

TABLE 2.2 Anxiety and Related Beliefs

1. It's incredibly difficult to let this run its course.
2. How am I going to get myself out of this?—avoid it!
3. I get thinking about—Am I going to make it through without anxiety?
4. There's plenty of things I need to do, shopping at the mall, restaurants.
5. Where did I park the car? Am I going to find it?
6. I must be damaged goods.
7. The church thing, sitting in crowds.
8. It seems—I need something to worry about.

by an anxious client in a single session. Each statement contains a belief or refers to a belief that is worth a challenge. Statement 6, in Table 2.2, is a metaphor for the belief "I'm defective; There is something wrong with me."

Clients often express elements of their belief system when they respond to a question such as, "What thoughts were running through your head when you said . . . ?" For example, Ed, the client portrayed in Table 2.2, said, "I'm afraid that I will get fidgety when I'm sitting in a crowd. People will laugh at me; think I'm weird. That would be awful." His thoughts in statement No. 7 led him to believe that he was in a threatening situation when he sat in church or other crowded places. Another question, "What did you mean when you said . . . ?" led Ed to respond to our reference to No. 4 with, "I'm not like other people. I can't do a simple thing like shop at the mall. I have to make excuses all the time. I'm sick of it. There's just no use." Ed's answers to these, and other questions in the session indicated that his avoidance techniques were no longer working for him, and that his beliefs of hopelessness and helplessness signaled depressed mood in addition to the anxiety he presented as the reason for his coming to therapy.

The Worlds We Live In. Ludwig Binswanger (1962) and other existentialist philosophers recognized that we act in multiple worlds that may appear independent but are constantly interacting. They coined this phrase to describe the way people shift behavioral patterns as they move from one situation to another. Some of those who come to therapy seem to have a one-dimensional set of coping abilities. We believe that optimum development includes building a repertory of behavioral skills that can be called upon as we attend to our career, relationships, and to our personal activities.

A long-haul truck driver was a loner at the truck stops as well as on the road. He seemed absorbed in TV and radio evangelism. On breaks, he lost himself in meditation. He said that the most important aspect of his life was working toward his own salvation. Feeling neglected in the atmosphere of Bible reading and prayer, his wife broke up their marriage. She thought he was crazy.

A Company CEO carried his bulging briefcase home from work. After a quick dinner he left the children and their nanny, climbed into bed, and read copies of all the correspondence his company generated each day. Another commuter picked up her children from day care, came home in time to accept a pizza delivery, and after she told her children to do their homework and go to bed, she would spend the evening on the Internet.

In addition to the varied DSM-IV characterizations of these clients, another way of describing their behavior is that they were stuck in their personal world, or to borrow from the existentialists, die *Eigenwelt* /dee ˋī-gen-velt/ (see Chapters 3 and 11 of this book for a detailed description of the concept of the three worlds). When it is balanced with the other worlds we live in, the *Eigenwelt* provides opportunity for growth, creativity, and expressions of our individually oriented competitive values. Rather than exclusive focus on their schizoid, workaholic, or digital-addiction characteristics, clients may do well to develop behavioral skills in their personal world. They can move from loneliness, to the reality of being alone, then to solitude in their personal world. They have the opportunity to learn balance in the world of relationships, *die Mitwelt* /ˋmit-velt/, and the world around us, *die Umwelt* /ˋúm-velt/.

We Act as if Our Beliefs Are True. We present this assumption in almost every session when we describe behavioral determinants and formation of attitudes and values. When we teach that we act as if our beliefs are true, we create a tautology that also declares, "When our behavior and associated feelings leave much to be desired, we are acting on beliefs that are not true, not in our best interests, or not good for us." The presumption that we act as if our beliefs are true leads directly to a notion that a revised belief system is the key to behavior change, to doing better, and feeling better.

This "as-if" concept allows clients to take responsibility for their own behavior. It gives them an opportunity to challenge and change beliefs and behavior that lead to destructive family rituals, useless habits, and stereotypical emotional responses that are not worth having. Clients are able to free themselves from faulty childhood lessons, cultural values that may be worthless, and notions that they are somehow defective if their performances leave a lot to be desired. They are responsible for making changes that reduce conflict in the world the way it is—with themselves, their community, and with others who are important to them.

Where Do Emotions Come From? This question has as many answers as there are friends and neighbors, self-help books, and experts in the field. Answers may reflect myths that feelings just happen or that they are wired into our genes. Some people believe that other people, places, and things cause negative and positive feelings. Clients often answer with a shrug when they face the question, "What leads you to break out in a sweat when your boss asks a question?" Their modal reply is, "I don't know." Their answer may be augmented with, "I just know he makes me angry. All he has to do is look at me." The challenge to the belief that other people can make us behave and respond emotionally is complex; it starts with recognition that we respond to our perceptions as if they are accurate. If we see another person or typical experience as aversive, we often attribute our negative emotional responses to them.

Developing a Practical Psychotherapy

We establish the notion that negative emotions promote misperceptions and trigger beliefs that are not true or not worth having. Because feelings have intensity and direction, their impulse often leads to harmful behavior. High emotionality restricts ability to make competent decisions. Clients learn that a sense of composure sets effective conditions for behavior change, and results in a higher success rate than admonitions to "Get a hold of yourself. You've got to fight it. Just do it."

Anger and the Addiction Cycle. The repetition tendency associated with anger leads clients to describe it in conflicting terms. They cite arguments that break up relationships, explosive encounters with children, and self-denigration as reasons for seeking therapy. They are quick to counter these observations with, "It gives me strength, courage. I like to feel the adrenaline flow. Anger lets me know I'm involved. It gets respect; it makes me feel good." Anger is progressive. Children escalate temper tantrums when they learn how far they have to go through the supermarket before their parents relent and buy the candy bar. Adolescents learn "If I get angry enough, I can win" and "Revenge, I can get back at them." Adults shatter important relationships when they seek competitive advantage with "When I'm angry, I have the power. I get what I want."

Clients report a scenario that is common to many angry confrontations. They begin with a perception such as, "She shouldn't mind such a simple request." The words seem reasonable, but they are often delivered as the first law of human relationships. The exasperated client turns livid as he assumes a moral obligation to change the situation. When he confronts relationships in shambles, he is likely to respond with "Don't I have the right to be a little upset?"

We agree with Carol Tavris (1982) who describes anger as the misunderstood emotion. Anger hurts. It is a strong motivational force. Anger puts a damper on inhibitions that help make reasonable decisions. We believe that behavioral characteristics such as equanimity, calm, and balance describe effective lifestyles. Clients often see a gain when they learn to diminish self-righteous, overbearing, and angry behaviors.

Another Way to Look at Fear and Change. A client who lives in fear comes to therapy with the belief "I've tried everything; nothing works." Clients express a single-minded crusade approach to fear and avoidance as "I've got to defeat this thing. I can't stand the loneliness." In the same breath they exclaim, "I'm terrified to think of going out alone—I hate the feeling."

We teach that attitudes about a crowded shopping mall or restaurant lead to rapid heartbeat, tight chest, and shallow breath. Self-downing attitudes lead to headaches and weak knees. Clients learn, in a paradoxical way, that their bodies respond normally and naturally to their shopping-mall attitudes and self-downing beliefs—as if they were true. Clients discover the idea that it would be in their best interests to accept, indeed, welcome, the physical feelings and begin to challenge their attributions of threat and danger in social situations. Clients have the option to extend their social involvement. They gain freedom to recognize when they are secure, safe, and free from threat. When clients accept responsibility for their physical feelings and behavioral choices, they are also able to define, expand, and explore their comfort zone.

It Feels So Good When It Is Over. A client described her decision to come to therapy as "I worry all the time. I can't get things off my mind. It's getting me down. I get depressed and I worry about that." When asked about a recent example of her concern, she said, "My daughter went on vacation and I spent those few weeks in agony. Terrorists. Plane wrecks. I just knew that something awful would happen to her." She also added, "I was so relieved when she called to tell me she was safe. We laughed and cried together. I loved it."

The last part of her description became a feature of her therapy; she heard about the Worry-Relief cycle and how the good feelings of relief served to increase her tendency to worry. At first, the client found it difficult to realize that her love for her daughter could be linked to her anxiety and depressed moods. She began to recognize that she frequently established a Worry-Relief cycle and exclaimed, "Yes, I worry all the time. I rehash everything—over and over." Then she added, "I hope you aren't telling me that I should cut her out of my thoughts and feelings, just let go of her. That I shouldn't love my daughter." How could there be a negative result, i.e., establishment of a painful process of repetitive anxiety and depression, from the strongest possible urge—a mother's love? Yes, the client's love for her daughter was coupled with beliefs that were not true, beliefs that she could foretell the future, and that the future would be awful.

Strongly held beliefs are often based on misperceptions, faulty suppositions, or information that is wrong. As this client worked in the therapy process, she began to realize that she often miscalculated the probability of danger to herself and others. She thought about disasters that were possible but improbable. The client was certainly aware of the joy she experienced when her daughter returned home safely. She was surprised to learn that those good feelings reinforced the Worry-Relief cycle and effectively increased worry frequency and intensity.

Mystery and Myth—Worry and Pain. A young man began his therapy session with "I had a miserable week. The pain. I've got to get it out of my mind. I've got to fight it." His pain is real. It radiates from hand to elbow. Its features are mysterious, unpredictable, and frustrating. In spite of many clinic visits, the young man has little promise of a successful intervention. He faces frustration in his work and household chores. A daily hassle, chronic pain is a likely factor in all of his future plans. A few of his myths about pain and its consequences include

The pain. I have to control it. To control it, I have to fight it.

Worry. I always worry. That's me. That's the person I am.

Frustration makes me furious—when I can't do things I should be able to do.

Worry activates me. It makes me a better person.

I worry a lot. It takes my mind off the pain.

What do other people think when they see this bandage?

Wouldn't anyone be angry about a thing like this?

We invite our readers, as we invite our clients, to consider this list of myths and challenge faulty beliefs or logic that they contain. Challenges include answers to

What beliefs are expressed in these myths?

Does the myth reflect the world as it is? If not, challenge perceptions and assumptions.

Does the myth work well for him in his relationships? Explain your evaluation.

Is the myth based on beliefs that are true, worth having? If not, provide alternatives.

Communication. As an integral part of a complex cognitive system, clients bring a well-rehearsed, often rock-solid, communication style to the therapy session. Clients often describe communication roadblocks that they experience within themselves and with others. Her expressions include, "He doesn't respond to a thing I say." He counters with, "She doesn't listen. When I have something to say, she just rattles on about something else." Together, they exclaim, "We never settle anything. Every little thing goes on and on until one of us blows up." They seek therapy because their relationship has gone downhill to "We don't communicate." Another way to look at problems of communication is to work on the assumption that people always communicate. They deliver a message when they seem oblivious to the other's voice. Body language often provides a withering reply that requires no translation.

The flow of information between people does not always come easily. In these introductory examples, the man who evades his partner's communications and the woman who redirects the conversation away from the other person's requests are helping to thwart the goals of their being together. Conflicts in these interactions may head toward acceptable resolution when one or both are able to clarify their wishes and wants. Unfortunately, the conflict can intensify with responses such as "You men are all alike." He adds fuel to the fire when he asks, "Why do women always change the subject?"

The escalating argument that seems to go on and on is common enough to have a name: The Game Without an End (Watzlawick, 1990). Individually, we are able to carry on a game without an end when we berate ourselves with thoughts and beliefs such as "I should have more self-confidence, more will power. I don't try hard enough. I ought to be making more money, have a better job." With others, we can clam up and keep the game going, or continually find exceptions to what the other person says. For a start, it is often valuable to recognize that arguments seldom work. In recognition of the complexity of human interactions, we add that powerful communication skills are flexible, tentative, and tested often for effectiveness.

We also teach that an inclusionary communication style, on an inclusionary-exclusionary continuum, is a valuable asset worth achieving. One who uses the inclusionary style responds or thinks positively, or at least in terms of reality-oriented events. To the question, "How was your day?" the inclusionary answer may be, "Good. I got a lot of work done this morning." An exclusionary communication describing the same day is likely to be "Morning was not bad, downhill after that—the usual hassle." Exclusionary communicators seem to search the horizon for negativity, faults, and gripes when they are greeted with, "How's it going?" Their most effusive positive answer seldom exceeds, "Not bad."

SUMMARY

This chapter describes features of counseling and psychotherapy theories that propose to help therapists and clients reach therapy goals of feeling better and doing better. From the many available theories, we limit this chapter to four that have discrete assumptions about sources of behavior and emotional responses. We describe behavior-modification treatments that assume that behavior originates in the environment outside the individual. The psychodynamic model attributes behavior to inside forces. Social Learning Theory and cognitive therapy models assume that behavior arises with combinations of the extremes along the outside-inside continuum. Rational Emotive Behavior Therapy is a foundation theory that places behavior-change responsibility in the client. In subsequent chapters, we will demonstrate practical theory-building as it applies to single-parent treatment. In therapy, clients have an opportunity to challenge and change that part of their cognitive system that produces dysfunctional behavior and adverse emotional response; the therapist teaches alternative ways to behave effectively.

EXERCISES

1. Recall a serious problem you faced and use Force-field Analysis to describe the problem. Discuss with a classmate.
2. With Sue's intake information, pp. 30–31, plus the suppositions and theoretical implications of a theorist you choose, respond to the following:
   a) What causes Sue's avoidance behavior?
   b) Describe three or four points for therapy intervention.
   c) Describe two or three therapeutic techniques that promise Sue substantial progress.

Choose one or two of the response opportunities. Limit your answers to a single page.

SUGGESTED READING

Bandura, A. (1997). *Self-efficacy: The exercise of control.* New York: Freeman.
  Bandura's recent book discusses how perceived self-efficacy operates within a broad network of sociostructural influences that people produce and at the same time are produced by.

Beck, A. T. (1988). *Love is never enough.* New York: Harper & Row.
  The book is a practical manual about handling marital communication based upon Beck's cognitive therapy.

Ellis, A., & Harper, R. A. (1975). *A new guide to rational living.* Englewood Cliffs: Prentice-Hall.
In this classic book, the authors present a theoretical basis for human behavior and behavior change.

3

Systematic Counseling Phases

OBJECTIVES

1. To provide an overview of a counseling process structured for work with single parents.
2. To describe the individual phases, their purpose, and their content.
3. To demonstrate different strategies that can be employed for the resolution of a particular phase.
4. To illustrate the natural progression of phases within the entire process.
5. To show how the counselor facilitates the client's work in a particular phase and transition to the next one.

PHASES

This chapter describes the various phases in the process of counseling single parents using a cognitive approach. During the development of each phase, opportunities for strengthening the individual's independence will be explored and emphasized. The counseling process is not fundamentally different from that used with individuals and families in general, but a shift in focus and emphasis is required when addressing the needs of this particular population. For instance, in divorce or separation, individuals experience conflicting emotions that are specific to their situations.

Eight phases are identified. Each will be briefly described with a composite case. These phases are:

1. Designating the problem area(s) to be addressed;
2. Identifying what does not work;
3. Introducing the idea of choices;
4. Starting and proceeding along the chosen path;
5. Reevaluating progress;
6. Generalizing learning onto other life situations;
7. Reconceptualizing the self; and
8. Coordinating and balancing the worlds we live in.

Each phase of the overall process will be described briefly, with connections to theoretical foundations as appropriate. To demonstrate the natural and logical flow of working through the phases, a single case study will be used throughout the counseling process. The continuity and interconnectedness of the different phases are demonstrated by following a single client from beginning to end. Later chapters will discuss underlying theoretical concerns in greater detail and connect with relevant research examples. Additional case studies will be used for the illustration of important points within a given phase.

Designating the Problem Area(s) to Be Addressed

As the client presents difficulties in handling daily responsibilities, difficulties in interactions with others, or experiencing frustration over unfulfilled goals, the therapist guides the client in choosing the order in which to proceed. In other words, which area of difficulty does the client want to work on first? The first area may be the most painful situation in the client's current stage of life, or it may be a less painful event that is emotionally easier to handle when attempting a new and untried coping approach. Leaving the decision to the client conveys the counselor's respect for the client's judgment. Thus, control over what to work on first remains firmly in the client's hands and ensures deeper client involvement in the counseling process.

Self-sufficiency is one of the major needs for single parents, and is best achieved when the counseling situation fosters independent, critical thinking.

When starting to work with a new client, the counselor needs to be aware that, for most people, the reason for enlisting the help of a counselor is that they are dissatisfied with one or several areas in their lives, but not all clients know exactly where to begin. In many cases the counselor knows little or nothing about the new client. One way of preparation is to have clients complete questionnaires, problem lists, and other forms requesting relevant background information prior to their first appointment. The counselor can use these materials for preparation and structure for the initial interview. Other counselors feel that a highly preplanned structure may interfere with the free flow of ideas that leads to problem solutions and, therefore, they opt for an unprepared interview (Brown-Azarowicz, 1986). Regardless of whether the counselor prefers a preplanned interview or a creative improvisation, it should facilitate the verbalization and definition of the problem area that needs to be resolved.

Case Study

Susan: Developing Priorities and Alliance

Susan, a young, White, middle-class American female, divorced mother of three sons and a daughter, came to her initial interview. When asked by the counselor about her reasons for seeking counseling at this time, she responded in a somewhat ambiguous way.

Susan:	I don't really know whether it is my ex-husband or whether it's me. I seem to be stuck in a no-win situation; no matter what I do, I come out losing.
Couns:	It sounds like you have frequent interactions with your ex-husband that are frustrating to you. Can you be more specific about the situations? Does it involve your children?
Susan:	Yes, that's it. My ex-husband is too busy to pick up or return the children. He insists I do that. What is more, he never lets me plan ahead. I have to wait for his call to tell me it's all right to bring the children over. Then I

	have to wait until he calls me again to tell me to pick them up. I cannot plan anything because he never knows how long he is going to keep them.
Couns:	Are you saying that there was no regular visitation schedule worked out at the time of the divorce, or is your ex-husband not adhering to a schedule and you are frustrated about that?
Susan:	He is supposed to have the children every other weekend and on some holidays, but he says his work will not allow this and after all, the divorce was my fault. Therefore, I should accommodate him. I don't really understand myself why I am going along with all that. There are other things, too, that I do what he tells me to. It is not that I am in love with him anymore. Those feelings have disappeared over the years.
Couns:	Let's clarify what you would want to have happen as a result of coming here.
Susan:	Well, that my ex-husband would want to spend time with his children and that I won't cave in and do what he tells me to do.
Couns:	You have identified two different goals here. The second one that concerns your actions we can certainly work on, but with regard to the first part—what would you be willing to settle for?
Susan:	What do you mean by "settle for?"
Couns:	Let's say, your ex-husband really doesn't want to spend time with the children, is there anything else that would be acceptable to you, such as just going along with the original agreement? You are frowning, what are your feelings right now?
Susan:	(hesitatingly) I think I am angry.
Couns:	At whom?
Susan:	My ex-husband, myself, and even at you!
Couns:	Yes, I can understand that . . .
Susan:	You can? Well, it is like you don't agree that my ex-husband should want to be with the children. Shouldn't parents want to be with their own children?
Couns:	If they did, that would be nice. Unfortunately there are parents in this world who do not like to have their children around and we have no power to make them want to be with them. Even a judge can only order them to adhere to specified visitation schedules, but cannot do anything

Systematic Counseling Phases 53

	about their wants and likes. This is a very difficult concept to understand, and we might as well work at it right at the beginning of the therapeutic relationship. Insisting on something that is not within our control most often turns out to be a waste of time and energy and leads to frustration. If we believe that things should be a certain way and it turns out they are not, we may ask ourselves what is wrong with the world? I don't understand it. Or we may even ask what is wrong with me that things don't go the way they should?
Susan:	That's right! I have asked myself that question. Something had to be wrong with me if I could not accomplish what seemed to be a natural thing.
Couns:	So you blamed yourself for something that you have no control over. If instead we focus on some aspect that we can exert control over, we have a better chance to succeed in getting what we want.
Susan:	Are you saying I should not worry about how I think the situation should be?
Couns:	I am saying to work on getting something that we have some input into or control over being successful. If I agreed with you that your ex-husband should want to spend more time with his children, how can we convince him to do so? We cannot make him want it. But if we instead direct our focus and energy to the things we can do, we might come closer to getting something we want or, at least, something that is more acceptable than what we have right now. Perhaps there is a way he would go along with the visitation schedule even though he might not want to. In other words, if I agreed that your ex-husband should want to do what we think is right, we both would be stuck. What have you tried so far to resolve the situation?
Susan:	That's exactly it! I am stuck! I discussed the situation with my friends and asked for their advice. They all agreed that Jeff should act like a good father and want to spend time with the children. They also agreed that he should be more considerate of my situation because I could not really plan a life for myself with the way things were. They said I needed to be more assertive and tell Jeff that he is wrong.
Couns:	Did you act on that advice? What happened?

Susan: I did and it didn't work; in fact, things got worse. That's why I am here.

Summary of Client-Counselor Interaction. The first session here is an intake interview, and leads to explorations of where to begin and where to set priorities. A therapeutic alliance between client and counselor is already established. During the interchange, the counselor gained a wealth of information about the client. Susan seemed to have some difficulty with anger and also with admitting it to the person she was angry with. She was hesitant to tell the counselor of her anger toward the counselor.

In the interview Susan acted as if her beliefs are a true reflection of reality. Such a way of thinking would lead to a constricted approach, due to the inherent tendency to disregard conflicting cues. Helping the client challenge beliefs regarding their basis in reality, and the possible consequences that would most likely occur if one were to act on those beliefs, is a significant part of the counselor's function within the cognitive therapy process.

The counselor's early awareness of a client's way of thinking greatly enhances the efficiency of counseling because the counselor also functions as a teacher. A person's particular style of thinking is most likely the path along which the person learns. It is the person's learning style as well. Generally, people choose styles of thinking that they feel comfortable with. Most likely, the preferred thinking and learning styles will be used repeatedly and habitually. Ways of thinking and learning are not innate abilities fixed at birth, but rather evolve as a function of a person's interactions with the environment; they can be developed and socialized (Sternberg & Grigorenko, 1997).

When Susan asked friends for advice and they agreed with her basic beliefs, she saw no need to change or even question her beliefs. She proceeded to act on her beliefs and became discouraged, angry, self-doubting, and depressed when her actions did not bring the expected results. Susan was now entering the second phase of the counseling process.

Identifying What Does Not Work

Before coming to counseling, most clients have already applied some strategies to resolve their difficulties. Some strategies may have been learned previously in trying to cope with similar situations. Some may have been passed on from parents, teachers, or friends. Other problem-solving approaches may have had their roots in folklore, legends, or popular folksayings. Some approaches may have been unsuccessful because the person was too angry to adhere to a reasonably self-enhancing strategy; still others may have been hindered by acting in counterintentional ways without being fully aware of the nature or direction of the client's own behaviors. The fact that the individual sought counseling to help with the resolution of the problem indicates lack of success achieved through the use of any of the foregoing approaches. The client's problems may have been too deeply rooted; the person may have followed advice inappropriate for the particular person or situation; or the folk wisdom that seemed to be based in common sense was also mixed with myths, superstitions, misconceptions, and beliefs that actually aggravated an unrealistic orientation. Whatever the reason for the lack of success, the counselor should use the opportunity to reinforce the client's initiative and to encourage behaviors that establish control and independence. Exploration of past problem-solving attempts frequently shows that parts of the approach could have been successful, but that a minor aspect of it may have rendered the strategy ineffective.

Case Study Follow-Up: Exploring Affect and Attempted Strategies

In her first session, Susan had described the difficulties that divorced mothers of young children frequently face when they are caught in conflictual situations regarding the children's visitation with their father. Susan experienced strong negative feelings as response to what she considered lack of consideration and unfair treatment by her former husband. Her friends' advice reinforced her negative feelings and recommended assertiveness. Fortified with suggestions from her friends, Susan confronted her former husband about sharing the responsibility for transporting the children and keeping to a regular visitation schedule. He did not agree with her and instead reminded Susan that it was her fault because she had initiated the divorce proceedings. Therefore, the responsibility for the children's visits with their father was hers and she better handle it without causing any more problems in everybody's life. With that he ended the discussion. During the next session Susan and her counselor discussed the event of her unsuccessful confrontation to learn what might have interfered with the attainment of her goals. What blocked Susan from acting successfully in her own best interest? Her intention had been to communicate to her ex-husband that she did not want to continue having herself and the children depend on his lifestyle, but instead to build up a life of their own. In the actual interaction with Jeff, Susan's behavior appeared counterproductive to her original intentions.

Couns: At our previous meeting you mentioned that you had approached your ex-husband with your wishes as encouraged by your friends, but you also indicated that your attempt was not successful. In fact, he seemed to have blamed you for the divorce. Did you agree with that?

Susan: I did start the divorce proceedings, that is true, but he gave me plenty of reason for it with his extramarital affair and neglecting his family.

Couns: When you think back, what was your overriding emotion in your meeting with Jeff?

Susan: I remember I was angry because he made me go through this confrontation. If he had been more considerate to begin with, I would not have had to do this. I only asked for what is right! That was when he blamed me for the divorce and told me I had caused enough trouble already.

Couns: Do you remember what went on in your mind toward the end of the discussion? What were you thinking? And feeling?

Susan: I was really confused. At the beginning I felt strong, I guess, a little self-righteous. I thought I was doing the right thing. When Jeff reminded me that I had started the divorce I thought he was right, I did file for divorce and he is a very important man in his profession. People need him and I should be more helpful and not just thinking of myself only.

Couns: Where do you think that came from? Here you went out to get something done to make your own life easier and then it seems you turned around to help Jeff.

Susan: I remember my mother saying that it is the wife's responsibility to help her husband and to protect him from interruptions in his work. My father was a teacher and just before he came home from work my mother would remind my brother and me to play quietly, so that our father would not be disturbed. His work always seemed so important. My father never scolded us. I guess he did not need to, my mother kept us in line. My mother also said it is unbecoming for a woman to be selfish. A good woman would think of others first and her rewards would be the happiness of her family.

Couns: Do you think that you might have acted out of that belief system at the end of your meeting?

Susan: Oh, I am sure of it. I may not have been actually aware of it but I often catch myself thinking whether or not a certain behavior would be reflective of a good woman. It's automatic.

Couns: When your mother taught you those values she was married to your father, and probably both of them were protecting each other in some ways. In other words, there was a mutual protection in which your parents cooperated with each other. You and Jeff are divorced, and from what you told me, he does not seem to behave in very cooperative ways with you. Who is protecting you now? Who is looking out for your best interest?

Susan: I should, but I am not doing a good job of it. Is that what you are saying?

Couns: Taking responsibility for yourself requires a lot of thinking and planning, and it helps when your planned actions are congruent with your beliefs and values. You might want to explore your underlying beliefs and values to see if they are serving you well or if they are in conflict with your current situation.

Susan: How do I know which values and beliefs are not good for me and how do I change them?

Couns: When in a given situation, our actions do not bring the desired results, and we wonder what went wrong, we sometimes do not understand why we behaved in a certain way. We can use the "as-if" technique to find out what underlying beliefs may have influenced our actions. Let's look at your encounter with Jeff. When you approached him, you felt strong because you knew you were asking for the right things. As you said, you were also angry. The anger may have helped you to feel strong, but it also may have clouded your thinking. Then, when Jeff did not agree with you, you were not able to shift your thinking but instead fell in with your previously habitual type of responding. In emotionally charged situations, we often resort to well-practiced habitual behaviors. In retrospect, if you wanted to know what happened with your actions, you could ask yourself . . . *what?*

Susan: I acted as if I believed that I had to help and protect my husband, and that I had done harm to my family by divorcing him.

Couns: You are right, that would explain how you may have lost sight of your own goals. Your coming to see me makes me think that you are not quite finished with this situation. You took the initiative to resolve the conflict with your ex-husband. From your description of your relationship with him, I can see that your initiative took quite a bit of courage. You can give yourself credit for that. The fact that your attempt was not as successful as you had hoped does not reduce your courage.

Susan: But I am still stuck in the situation. Nothing has changed for me. What can I do about this?

Couns: Yes, your former husband is still not cooperating with your wishes; that means our work is not completed. For our next session I would like to give you a homework assignment. Please make a list of other possible strategies that you can think of to resolve this conflict. Please write down as many different ways as come to your mind.

Summary of Client-Counselor Interaction: Exploring Affect and Attempted Strategies. As we have seen, Susan's attempts to assertively negotiate different visitation terms, as suggested by her friends, were opposed by her habitual thoughts of being responsible for the peace and harmony in her family and being a helpmate to a man who had ceased to be her husband. She felt intimidated and seemed to accept his line of reasoning instead of keeping track of her own. The counselor assisted the client to see that her anger and self-righteous attitude had prevented her from preparing herself sufficiently for the encounter with her ex-husband. Her friends' moral support made her believe that her former husband would recognize that she was right. When he instead accused her of causing all the trouble, she habitually responded out of a long-standing belief system that was not appropriate to her current situation (Maass, 1995) and, in fact, blocked any behavior that would lead to fulfillment of her original goals.

As long as she felt intimidated, Susan failed to realize that her ex-husband had an equal responsibility for the children's welfare because he had fathered them. How he wanted to relate to them was his responsibility. By protecting the children from knowing how little effort their father made to be with them, she also protected her ex-husband from her own wishes. Susan had not yet made the transition in redefining her role from a combination of wife, mother, and homemaker to that of head of household and mother. Redefinition of her role also required redefinition of boundaries between herself and her former spouse. Another emotional difficulty emerged when Susan expressed her concern that if she considered her own wishes she would appear as less nurturing and would feel guilty in turn.

The work of the counselor in this session was to reinforce the client for assuming responsibility for desired changes and to uncover some of the reasons for the unexpected outcome. The main points for the client to remember in similar situations were: (a) Once a particular problem-solving strategy was decided upon, it would be wise to have a plan of action beyond just being in the situation; (b) make sure that the intended actions and behaviors are congruent with the individual's underlying belief and value system; and (c) be alert and aware of strong emotional forces within oneself during the interaction and how to avoid perceptual distortions resulting from these emotions.

Whether we consider them to be blocks or mistakes, the reasons for not succeeding vary. Rather than hide them from awareness, the counselor is instrumental in teaching the client to regard them as important data and record them as such. The more we know about a situation, the more creative we can become about solutions. The identification of reasons for not achieving the desired results in clients' past problem-solving approaches moves the counseling process logically and smoothly into the next phase, the notion of choices.

Introducing the Idea of Choices

In contrast to earlier times, when the biological instinct hypothesis attributed most of man's behaviors to preformed, naturalistic, instinctual, and unchangeable forces, in the last century human behavior has been regarded as a complex integration of basic biological needs and essential cultural adaptations. The idea that human actions were predetermined and occurred without choice or decision has given way to the concept of intention and choice in human behavior, although the individual may not always be aware of available choices or the decisions actually made in a given situation (Salzman, 1976).

Listing Different Approaches. Susan had been given the assignment to develop a list of possible ways to resolve her situation with her ex-husband. The assignment had kept her actively involved in the problem-solving process between her sessions. As the client is exposed to various problem-solving approaches, no demand is made for making a commitment to follow any particular path at this point. The process in this phase can be likened to studying a road map with different paths leading to the determined destination. Choosing a particular path may take some time. When to move and along what path to proceed are decisions made by the client. The purpose here is to convey early on in the counseling process that choices are within the realm of possibilities. Just because we have done things a certain way in the past does not mean we have to continue doing them the same way for the rest of our lives. Another aspect to consider is that a direct path does not always yield the best results in the most efficient ways.

Estimating Consequences. Problem-solving processes include various aspects of judgment, such as judging the frequency of events or judging the likelihood of events or outcomes. The problem-solving process can be viewed as a chain of events (imagined by the problem-solver) that occurs between the initial awareness of the problem and the point of resolution, unless it is assumed that no solution is possible (Sanford, 1985).

The current state is the start-state, where the individual becomes aware of the problem. The goal-state represents the solution to the problem. Various transactions or steps are possible between the start-state and the goal-state. Theoretically, all the different paths between start and goal could be explored, but in real life the process would be rather time-consuming and inefficient. How people make decisions in the face of uncertainty and without the use of formal models of probability and decision theory is the concern of the psychology of intuitive judgment. Estimates of the likelihood of an occurrence are largely dependent on how readily it comes to mind. The decision-making person is clearly influenced by memory. As the person remembers the general frequency of a given behavior or outcome in connection to similar situations, the person most likely will assign weights to the probability of occurrence of several outcomes. Questions asked when exploring the possible outcomes of different approaches are: What path holds the most promise for reaching the desired goal? What approach includes the lowest risk factors for possible negative outcomes? How much energy or resources is the client willing to expend in the attempts to reach the goal? As always, it is the client's decision.

Case Study Follow-Up: Being Nonjudgmental

Susan's written list consisted of three possible solutions: (a) Enlist her father's or her brother's help because her ex-husband tended to listen more readily to males than to females; (b) ask her mother-in-law to intervene because as the children's grandmother she would be expected to want to keep the relationship intact; and (c) take her ex-husband to court for not following the agreement regarding visitation schedules. When Susan presented her list the counselor asked her to estimate the possible consequences of each approach.

Couns: I see you have worked hard on finding solutions to your situation. Is there any one of the three approaches that you find promising enough to start with?

Susan: No, not really. Asking my father to intervene for me and talk to Jeff does not look like a good idea because my father had discouraged me from divorcing Jeff in the first place. He expressed the opinion that it would be safer for all concerned if I kept the family intact despite Jeff's extramarital affairs. I should have been willing to "forgive and forget" for the benefit of the children. "Sometimes women have to make allowances for their husbands." As much as he would like to help me, if I asked him now, he would probably remind me of his previous advice. Asking my brother would be equally bad for the same reason. He would eventually tell my father and I would get the same response, only delayed in time.

Couns: How did you assess the consequences of following your second idea?

Susan: I am not sure that would work out for the best either. In the past, my mother-in-law always seemed happy to have the children with her for her own enjoyment, but I don't think she would be willing to interfere with her son's life. She spoiled him as he grew up and now she is actually intimidated by him. She would not be willing to risk his displeasure by talking to him about being more consistent with the visitation schedule of his children. Since the divorce, we are not as close as before.

Couns: You seem to sense that asking Jeff's mother might place her in a position where she would seem to be taking sides and she would not want to do that. Your perception certainly appears reasonable and realistic. How do you feel about the third option on your list?

Susan: This would be the very last resort. For one thing, I do not have the financial resources to hire a lawyer again. Jeff's finances allow him to employ the services of the most successful expert in the field. That is the reason for my own current financial limitations. In addition, taking him to court would probably aggravate the situation to such a degree that the children would be affected. Before doing that, I would rather approach him again by myself or learn to live with the situation as bad as it is.

Couns: You have done a great job of looking at the consequences of the three possible solutions on your list, and they seem to reflect realistic evaluations on your part. Unfortunately, none of them have found your approval, but your last statement contained two approaches that you had not mentioned before. They seemed to have evolved as part of the options you saw and the likelihood of success you assigned to each of them. Now you have two more options to add to your list.

Susan: Well, learning to live with the situation as it is seems like giving up. Before I do that, I will try to talk to Jeff again.

Summary of Client-Counselor Interaction: Being Nonjudgmental. The above interchange demonstrated that when Susan discarded her earlier options, she also automatically decided between the two new alternatives. Learning to live with the situation was interpreted by her as "giving up." Although this would not necessarily be true, there was no need now to argue the point. It was her right to decide what to do. It was also part of her value system what constitutes "giving up," and because she had already decided what option to implement, this would not have been an opportune moment to address her value system. The counselor is fostering an atmosphere of freedom for exploring options and selecting those that appear most promising to the client. Through the process of elimination, Susan had seriously considered to exercise one of her additional options. Her decision to approach her ex-husband again was the transition to the next phase.

Starting and Proceeding Along the Chosen Path

After the client has ranked choices and selected a particular approach, various skills and techniques to facilitate the success of goal-directed behaviors are explored and taught if needed. Techniques include written homework assignments that are particularly important here. Underlying thoughts and beliefs are to be explored, challenged, and replaced by more rational alternatives that lead to alternate actions if the new desirable behaviors are to be successful.

Unresolved Affect. Behaviors are rooted in deeply felt emotions and deep-seated values and beliefs. As was demonstrated earlier, many of the behaviors needed for survival in the new lifestyles of single parents are in direct contradictions to actions and behaviors that were appropriate in their previous circumstances. During the time of marriage, a spouse's actions were influenced by warmth, fondness, and trust, now feelings of guilt, abandonment, loneliness, fear, distrust, and anger toward the absent spouse may be flooding the single parent. The new feelings are often in sharp contradiction to the values held by the person. Intensive work is required to manage conflicts and resolve contradictions. Often, in the phase of proceeding along the chosen path, unresolved feelings of guilt, shame, anger, or self-doubt emerge and need to be resolved.

Mental Imagery, Behavior Rehearsal, and the Skillful Will. Mental imagery is a valuable skill to be used in planning and rehearsing new behaviors. In imagery, the individual simulates what might happen in a given situation if one acted in a particular way—without actually being in the situation. If imagery is to be of any use, the details of the simulation must be like those that truly exist in the physical world of the situation. Thus, in order to have a good fit between the simulated mental model of the situation and the situation itself, the person must possess rather detailed knowledge of the actual situation (Sanford, 1985).

Roberto Assagioli's (1973) idea of the "skillful will" describes how images or mental pictures can bring about or intensify emotions and behaviors that correspond with those images. As individuals intensely imagine themselves acting in a certain way in a given situation, they can actually experience the emotions that they can expect to feel in the real situation. They also become aware of an internal push to action. Body muscles or facial muscles can be felt and observed to move according to planned behaviors. Repetition of the process will intensify the urge to act out the imagined behavior. (More recently, this idea has found significant application in the field of sports psychology [McLean, 1988].)

Case Study Follow-Up: Guiding Reality Check

Susan had made her choice about how to work on resolving the visitation problem with her ex-husband. Because she had decided to refrain from enlisting the help of others and instead to approach Jeff again on her own, it was important to explore why her first attempt had not been successful. Repeating the confrontation with Jeff raised a wave of negative emotions through anticipation of his rejection. These fears made it all the more important for her to stay with the reality of the situation and focus on her own potential resources.

Couns:	When we first discussed your confrontation with Jeff, the way you described it to me indicated that you had expected some degree of cooperation from him. Is that correct?
Susan:	Well, yes, as we discussed it in the first session, I thought I was right and he would understand that, but he didn't.
Couns:	In the past when you were still married, was your husband more cooperative then?
Susan:	No, not really. In fact, Jeff has never been very considerate of others' interests. He is really quite selfish. I shouldn't

	even have expected any help or understanding from him.
Couns:	Can you think of any other way to approach him that would be more promising?
Susan:	There would have to be something in it for him! Why didn't I think of that before?
Couns:	You mean if it would be advantageous for him to be more cooperative with your wishes, you would have a better chance. As you know him, what might be appealing to him?
Susan:	Jeff is very ambitious. He always wants to look good in the community, both socially and professionally. I think he may even run for political office some day. That was probably the main reason why he did not want the divorce. He would not like to be known in the community as a father who does not care about his children.
Couns:	How does that fit in with your plans?
Susan:	It made sense to me when you pointed out that Jeff has a responsibility as the father of the children and that it was up to him what kind of a relationship he wants to have with them. I thought about that a lot. By trying to protect my children from knowing how their father really is, I also protected the wrong person—Jeff!
Couns:	Yes, as we discussed earlier, you acted on your old values of taking care of those around you. The values you had learned from your mother. It is not a question of whether those values are good or bad, but of how well they work for you now. As you seem to realize, in this case they did not work well for you. How do you want to proceed now?
Susan:	I think I need to stop protecting him and start thinking more about what is good for me and the children. How can I get all this visitation routine changed?
Couns:	What would you feel comfortable with as a first step?
Susan:	I think I can try to work on the transportation part. I still believe we can share it. Should I give him the choice to pick them up or to return them? What would be better for me driving the children to his house or picking them up?
Couns:	What would be the consequences in either case—as you can see them?
Susan:	If I were to bring the children to his house, I might run the risk that he is not there, and I could not just leave them out in the street.

Couns:	How do you see the consequences if you let him pick up the children?
Susan:	If I let him pick up the children, he most likely would not be on time, and I may have to make the children wait, and I could not leave either. If I let Jeff return the children to the house, he may bring them back earlier and if I was not at home to be with them, I would worry wherever I am. Perhaps it would be better if I ask him to pick up the children at the beginning of the visitation. I would have to work out something to overcome his unpredictability. Oh, I know, I will tell him that we will wait no longer than 1 hour for him. If he is not there by then, the children and I will go to a movie or to visit someone. Because they are already dressed to leave the house, we might as well go.
Couns:	When you think about actually saying these words to Jeff, how do you feel?
Susan:	I am already getting anxious about it.
Couns:	Where do you think the anxiety is coming from? What thoughts and beliefs are operating here?
Susan:	I think that he will not go along with it and will try to put me off as he did before.
Couns:	Based on what you told me, that seems to be a reasonable assumption on your part. We can very much expect Jeff to act as he did in the past. Now comes the part where you can change your behavior from what you would have done in the past, isn't that right? Your next step is different from what you did before. Because you already have a good guess on how he will respond to your opening statement, you can focus more strongly on what you want to do and say next, and on how you want to feel while you are continuing with your actions.
Susan:	I want to feel confident when I talk to him.
Couns:	Confident in what way? Where would the confidence come from?
Susan:	Confident that I am doing the right thing for myself and my children. And confident that I will not cave in again because I am afraid of his anger and disapproval. I need to remind myself that I have to act on my own behalf whether he agrees with it or not. He is not going to help me or make it easier for me. Actually, if I can work through the first part—it being the right thing—I believe I can

	handle the second part.
Couns:	Excellent! You have come down to the fundamental issue; if you are comfortable in the knowledge that your actions are congruent with your values, you are stronger in your behavior and have a much better chance of succeeding. When you first approached Jeff, you were confident that you were doing the right thing based on what others thought who were in agreement with you, but that confidence was not really congruent with your real beliefs at the time. Now you can feel confident in doing the right thing because you know it is right for you and your children, no matter whether others agree with you or not.

I would like to add something to your earlier explorations regarding the choice between delivering or picking up the children. If you are willing to say to Jeff that the children will not wait longer than 1 hour for him, you can probably use a similar approach if you end up with the task of delivering the children to him. You may not want to wait a whole hour outside his home, but I am sure you can devise some other strategy, such as waiting a short period of time and possibly come by again after running some errands. Thinking about that gives you more options in case your first choice of having him pick up the children is not workable for some reason. |
Susan:	That is true, if I can handle the situation one way, I should be able to cope with it in a similar situation.
Couns:	How can you prepare yourself for the actual event?
Susan:	I am glad you asked me that question. I thought that I need to be very careful that I do not repeat my previous performance. So I have actually started to write out a kind of scenario with the actual words I am going to say to him. It helped me a lot when I thought back about the earlier assignment you gave me about writing down the different approaches I might try. Then the assumption of possible outcomes or consequences actually helped me to decide which approach to take. I used a similar way of thinking when I asked myself: How would Jeff respond to this? In a way, I made up several conversations in my head and I wrote them down, so I would not forget them. It took a while to find the words for statements that I felt comfortable with. But I am not finished with it yet.
Couns:	You did excellent work! It was probably not easy to start

working on that future interaction with the negative anticipations you had. To experience negative anticipations is natural and understandable in your situation. But you recognized that it would not help your cause and instead you went beyond that. You wrote a variation of the old scene with you being in control of what you want to say. By anticipating what Jeff would most likely say in his response, you already prepared yourself for your next step. You are doing wonderful work in assuming responsibility for the direction of the next interaction with Jeff. You can strengthen your part through repeated actual behavior rehearsal and imagining yourself in the situation thinking, acting, and feeling the way you want to.

Summary of Client-Counselor Interaction: Guiding Reality Check. Earlier in the counseling process the counselor had become cognizant of the client's particular style of thinking. The counselor used the knowledge when guiding the client to check the evidence for her beliefs. Confronted with the contradiction between her idea about how a parent should behave and Jeff's actual behavior, Susan understood how her earlier efforts had been doomed to fail. She had forgotten to consider reality. As her statement indicated, she now realized that in order to be successful, she had to find an approach that appealed to Jeff's way of thinking, not just her own. Now instead of focusing on what Jeff could and should do differently, she shifted attention to what she herself could do differently. The counselor also emphasized that now her self-confidence would be firmly grounded in her own belief system and not be based on what her friends considered to be right, even if her friends were in total agreement with her. In general, the shift signifies a more promising alternative, because it will put not only increased responsibility but also increased control into her hands.

Techniques for proceeding with actions along a chosen path are behaviorally based, but the emotions accompanying actions are closely related to underlying values and beliefs. Incongruity between behaviors and values results in emotional dissonance and significantly jeopardizes the achievement of goals. The counselor emphasized the importance of congruence between Susan's actions and her basic values as a determining factor for her success. When Susan had arrived at a strategy that she felt reasonably comfortable with, it was time for behavior rehearsals.

A discussion about events that could be expected to occur was included in the session to prepare the client for some future difficulties. Jeff's testing the limits of Susan's new behavior, and her own possible occasional regression to previous behaviors, would be examples of difficulties that could be overcome with time and repeated practice. Mentioning the possibilities of setbacks and emphasizing the fact that Susan would have ample opportunity to strengthen her new behaviors softened the sting of failure from the beginning.

Reevaluating Progress

So far, the counselor's basic task has been in assisting the client to gain awareness of possible misconceptions inherent in the client's thoughts and how the misperceptions are related to the client's underlying beliefs and values. To bring about lasting behavior change, a change in the client's unrealistic conceptions is necessary. As the client works through a given problem situation, there comes a time when it seems reasonable to evaluate the gains or losses experienced up to that point. Has there been improvement in the client's situation as a consequence of changed behaviors? Or have there been setbacks? Did the client have difficulties maintaining the new behaviors? Perhaps they were not yet congruent with the client's values and beliefs. Are further explorations of how underlying beliefs still hampered or blocked self-enhancing actions needed? Both counselor and client need to realize that change is not easy to achieve. At times, despite their best efforts, clients do not experience the desired results without delays or detours. Clients may become discouraged and want to give up: "It's just no use, I can't be different from the way I am." When people are disappointed by the lack of expected success, they tend to exaggerate the degree of needed change and escalate it into the overwhelming fear that the whole person has to change in order to be successful. A beneficial shift in thinking occurs when emphasis is placed on the importance of smaller successes to be used as building blocks for future greater achievements, instead of focusing on the overwhelming work yet to be done. Reevaluating is also an opportunity for the counselor to monitor progress for accountability purposes.

Case Study Follow-Up: Emphasizing Coping Skills

In working with Susan, the counselor considered the appropriateness of evaluating and summarizing the results of Susan's work in counseling. Single parents more than any other clients need episodic feedback about their increasing coping skills. They also need reminders of their successes in handling by themselves many responsibilities that usually are shared between two people.

Couns: Today, unless you have an urgent matter to discuss right now, I thought we might spend some time looking at what has changed in your life so far as result of coming in to counseling. What has changed, and is it better or worse?

Susan: Do you mean like taking stock of what I have done? Well, in the beginning I thought I would not be able to make any headway. Do you remember when I told you my first attempt to institute a regular delivery and pick-up schedule for my children's visitation with their father? The very first time it did not work out as I had planned. He had to be out of town and did not know when he would come back, so he did not or could not accept the 7:00 p.m. deadline for getting the children.

Couns: As I remember, you suggested that you trade weekends with him at this particular time and that worked out quite well.

Susan: Yes, that is true, but the self-torture that I went through, putting myself down for having given in again ... although there were times when I thought I had done right, because I did not really need to be inflexible about getting what I wanted. Your reminding me that I always had another chance to be assertive helped a great deal then. I must have been more convincing than I realized, because the next weekend my mother-in-law called and asked if it would be all right if she picked up the children instead of Jeff. My first thought was "He is doing it again, letting others do his chores" but I got over that when I remembered it was an issue between Jeff and his mother. It was none of my business how he handled his obligations as long as it did not interfere with our lives.

Couns: That was quite a learning experience for you. How did you feel at that time?

Systematic Counseling Phases

Susan: It was a great learning experience! When I realized that I did not have to worry about Jeff's problems anymore, that almost gave me a feeling of freedom. I also felt relieved because I thought I could focus more on what I wanted. There was a little bit of hope in there, too. I had accomplished something that was of value to me. Perhaps I could do more, but then, of course, there were some setbacks when Jeff was angry because the children and I were gone when he came to get them. That was the weekend his mother had gone away to Las Vegas with her friends. He was in a rage and kept calling most of the next day. It was so bad that the children and I finally took off and went to the zoo.

Couns: You stood your ground, as I remember, without arguing or complaining, and Jeff seemed to realize that you were determined to stay with your decision. How did the children respond to the situation?

Susan: The children took it pretty well, except Becky, my youngest, she wanted to wait for her Daddy. She misses seeing him the most. The boys are more used to his lack of attention to them. After a bit of crying, Becky was all right. Actually, I was lucky the way it worked out. A friend of mine has this wonderful aunt who comes to visit every once in a while. Aunt Lucy is a great storyteller. My friend's children just love her. On this particular weekend, Aunt Lucy was in town and my friend had invited me and the children to come over on Friday evening. I had not told my children about it because it was Jeff's weekend with them and I did not want them to be disappointed that they could not go. So when Jeff did not come to pick up the children I called my friend and told her we were on our way. I told the children that I had a surprise adventure for them. It was a wonderful evening and the children really enjoyed this special treat. I know, I will not always be so lucky, but it really worked out well.

Couns: Overall, how would you rate your work so far?

Susan: I am very grateful for having had some success, but I think I need more practice and more training. I still have moments when my first impulse is to act in my old ways, just being nice to everybody and agreeing with what they want. Sometimes I can pull myself away from that before I make a response, but sometimes it is too fast and I don't take the time to think of what would be in my best interest.

Couns: You are right, it does take quite a while for your new way of thinking to become as natural or automatic as the old way. At this point, it is often helpful to think of other areas of your life where you can apply your new way of thinking. Any additional practice is bound to strengthen your new thinking, behaving, and feeling. Perhaps before our next session you can think of another situation where you would like to make changes.

Summary of Client-Counselor Interaction: Emphasizing Coping Skills. While helping the client to summarize the effects of her work so far, the counselor used every opportunity to reinforce the client's initiative and behavioral consistencies that led to her success. The counselor purposefully encouraged the client to report on her successes in her own words. Having Susan describe her experiences served to strengthen in her own mind the connection between her actions and the outcome, reflecting the control she had exercised in the situation. Susan also learned that being flexible (as in trading visitation weekends with her ex-husband) is not the same as giving up control or losing track of one's goals. Another revelation came when she realized that by leaving the responsibility for handling his part of the visitation to her ex-husband, she had more time and energy to plan her own life. The confidence and good feelings that accompanied her report inspired Susan to continue with her work by applying her new learning to other areas of her life.

The structure of the counseling session was designed to confront the client with the evidence that actions congruent with her values had an increased chance of succeeding, especially when events did not occur exactly as she had planned. Additionally, avoidance of assuming other people's responsibility for what is their own business not only conserves energy for one's own planning, but also reduces confusion in the decision-making process regarding one's own goals. Finally, the realization that additional practice is likely to enhance skills for managing future life circumstances persuaded the client to target another area for improvement. There is nothing better than success to facilitate additional training and practice.

Generalizing Learning Onto Other Life Situations

The phase of generalizing learning has a double impact. First, repeated applications of newly learned skills of thinking and acting serve to strengthen their effectiveness. Through frequent practice, the skills become easily available to the person and, in turn, the person feels more comfortable in using them. The second aspect is that repeated application pervades more and more life areas and eventually the person's whole quality of life will improve.

Broadening Applications of Learning. Essentially, the generalizing phase constitutes a series of repeated progressions through phases One to Five. Depending on the nature of the new problem situation, the length of work through the different stages is not necessarily the same for each phase and may be significantly shorter with consecutive repetitions.

As was done with the initial problem, the situation to be worked on needs to be defined in terms of the desired changes and outcome goals. Additional information can be obtained by examining previously attempted solutions that did not work out to the individual's satisfaction. Underlying beliefs and values can be explored as possible blocks to achieving success. Where necessary, challenge and modification of self-defeating beliefs can lead to a new plan of action. Imagery and behavior rehearsals to practice and strengthen new behaviors follow in the cycle. Working repeatedly with success through the cycle equips the person with a repertoire of self-enhancing behaviors and problem-solving skills that can be seen as similar to the learned resourcefulness described by Rosenbaum (1983). If resourcefulness can be learned, then the counseling environment is an appropriate setting for teaching this skill repertoire.

Case Study Follow-Up: Reinforcing Initiative

The improvement Susan experienced in her part of the children's visitation schedule with their father led her to consider taking active control in other areas of her life as well. In handling the situation with her ex-husband, she had learned that in order to reach her goal, she had to strongly commit herself to act in her own best interest. She could not expect others to do that for her. The next area of application Susan decided should be her professional life. In order to obtain a better-paying position, she knew that finishing her college degree was an absolute necessity. Susan was grateful for the job she had right now and gave a lot of her time and energy to her employer. There were opportunities for advancement within the company that she could strive for if she had the college degree.

Couns: Now that you feel good about the success you achieved with your ex-husband's visitation schedule, what other area of your life have you considered to improve on?

Susan: I thought about my work situation. Although Jeff pays a reasonable amount in child support for the children, being single means I better think about supporting myself in the future. I like my part-time job and I like the people there, but it does not pay enough for me to live on comfortably. Even if I were to work full-time, it would not be sufficient. I am on a dead-end path. Without my college degree, there are not many opportunities for advancement. Some of my past college credits are obsolete. I have made some inquiries at our local colleges and the best opportunity that I found would require a year of taking classes on a part-time basis, including summer classes. There is a chance that finishing my degree would make me eligible for advancement within the company. My boss may even pay for some of the courses if I get good grades.

Couns: As usual, you have done your homework well. Not only have you decided on another area to work on, you have already defined your goal and collected information regarding the requirements for your goal. I am impressed by your determination.

Susan: I have to admit, it was not that straightforward. For a while I felt sorry for myself when I considered the need to be self-sufficient in the future. Here I had invested so much time and energy into being a good wife and mother and now I have to start all over again. I really had a pity-party for a couple of days. Of course, that did not change the reality that there was nobody else to take care of me. There is a possibility that in the future I may find another husband, but that is only a possibility. I am not even ready to date again. So I finally got my transcripts together and started on my round to the local colleges.

Couns: It is natural to feel the way you did. You have been through a lot of changes and a lot of stress that is associated with the changes. What is important to remember, however, is that you kept a firm hold on reality and on what would be in your own best interest under the circumstances. The mere fact that you were able to get yourself away from feeling sorry for yourself and start acting in your best interest is the important thing. We will always be able to experience feelings of self-pity and other self-defeating emotions, but we do not have to feel helpless and out of control if we remember that we have been there before and have managed to change our thinking and, with that, our feelings and actions. Now that you have taken a step toward your goal, how would you like to proceed?

Susan: I guess I have to talk to my boss about it. Even on a part-time basis I would need flexibility of work hours to take all the required classes when they are offered. I probably need more money for child care, so I definitely have to keep my job. I wonder how I should approach my boss.

Couns: Do you remember how you resolved to approach your ex-husband about his compliance with the visitation schedule? You realized that your best chance would be if you could come up with a suggestion that had something in it for his interest. Is there anything you can offer your employer that would be of interest to him in his business?

Susan: That was a great idea then and it worked like a charm. You are saying that this approach might work again?

Couns: In general, people are more agreeable to help you if there is an advantage for them too. It makes them think that they get something valuable in return for their assistance.

Susan: One thing that would be of benefit to my boss is an offer to work on Saturdays. In the nature of his business it would be helpful if somebody would cover on Saturdays. Most of the other employees have families and do not want to give up their weekends. So it is always a struggle to find somebody when it is absolutely necessary to be there on a Saturday. If I offered to work every second Saturday when the children are with Jeff, my boss might like that idea. Also, I could fill in emergencies on other Saturdays if I would be allowed to bring my kids along. My children are pretty good in entertaining themselves for a while. Of course, I would not want to do that every Saturday, but I could certainly do it in an emergency.

Couns: It sounds like you have come up with an offer that your employer can hardly refuse in the best interest of his company. Are you thinking of rehearsing your speech

	again as you did before when you were so successful with your ex-husband?
Susan:	Absolutely! That was really helpful. I felt so strong when I noticed that my preparation helped me control the direction of the interaction with Jeff. That was one of the best skills I ever learned. With my boss, I think I will in addition write a little proposal, accounting for my work hours under the new plan. The proposal should show that he would not lose any of my work hours when I would have to leave earlier for my classes. He likes to have things down in writing, so he knows what he is agreeing to. It also would let him know that I am preparing myself for an advanced position in the company.
Couns:	Great! You are on your way. I don't think I need to wish you good luck. The way you are handling your situations, luck is not a factor.

Summary of Client-Counselor Interaction: Reinforcing Initiative. Encouraged by her previous success, the client had decided to address another area of her life that seemed problematic. When she entered the session, she had already defined her goal for the situation. The counselor reinforced her for her work and the steps she had taken on her own initiative. The counselor's reinforcement for her actions facilitated the client's admission that she had encountered some negative feelings in contemplating her next step. By reassuring her that those feelings could be expected to surface at times, the counselor took the opportunity to point out that she was not alone in experiencing those emotions. The counselor also reminded her that in spite of those feelings, she had been instrumental in turning herself around to continue with her plans for a solution. No matter how she had felt, she had not been helpless. When it came time to define a plan of action, the counselor subtly assisted the client to consider her previously successful approach of planning her actions. Susan had learned to value the effects of the behavior rehearsals in her past endeavors and was ready to use again those skills that had worked for her before. The main focus of the interchange was centered on reinforcement for the client's past successful behaviors and direction toward future goals that would emphasize the client's resourcefulness.

The results of her actions demonstrated to Susan that she was doing the right things for herself. Her skills in managing demanding situations in her environment improved with repeated applications. The validity of her new beliefs was reinforced and solidified by the consequences of her new behaviors. The change in her way of thinking resulted in another outcome, a change in Susan's perception of herself.

Reconceptualizing the Self

When new beliefs and behaviors have become somewhat stabilized within the client's cognitive set, the time is right to look at the whole person. How does the new set of thinking fit into the client's overall lifestyle and picture of self? The therapist encourages the client to engage in self-exploration, leading to discovery of possible changes that the client may have observed in herself. Most people have images of themselves. Some self-images may be realistic and others may be less accurate; either way, they influence their interactions with others. Misconceptions or misunderstandings of the self often have a negative impact on the person's successful personal and social adjustment.

Self-Perceptions, Emotional Investment, and the Threat of Change. Awareness of the effects of self-image on the client, as well as on others with whom the client interacts, is important to the client's overall functioning. The therapist needs to consider the appropriate timing for such explorations. With a single-parent client, the most advantageous timing may not be early on in the therapy process. People in general feel threatened by the need for change and clients are no different. While they can accept the notion of modifying some behaviors, exploring the whole self for possible change is often too overwhelming to contemplate and may lead to initial resistance. Most people tend to have a considerable emotional investment in how they perceive themselves. As one client in her first therapy session inquired, "In coming here, does that mean I have to change my whole person to get better?" Postponing the self-exploration for later on in the therapy process makes it less threatening because there has been sufficient time to build a supportive client-therapist relationship. The client has developed trust in the relationship to the counselor and is much less resistant to such explorations. Successes that the client has already experienced also help to reduce resistance.

Case Study Follow-Up: Acknowledging Changes in Self-Image

Earlier in the therapy process, Susan had described herself as a gentle, loving woman who places the needs of significant others in her environment (spouse, children, parents, etc.) before her own needs. She was raised to see herself that way, and she continued to hold on to that picture. Even though she had already acted differently in the situation with her ex-husband and her own vocational planning, she had not actually acknowledged the change to herself.

Couns: The other day when I asked you to describe yourself as you perceive yourself, you gave a description of yourself as you had been in the past, operating on your old values of taking care of others before considering your own needs. You seemed surprised when I pointed out that you had actually learned how important it is to consider your own needs as a priority in many situations. After all, your success in coping with the visitation schedule and your career plans is evidence for the significant change. You have worked so hard when planning your approaches to solve the problems and spending your time and energy in behavior rehearsals. What made you hesitate to acknowledge it? How did you feel when I brought up the evidence of your hard work and the well-deserved rewards?

Susan: I remember feeling a shock, almost a fear for a moment.

Couns: Are there any thoughts you remember having at that time?

Susan: Yes, I remember very clearly thinking that if I do take care of myself and do things well, then I will always have to do it and nobody is going to help me when I need it. People won't like me! What if I cannot do it? It's like losing part of me.

Couns: I can see that you would be frightened with those thoughts. You have accomplished a lot in a short time. For many people, it takes longer to make such substantial changes as you have done. That you have difficulty believing it and trusting yourself is not surprising. There is a change insofar as you have expanded yourself rather than losing part of yourself. You have added to yourself by increasing your coping skills. When you work as intensely as you did, there comes a point when your thoughts are not congruent with your feelings. Your thoughts reflect your new learning but your feelings are lagging behind, still according to your old ways. You can think of it as a dissonance between your new thinking and your old way of feeling. With time and continued work the dissonance will shrink and you will feel more comfortable.

Susan: Although I felt somewhat uncomfortable last time, later on my way home I started to feel excited, almost giddy. I kept thinking of how many areas I could make changes in to improve my whole life. It seemed so powerful. I know this sounds silly, but I thought little by little I could redesign or reengineer my life. Perhaps I am getting carried away, but I felt in control and at the same time it was like starting on a new adventure. It will be interesting to see if people will respond to me differently, depending on how I act toward them.

Couns: That is a wonderful way of expressing your experiences! And you are quite right, you have many tools that you can use to reengineer your life. You can measure and evaluate realistically by collecting and assessing evidence. Then you can contemplate what you want to be different. By considering consequences and chances of success, you can design and practice the approach that seems to be the most effective to you. And you are wise to consider the effects of your own actions on others as you are planning your strategies. I think I would like to borrow your expression. For our next session it would be beneficial to take a comprehensive view of your current life situation as indication for a possible termination point of our current counseling.

Summary of Client-Counselor Interaction: Acknowledging Changes in Self-Image.

When faced with the evidence that she could and did act in her own best interest without feeling guilty or being punished in other ways, the client was surprised: "I didn't know I had it in me!" was her response. The counselor reminded her of her efforts in selecting and planning the various approaches she had employed in the different situations and the time spent in behavior rehearsal techniques. The favorable outcomes were well-deserved. With the counselor's guidance, Susan was able to incorporate exploration of her own needs and goal-directed planning activities into her concept of herself. She recognized herself as a much more independent, determined, and capable person than she had given herself credit for in the past.

A significant aspect in the session was Susan's emotional transition from fear of losing part of herself to the excitement of considering the almost limitless possibilities of creating a new person and life around herself. Although the individual's exploration of the self-image is essentially a process of inward looking, it is in part a function of social values and expectations that are transmitted through the individual's relationships with others. Because of our connectedness to the society around us, we need to consider caring, respect, and esteem for those around us. Well-adjusted individuals will strive for a balance between self-esteem and other-esteem while creating a harmonious existence within themselves and the world around them. With the focus on successful integration of the individual into the surrounding world, the counselor prepared the client for the event of termination as a logical conclusion.

Coordinating and Balancing the Worlds We Live In

The termination part is especially important in working with single parents. The work on one or several problem areas has been completed, the client's competence and independence have been emphasized, but the possibility for return to counseling in the future needs to be kept in mind. The larger the area of change and improvement achieved, the more likely it is that some of the changes will bring with them a further need for exploration.

Self in World. Ludwig Binswanger's (1962) concept of the human existence occurring in three worlds is useful here. The three worlds are the *Eigenwelt* \'ī-gen-velt\ or personal world, constituting the individual's self-world of inner feelings, thoughts, and bodily experiences; the *Mitwelt* \'mit-velt\ or interpersonal world shared with significant others; and the larger environment, the world around us, is the *Umwelt* \'úm-velt\, including both animate and inanimate features of existence. The three worlds can be independent but they frequently overlap and interact. A healthy balance of the client's existence in the three worlds is the goal in therapy and the culmination of the successful counseling process.

In single parents, more than in any other living arrangements, great changes occur in all three worlds. As the individual separates from significant others, such as spouse or children, the *Mitwelt* (interpersonal world) is influenced as well as the *Eigenwelt* (personal world) as the person takes on different roles and responds to different needs. Often, the *Umwelt* (environment) changes as the individual may seek new employment or move away from the long familiar neighborhood.

Case Study Follow-Up: Validating Interconnectedness

Susan had to conceptualize herself in a different personal role. Suddenly she was head of her household. She also had lost her spouse from her interpersonal world. Her relationship to her children had not changed greatly, because she had been more involved in their lives than their father had ever been. Even though he was fading out from Susan's interpersonal world after the divorce, she initially experienced greater interference from her former husband until she had learned to resolve the situation to her satisfaction. The need for an independent career and full-time work gave rise to additional changes affecting her worlds of living.

When termination approached, Susan reported one other pleasant outcome. During one of those occasions that Jeff's mother picked up the children for him, they spent a considerable amount of time with her. As they were attempting to entertain themselves, the oldest child started to draw cartoon figures. He was quite talented and his grandmother asked him about the situations that were depicted by his drawings. They seemed to tell a story. While waiting for his father, he had remembered stories that Susan had told the children as bedtime stories. Many of the stories had begun as popular fairy tales, but Susan had often used her own imagination in continuing the stories until they had become quite different from the familiar fairy tales in their content and ending. Susan had not written down these stories but her children remembered many of them. Seeing the talent of her grandson, Jeff's mother encouraged the children to help their mother remember the stories well enough to record them on paper. The cartoon drawings would provide illustrations emphasizing different parts of the stories. Grandmother suggested this as a project that they could use for making Christmas gifts for friends and family members. The project turned out to be successful. Susan, her children, and her former mother-in-law are currently involved in negotiations with a publishing company.

Susan's way of resolving the difficulties with her ex-husband's noncompliance with the visitation schedule had actually resulted in a closer bond between the children and their grandmother. Susan's relationship to her former mother-in-law also took on a different meaning. Both women respected each other as persons rather than as relatives. They became partners in a new venture that provided an outlet for meaningful activities to the grandmother as well as to the children. While the grandmother encouraged the children to engage in the artistic activities of illustrated storytelling, she had the time and the resources to organize the work to a level where it could be presented to a publisher. The close relationship between grandmother and grandchildren also benefitted Susan, because it freed up time for her own studies.

Couns: As we talked about the different parts of our lives the other day, how do you see this applied to your life since you made all those changes?

Susan: What you called the *Mitwelt* has certainly changed for me. There is no spouse in there now. Perhaps in the future there will be somebody again, but now that space is empty. I think, in a different way, my mother-in-law has a larger place in our lives. In the past, the relationship was one of getting advice, asking her for favors, and doing things like taking her out for Mother's Day because she was Jeff's mother. Now we are more like partners since we started working on the children's stories. I don't have to ask her to babysit as a favor. She and the children are working together and enjoying it. They have a special relationship. The other day I overheard my oldest son talking to a friend about being away from home that weekend. The other boy said something like, "You are going to be with your father and grandmother again." My son answered, "Yes, but we are also working on our business. My grandmother bought a new computer for the business and we all have to learn to use it. She is not just a grandmother; she is a business manager." I was so proud of my children and my mother-in-law too. I had to tell her about it.

Couns: What you described is a special and unusual relationship

Susan: between children and their grandmother. What else has changed for you when you think of your worlds?

Susan: I guess, you could say the *Umwelt* has become larger for me. It is not just the shopping, the neighbors, and my part-time job anymore. Now it includes school, and some of it feels like it belongs to me in the *Eigenwelt*. Some of the things I am learning have a personal meaning for me. I can't clearly distinguish between three separate worlds. They overlap in some areas.

Couns: A good observation on your part. There are not always clear and well-defined boundaries between these worlds we live in. There are overlaps and intersections from one to the other. The boundaries are flexible, accommodating to ongoing growth and changes. What we are trying to achieve is a healthy balance. When people spend most of their lives in just one or the other part, they miss out on a lot of things that could be theirs if they participated more extensively in the second or third part of their life spheres. A life balanced in all three, the *Eigenwelt*, the *Mitwelt*, and the *Umwelt* is a rich life, filled with meaningful interactions in all of them. Although balance is the goal, it is usually not a static balance. As situations change, continued readjustments to the balance will be required.

Summary of Client-Counselor Interaction: Validating Interconnectedness. The function of the session was largely one of integrating and summarizing the outcomes resulting from the changes the client had made in her life during the counseling process.

As Susan's relationships changed with her husband and his mother, so did the relationship of her children with their grandmother take on different meaning. The boundaries and spaces of the family's interactions were fluctuating and settling into different configurations. The counselor confirmed and validated the client's observation of the overlapping and interconnected nature inherent in the process of balancing our worlds (see Figure 3.1). It is important to stress the aspect of repeated flow and settlements because the process is a dynamic series of events occurring over a person's lifetime. Once a balance is achieved, it does not necessarily remain static, because relationships may change over time in levels of meaningfulness and significance. New people may enter our lives. The counselor acknowledged the client's achievements along the way of balancing her worlds

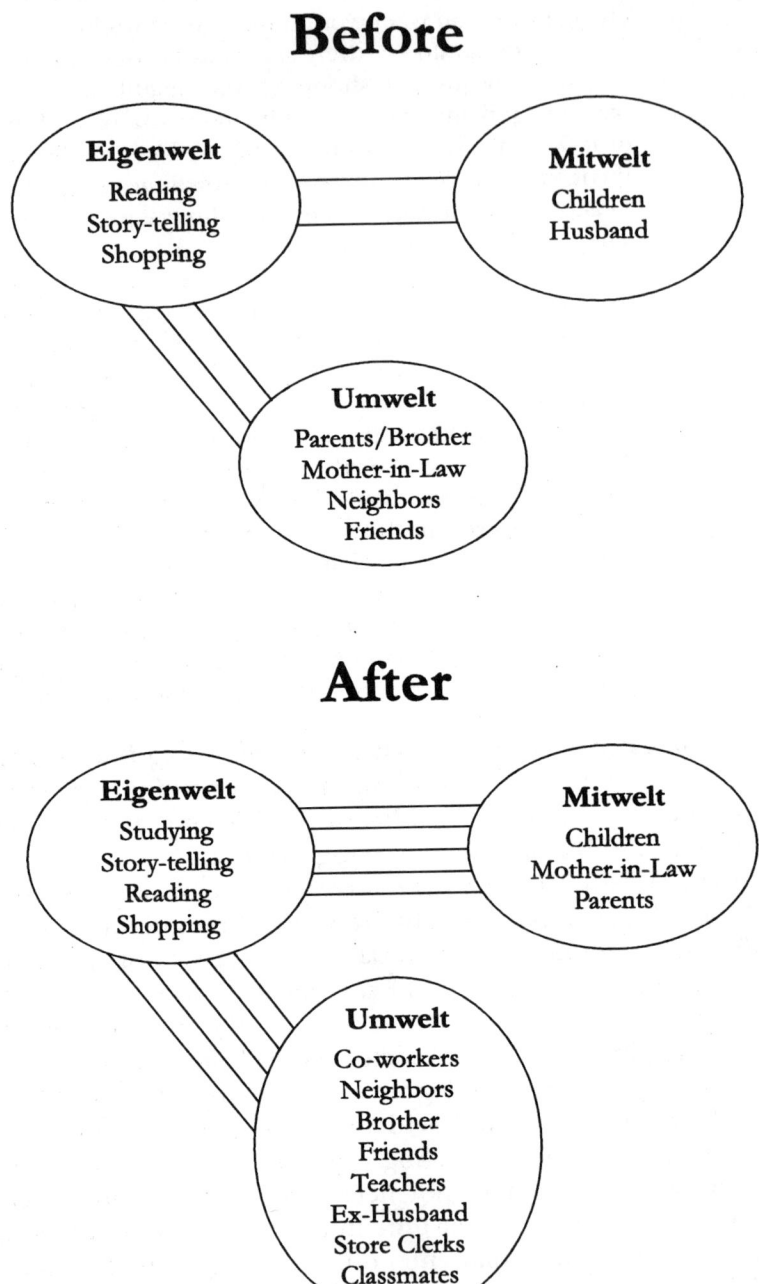

FIGURE 3.1 Susan's three worlds are depicted before and after therapy.

while at the same time emphasizing the fluctuating nature of an ongoing adjustment process.

SUMMARY

Different phases of a counseling process, modified especially for work with single parents, are described. The logical and natural flow of the individual phases within the entire process is demonstrated by following the work of the same client, who is representative of the population of single parents, through the succession of phases. Actual dialogue between client and counselor illustrates the counselor's facilitation of progressing through a given phase, its resolution, and the transitions from one phase to the next. As the steps of this comprehensive counseling approach logically follow one another, the client's growth occurs in a systematic progression. The progression often starts from a single painful situation to the acquisition of new coping skills, resulting in a different view of one's self and one's abilities, and finally in a successful adjustment and harmonious existence within one's worlds.

EXERCISE

Assume you are working for an agency that prescribes brief therapy, or that you have a client like Susan whose insurance benefits consist of six authorized therapy sessions. She has no financial resources of her own. The described program takes at least eight sessions (without need for additional repetitions). How would you structure this counseling program? Would you resort to the use of questionnaires? If so, what questionnaires would you want to use? There are no right or wrong answers because every counselor works differently.

SUGGESTED READING

Sanford, A. J. (1985). *Cognition and cognitive psychology*. New York: Basic Books.

This book is a comprehensive introduction to cognitive psychology as set within the broader cognitive science framework. The emphasis is on research, attempting to simulate human cognition through computer programs.

Sternberg, R. J., & Grigorenko, E. L. (1997). Are cognitive styles still in style? *American Psychologist, 52,* 700–712.

The authors discuss the concept of cognitive styles and describe its significance for theory and research considerations. The authors also present their own theory and research.

4

Designating the Problem Area(s)

OBJECTIVES

1. To acknowledge client's distress and reasons for entering counseling.
2. To determine if the client's presenting problem is the main source of distress.
3. To guide the client toward recognition of the real problem if appropriate.
4. To facilitate accurate identification of problem if the client has only a vague conceptualization.
5. To transfer responsibility for decisions, actions, and outcomes to the client.
6. To facilitate transition to the next phase of the counseling process.

PROBLEM AREA(S)

Clients seek counseling because they feel distress. They realize that things in their lives are not the way they want them to be. Aware of an existing problem, they may have seriously thought about possible resolutions, but not yet made a commitment for action. Prochaska, DiClemente, and Norcross (1992) considered this the contemplation stage. For some people, the contemplation stage can last quite some time as they consider pros and cons of the problem and its possible solutions. They may think that they have to work on the resolution by themselves. Others may be more eager or ready for action, and shorten the duration of their contemplation stage by immediately seeking the assistance of a professional.

Regardless of the length of time spent in contemplation, when clients enter counseling more than one area of their lives often is affected. Sorting out the various parts of one's life that could benefit from change is an awesome task for most people, especially when they are already overwhelmed by their misery. Single-parent families have the potential for an aggregation of difficulties stemming from chain reactions of smaller setbacks. For instance, financial strains may result from delayed child-support payments. Insufficient funds for the purchase of clothing or school supplies may cause difficulties with the child's functioning at school. The lack of money may severely limit social functions because money is unavailable to pay for reliable babysitters or for entertainment-related expenses. In tight situations, single parents are tempted to rely on the use of their credit cards, thereby laying the grounds for future financial, mental, and emotional stress.

Starting the Process: Identifying and Prioritizing Problem Areas

At the beginning of counseling, many clients feel the urge to ventilate their feelings. Emotional ventilation provides relief for the moment and may even have an energizing effect. The experienced counselor will use the momentum of the combined relief and energy and direct it along constructive channels that will in turn facilitate the process of resolution. The therapist who assumes that the client will begin with the most pressing issue is ill-prepared. Clients' decisions on where to start are respected and encouraged, but the therapist can and should assist in the process of prioritizing.

Clinicians use different strategies for the purpose of prioritizing. Clients first complete intake informed consent/contract forms. Then, additional information may be obtained by paper and pencil means. Some therapists (Beck, 1988) obtain clients' descriptions and responses to questionnaires. Multimodal therapy clinicians utilize a Multimodal Life History Questionnaire (Lazarus, 1984). At the end of the second session, clients receive a 12-page printed booklet with questions about past and ongoing problems. At the beginning of the third session, the therapist has sufficient information from the previous two sessions and the questionnaire to construct a preliminary Modality Profile.

Interpersonal/Intrapersonal Growth Scales

Featherstonaugh and Maass (1979) (see also Maass & Featherstonaugh, 1981) have developed the Interpersonal Growth Scale (IGS) (see Figure 4.1) and *Intra*personal Growth Scale (see Figure 4.2), depending on the range of application. The instrument consists of a system of rating scales representing various major life areas. The scales were originally designed for use in marital counseling, but they can easily be adapted to work with individual clients or clients and their children. Dimensions on these scales range from 1 to 10. The numeral one (1) reflects the area of lowest or no concern and ten (10) denotes a significant problem. In completing the scales, clients have an opportunity to express values that operate implicitly, describe their function, and make estimates of their strength in a particular situation.

The scales are used to reflect various life situations at different times in the client's life by simply marking the scales with different symbols. For instance, one set of marks (squares) describes the current situation, another (triangles) expresses goals for the future, and a third type of notation (circles) reflects a past situation when this particular life area was not problematic.

Transferring Responsibility to the Client. After introduction and explanation of the overall process, the responsibility for completing and using the IGS shifts readily from counselor to client. The flexibility of the instrument allows for easy substitution of life areas as needed for a particular client. The highest ratings on individual scales usually denote the degree of discomfort experienced by the client. These ratings will facilitate the process of prioritizing the different problem areas. In summary, working with the IGS provides an objective record where individuals express perceptions and goals.

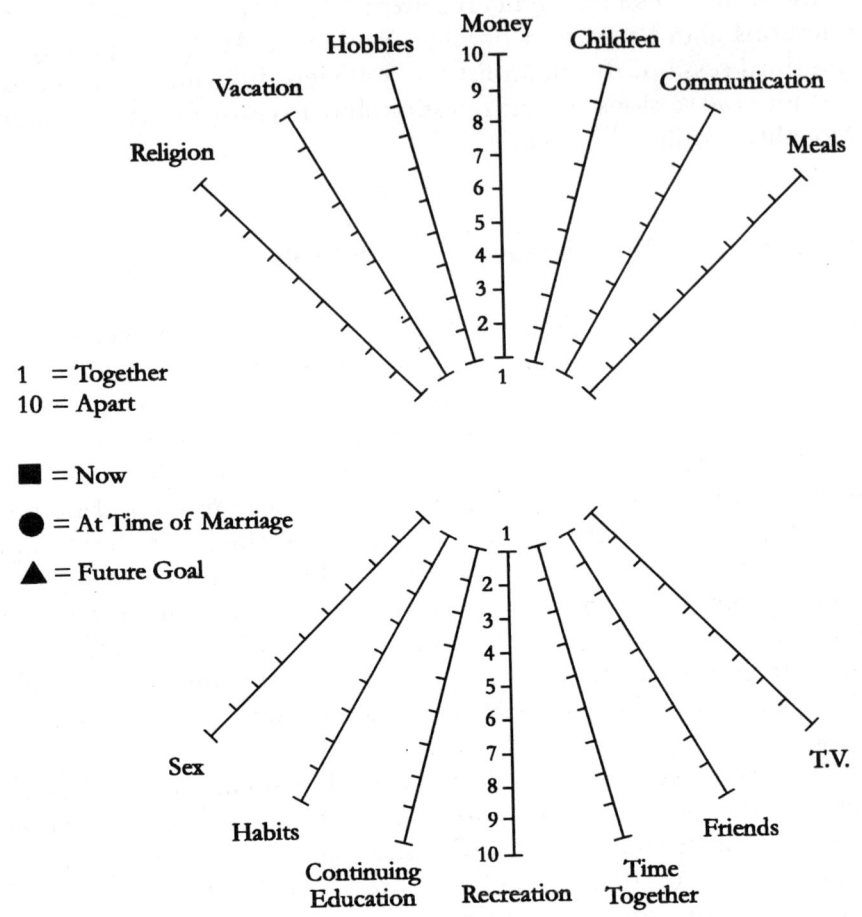

FIGURE 4.1 Sample of the Interpersonal Growth Scale (IGS).

Achieving Consensus. Areas where changes would be beneficial are emphasized; unrealistic expectations are identified; and, continuous explorations of problems are encouraged through use of the instrument. On the basis of the completed IGS forms, clients and counselors achieve agreement on targeted work areas and goals expected as consequences of working on those areas. Thus, the instrument serves

Designating the Problem Areas

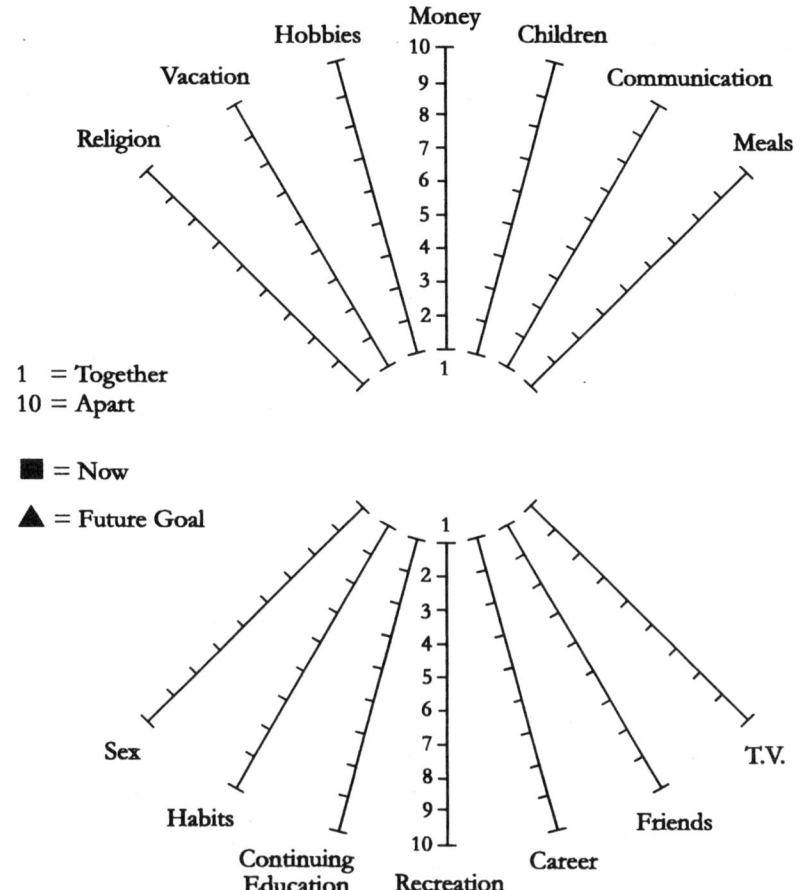

FIGURE 4.2 Sample of the Intrapersonal Growth Scale (IGS).

as an informal contract and treatment plan. The instrument is contained on a single page, and prevents clients from feeling overwhelmed when presented with it. During the counseling process, different scales can be developed for detailed exploration of particular problem areas. As the time for termination approaches, clients may again complete a set of the IGS to measure progress made toward previously specified goals.

Case Study

Bill: Unwanted Divorce

Bill, a 39-year-old, separated and then divorced, father of two sons, was referred by his friend and co-worker. Bill's depression interfered with his work performance. As foreman of a 12-man mechanics crew, he carried significant responsibilities. His boss was concerned. Bill's opening statement to the therapist was: "I want you to help me get my wife back." Bill and his wife Linda had separated 2 months before. Currently Bill was living with his parents.

At the beginning of their courtship, Bill and Linda had many interests in common. Their values seemed compatible. Both enjoyed being close to nature. They took long walks together discussing their future. One of their favorite dreams was to buy a recreational vehicle and travel to campgrounds in national parks where they could enjoy the wonders of nature. Their first son was born almost 2 years after their wedding. Three years later, when their second son arrived, they considered their family to be complete. Both agreed that Linda should stay home to raise their sons. Bill worked hard. Instead of taking vacation time, he worked overtime to provide a house for the family.

In the Southern part of the state—away from all the hustle and bustle of the city—they found the perfect place to bring up their sons. Bill did not want to leave his job in the city. He had been promoted to foreman, his workers respected him, and his future seemed assured. The drive to work took 90 minutes. To be at work on time, Bill had to get up at 4:00 a.m. The 3 hours of driving time stretched his workdays to 11 or 12 hours. Very little time was left for Bill and Linda to enjoy by themselves. Occasionally, they talked about the time when the children would be grown. They were still dreaming about traveling in their own camper to national parks.

As their sons became more involved with school and their own activities, Linda looked for a part-time job. Opportunities were limited, but the only restaurant in town needed a waitress for two evenings a week. One of the two evenings was to be on the weekend and the other during the week. Initially, Linda did not want to work in the evenings, but she rationalized the situation. She would be at home for her sons during the day, and the one evening during the week

Designating the Problem Areas

Bill would be able to return home just before she had to leave for work. It seemed like a perfect opportunity to make a little extra money without having to neglect the family's needs.

When one of the other waitresses became pregnant, the restaurant owner increased Linda's working hours. Soon, she worked four evenings a week with at least one of them on the weekends. Her boss was pleased with her work and her eagerness to help. Prior to her job Linda had made some remarks to Bill about their inability to go out or visit with friends. Occasionally, she had mentioned that their sex life was not all she had expected. During the last couple of years she appeared calmer and did not complain about anything that Bill could remember. Then, on her birthday, she asked for a divorce.

Couns: As you described your situation, you seemed surprised about your wife's wish for a divorce.

Bill: I was absolutely shocked! It all seemed so perfect. Our boys were visiting with their aunt in Canada for the summer. I thought this would be a good opportunity for a short trip for the two of us before picking the boys up from Linda's sister. We had talked so long about getting a recreational vehicle and finally had enough money for a down payment. If I continued to work overtime, we could afford the monthly installments. With her birthday coming up, it seemed like a wonderful surprise. I used my lunch hours to shop around for a camper. I found one perfect for us and arranged for all the paperwork. The camper was ready for pick-up on Saturday morning, the day after Linda's birthday. I even took a picture of it to include in the birthday card.

Couns: You worked hard on your surprise, but this was the birthday when she mentioned the divorce.

Bill: Yes, I was disappointed when Linda told me that she was going to work on Friday evening, but I dismissed it and planned around it. On the way home from work I bought the card, some flowers, and a bottle of her favorite wine and arranged everything on the table before driving over to the restaurant. Fred, the owner, seemed surprised to see me. He told me Linda had left earlier because of her birthday. When I returned home she was not there. More than an hour later I heard her car turn into the driveway. She cried when she saw the picture of the camper. She said she liked the camper, but it was too late. The thought of divorce had been on her mind for some time. A customer at the restaurant had been very attentive to her. With me gone so much she felt lonely and had become involved in an affair with the young man. She felt sexually more fulfilled with him. After the shock wore off, I begged her to give us another chance. She refused, saying she had given me many chances, but I had not listened.

Couns: Linda told you she had not been happy for some time, but you were apparently not aware of it. When you thought she had calmed down, she had actually given up on the marriage.

Bill: I guess so. I never meant to neglect her, but I usually was too tired to do much after coming home from a long workday. Can you help me get her back?

Couns: Your wife seems quite determined. How much has she acted on her decision?

Bill: She has not wasted much time. The Monday after she told me about the divorce, she had her lawyer file the papers. She told me she already found a house to rent for herself and our sons because she knew we would have to sell our house. In fact, she had contacted a real estate agent about putting our house on the market. Who knows what reason for selling she gave the agent. It seems strange to have these things going on without me knowing anything about it.

Couns: From what you are saying, it appears your wife had considered a divorce for some time and was determined to go through with it when she told you. I don't know what would persuade her to change her mind now. It would be nice if you had another opportunity to talk to her and propose any changes you might want to make to save the marriage. You can certainly try that. In the meantime, I would like you to complete this set of rating scales about some areas of your life, such as your marriage, your job, different relationships in your life, and other interests. This will give us a better picture of your overall life. The scales go from 1 to 10, with 1 denoting "no problem" and 10 being the most conflicted. Please go over the scales three times, marking where you see the situation right now, another time reflecting the state of affairs at the time of your wedding, and a third time showing your

Designating the Problem Areas

	future goals. If you can, please send me the scales in the mail, so I have them before your next appointment.
Bill:	I don't think it is necessary to go through all that. I know what I need. All I have to do is get my wife back and I am willing to do whatever is necessary to accomplish that.
Couns:	I agree with you, it would be great if you could get what you want. In order to determine how to proceed, it will be beneficial to know more about some significant areas of your life.

Summary of Client-Counselor Interaction: Unwanted Divorce. Initially, this client's behavior indicated that he thought he needed a coach rather than a therapist. He was reluctant to consider any other solution than getting his wife back. In his opinion, the achievement of his goal would resolve all his problems. The wife's determination for a divorce was not lost on the counselor. Considering the client's unawareness of his wife's feelings about the marriage, working on a courtship schedule appeared premature without additional information about significant areas in the client's life. The Interpersonal Growth Scales were intended to obtain the desired information. Although Bill was irritated with what he considered a waste of time, he reluctantly agreed to complete the instrument.

Case Study Follow-Up: Rethinking Counseling Goals

The initial set of rating scales Bill completed and mailed to the therapist included areas pertaining to marriage, such as sex, communication, time spent together, recreation, and vacation. Most of those areas received high marks, reflecting difficulties (see Figure 4.3). Children, parents, hobbies, vacation, money, and religion were additional areas presented on the scales.

Couns:	I am glad you were able to complete the instrument. You have a good relationship with your sons and you seem determined to make it even better in the future. What was surprising is how you rated the different aspects of your marriage. Your ratings do not seem to reflect a very happy marriage.
Bill:	Well, I have to admit it, you made me look at it in more

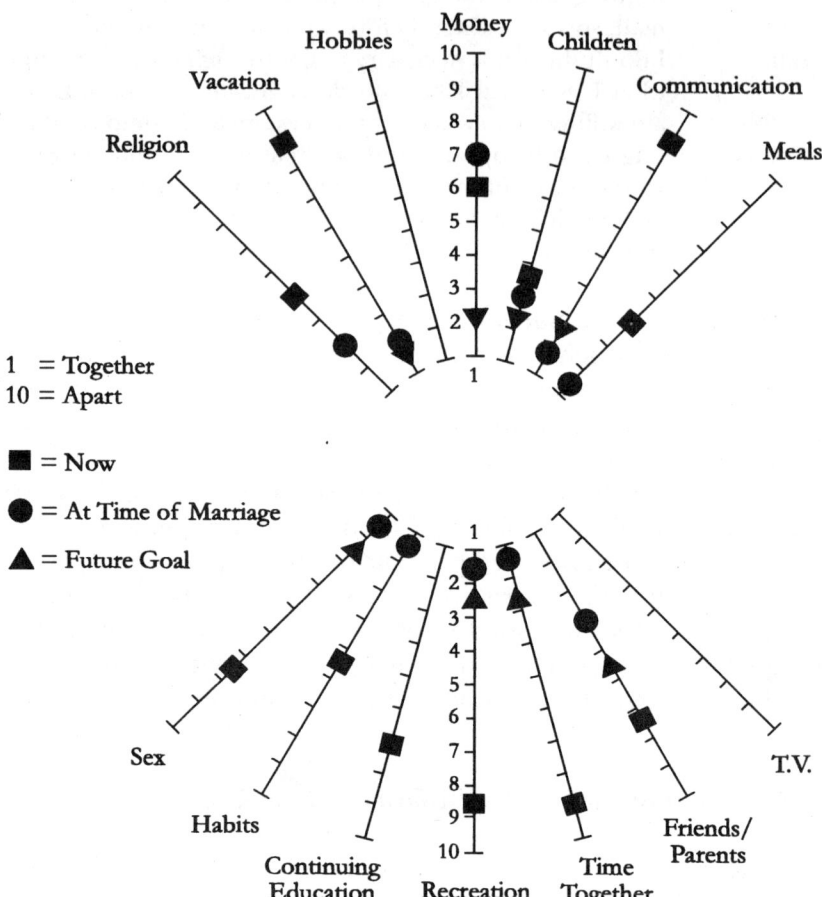

FIGURE 4.3 Ratings from Bill's Interpersonal Growth Scale (IGS).

depth. In retrospect, it seems that except for the children we don't have much in common anymore. I can't remember when we last talked about joint decisions. Our sex life has not been very active either. We have not gone out with friends or gone on vacation. We don't spend much time together. Most of the time we don't have breakfast together because I have to leave so early. Perhaps Linda is right, we let our relationship deteriorate. She thinks it

	is all my fault, but she could have been more insistent in making me listen. Her going to work did not help either because it took even more of the evenings and some of the weekends away from us. To think that she may have used some of the time when I thought she was working to meet with this young man. They may have made love while I was at home with the boys. When I think about that I get angry.
Couns:	It sounds as if you feel betrayed or taken advantage of. How is your anger going to help you in convincing Linda to take you back? And if she did, how are you going to feel in the future?
Bill:	Right now, she is not giving me a chance. She has made it clear that she will only talk to me about the divorce settlement, the custody arrangement, and visitation schedule with my sons. The day after my session with you I got a registered letter delivered at work. It was from Linda's attorney, telling me that no other communication was wanted by Linda. Your assignment was actually quite helpful because it made me realize that our marriage had not been very good for me either lately. I had not wanted to look at that and admit it. I still would want to continue with the marriage and try to make it better, but it would be mostly for my boys. I am lonely for them and I feel guilty about having to leave them.
Couns:	How are your sons responding to the changes?
Bill:	They were quite upset. I told them that I did not want to leave, but had no choice. At first they could not understand why I did not stay in town. When I explained to them that my moving in with their grandparents was a temporary solution, they felt a bit better. It breaks my heart to not see them every day. For now, when they come for their weekend visits, we stay at my parents' home. If Linda insists on the divorce, I have to wait and see what my financial situation will be before I can look for a new home.
Couns:	You sound more accepting of the possibility of a divorce. With the emotional turmoil you have been experiencing, your parents' support must be a great comfort to you.
Bill:	They have been wonderful, my sister too. I don't know what I would have done without them. I told my sister about the homework assignment that you gave me. She

	thought it was a great idea because it made me face reality. I think she suspected that Linda had some other interests, but did not want to get involved in our marriage. Somehow, my sister and Linda never became as close as I had hoped. I respect my sister's position and I told her so.
Couns:	Although you are in an unsettled situation, you seem to have achieved some sense of stability for now.
Bill:	Yes, that is true. I miss my boys and I spend as much time with them as possible. Linda is not interfering with that. She wants the divorce to be over with and, I guess, I will have to get used to that. I remember the last time I was here, I was so convinced that I had to get Linda back. Actually, I was upset with you when you gave me those rating scales. I thought it was a big waste of time when I needed every minute to win my wife back.
Couns:	I was aware of your feelings and I appreciated your politeness when you went along with it, even though you may have considered my request to be unreasonable. Your willingness to look at the situation more objectively undoubtedly caused you pain, but it also gave you a different level of awareness of your own feelings. What are your plans now?
Bill:	As you said before, I am in a somewhat stable holding pattern, if there is such a thing. My job and my family are my support systems. I will be looking around in different neighborhoods for a new home. I cannot make a definite decision, yet because I don't know how much money I will have left after the divorce. I don't want to move that far away from the city again. My job is my financial security. Driving all that distance takes too much time out of my life. What I would really like to do is to move closer to my sister. I like her husband, and their two children would be great company for my boys. Even though I want to spend every minute with them, I know that they need to have friends their own age on their weekend visits, too.
Couns:	In spite of your pain you have done a lot of thinking leading to some preliminary decisions.
Bill:	Some pieces are beginning to fall into place. Do you think I can take a break from counseling now? I am sure I will need your help again after the divorce is final.
Couns:	You probably need time and money for the divorce process. With the support of your family and your job you

seem to be doing as well as can be expected. If anything comes up that you want to discuss with me, I am just a phone call away.

Summary of Client-Counselor Interaction: Rethinking Counseling Goals. The rating scales had shown Bill that his primary goal for entering counseling had not been a realistic one. While acknowledging the client's painful struggle, the counselor gave feedback regarding the client's current situation, and expressed appreciation for the client's compliance with the homework assignment. The therapist was sensitive to the client's adjustment and shift in immediate goals that made current counseling appear less urgent. The counselor's closing statements provided a comfortable atmosphere for the client's possible re-entry into the counseling process at a later time.

Single Fathers as Primary Parents

The essential skills for functioning in the role of primary caretaker can be developed by female or male parents. They are not personality traits particular to any gender, as previously believed by psychoanalytic and sex-role socialization theorists. Risman (1987) proposed that single fathers placed in the role of primary parent not by their choice (i.e., widowed or deserted by wife) will demonstrate parental behavior more closely resembling that of mothers than that of married fathers. When single mothers and single fathers were compared regarding time spent with their children and spent in doing household tasks, increased levels of involvement were found for fathers in situations where mothers were absent (Hall, Walker, & Acock, 1995).

As part of a larger study, Cooksey and Fondell (1996) looked at different categories of family structure for effects of fathers' time spent with their children and the children's grades. Of interest here are the categories of family structure, where a particular child lives with the biological father and a stepmother, as compared to the child living with a single parent. Time spent was measured in the frequencies of father-children involvement in various activities. The activities ranged from leisure activities, to working on a project, to meals shared.

The conclusions were that single fathers are quite involved in their children's lives, and engage more in a variety of activities than do fathers in more traditional family settings. In father-stepmother families, fathers spent more time with their children than fathers did in families where the biological mother was present. Overall, children whose fathers shared meals with them and were involved in a variety of activities with them tended to have significantly better academic performances than children whose fathers were less involved in their lives. In this particular study, children from two-parent biological families performed better in school than children from all other types of family structures, even though fathers in two-parent families were less involved with their children than the single fathers. Children from single-father households tended to show significantly poorer performance, and teenage children living with single fathers had the lowest grades, despite higher level of paternal involvement. Although paternal involvement is thought to be an important predictor of children's academic performance, it seems to play only a small part. As Hetherington et al. (1998) summarized, the differences in behavior in children of divorced parents and intact families are less when the pre-divorce mental health of the family is taken into account.

Individualist vs. Microstructural Theories

Risman and Park (1988) contrasted two different theoretical explanations, individualist and microstructural, and tested the strength of each by comparing single custodial mothers and single custodial fathers on a variety of dimensions. The individualist view holds that sex-role socialization accounts for sex differences in parental behavior. Preferences for sex-typed parental roles are assumed to be internalized as personality traits. Microstructural theory argues that contextual factors in the everyday environment, such as differential opportunities, bring about sex differences in parenting. Parenting behavior is not thought to be primarily fixed by biological predisposition or sex-role socialization, but is viewed as an ongoing adaptive interaction of social expectations and children's perceived needs.

Subjects in the study were mailed questionnaires. Out of 281 single fathers, 54% responded, and 58% of the 126 contacted single mothers responded to the questionnaires. The study focused on measuring the relationship between the single parent and the youngest child (under age 14 years) living with the parent full-time. Family structure and extrafamilial societal position were considered as the main microstructural factors. As dependent variables, three dimensions were analyzed: Intimacy (parent's assessment of the child's self-disclosure and level of affection that the parents reported feeling for this child); child development (parent's ratings of the child's personality on 14 traits and the presence of academic, school discipline, and mental health problems); and housework (varying degrees of reported responsibility for different household tasks taken on by parents and children).

The results showed a positive relationship between parent's sex and reported level of children's self-disclosure. Women were significantly more likely to report higher disclosure from their children than men. Surprisingly, parents with more education were less likely to rate high affection for the children. When sex and microstructural variables were analyzed together, parental employment status accounted for significant differences. Parents who worked full- or part-time experienced more disclosure from their children than did parents who were not employed at all. Working parents also reported fewer problem traits in their children than did those who were at home full-time. On the dimension of housework, the results showed that women were less likely than men to have other persons assume responsibility for their household labor.

In their discussion, the authors concluded that both men and women could function equally well as primary caretakers, but parents who most closely resemble the traditional caretaker role reported the most problems with their children's development. As an explanation, the authors suggested that many of the at-home parents may really be seeking employment, and thus would be better described as unemployed workers than full-time homemakers. How the investigators arrived at this consideration was not made clear. An equally likely explanation would be that the higher degree of exposure parents and children have in situations where the parent is not employed outside the home leads to an attitude of taking each other for granted and resulting in deterioration of behaviors. Moreover, the fact that the data came exclusively from the parents' perceptions is a serious limitation. Information from schools and the children themselves would have added some level of objectivity to the study.

Subjective Perceptions of Problems and Their Resolutions

Problems as perceived by clients can have different sources of development, such as being externally imposed on the client or originating within the client (Heppner & Krauskopf, 1987). Whether a problem is created by external forces (actions from people or events outside of the realm of control of the individual) or by factors residing within the individual (feelings of dissatisfaction or vague unhappiness about one's current life situation), the difficulty is further complicated by the individual's subjective perception of the problem area and its possible solutions. Knowing how the client views the nature of the problem situation can be of benefit in deciding where to direct the focus.

In the previous example, the client was faced with a problem seemingly brought on by outside forces (wife wanting a divorce). Initially, the client saw reconciliation with his wife as the only solution. In other cases, the immediate problem may have been caused by an external event, such as the death of a spouse, but the path to a solution is often obscured by contradictory feelings interfering with the actions and decisions to be made by the person. Beliefs about what the person should do and what the individual might want to do can create a subjective perception of helplessness and confusion in the individual.

Horizontal and Vertical Loyalties

In discussing loyalty and loss, David Seaburn (1990) distinguished between vertical loyalties and horizontal loyalties. Vertical loyalties span the person's connectedness to previous and future generations, such as parents, grandparents, and the person's children. Relationships with spouses, friends, and peers are characterized by horizontal loyalties. At times of widowhood, horizontal and vertical loyalties can contribute to conflicts. The individual confronted with conflicting loyalties may have great difficulties sorting out and prioritizing loyalties. Seaburn failed to consider the effects of the individual's loyalty to the self that complicates the situation further. The individual's personal world is impacted by and, in turn, impacting upon both horizontal and vertical loyalties through the system of cooperative and competitive values, as pointed out by Adkins (1960).

Case Study

Kent: Sudden Widowhood

Kent, a widower with two children, had called for an appointment. His wife had died suddenly after a car accident, and he wanted to be seen as soon as possible because he had to make some serious decisions about his family's future.

Couns: You sounded like you were in great distress when you called. I am very sorry about your wife's death. How can I be of help?

Kent: I am grateful that you could fit me in so quickly. I don't think I can allow myself the time to mourn over my wife's death right now. Decisions have to be made and my feelings cannot interfere with making the decisions.

Couns: What are the urgent decisions you are facing? Are they connected with your wife's death?

Kent: The decisions involve our children. Heather, my daughter, is almost 15, and my son Tim is 11 years old. How can I take care of them when I work full-time? Having just lost their mother, they need special attention and support now.

Couns: Taking care of two children is a big responsibility for a working person. How do you see your options at this point?

Kent: The easiest solution would probably be to have them live with their maternal grandparents. We moved to this town almost 2 years ago, and the children still have ties with friends and relatives there.

Couns: What are your feelings when you think of this possibility?

Kent: I have mixed feelings about sending my children back. I would sure miss them, but, as I said, feelings should not enter into the decision. I should decide on what is best for my children.

Couns: How do you see the benefits to the children? Have you consulted them about the decision?

Kent: I have asked them. My daughter does not want to go back to our hometown. Heather wants to become an architect and we think that she is quite talented. She likes the schools here. One of her teachers has helped her to get

	into some special drawing classes that will be a good preparation for her. Tim would just as well go back, but he doesn't want to leave me. The benefits in moving the children back would be that they would be well taken care of by their grandparents. My mother also lives there and would be an additional support for the children.
Couns:	Apparently, you have not made that decision yet. That leads me to believe you are not quite happy with it or you have some other options that you are considering.
Kent:	My mother could come and live with us, but she has arthritis and it is difficult for her to get around. She would come and help us for our sake, but it would be a sacrifice for her. She likes her home and the community. She probably would not be as happy here and I hate to ask her to leave her comfortable life. Another possibility would be for all of us to move back.
Couns:	How would that impact your life? You had a reason to come to this town in the first place.
Kent:	Moving here was a big step toward my dream for the future. In college I had a double major, English and History. I have a strong interest in history and always wanted to write historical novels. I thought working for a big publishing company would be helpful and give me more understanding of what I need to do about writing. My job for the local newspaper back home was good, but had no room for further development. When I got the offer from this major publishing company, I thought it was the chance of a lifetime.
Couns:	How do you like your job now? Has it worked out for you the way you had hoped?
Kent:	It's a great job. I like the editing work; it actually helps me sharpen my own writing skills. Sometimes there are tight deadlines, and tension builds up. But overall, I think it's the job for me. Before my wife's death, I had even been able to think of a new twist to the novel I had started back home. Of course, I can't concentrate on anything right now. Even on my job I have difficulty concentrating. That's why I have to make the decision about our future.
Couns:	With the recent traumatic event in your life, it would be difficult to concentrate on other things, especially with the unsettledness of your current situation. Because you like your job so much, have you thought of a way to stay

Designating the Problem Areas 105

Kent:	here and keep your children with you? I don't see that as an option.
Couns:	Perhaps not. It might help if you made a list of your options as you just outlined them for me today. With every one of the options, please list the reasons why this would be a good solution and the reasons why it might not work in your opinion. In other words, list the pros and cons for every option you are considering. There may be something that we have not addressed yet, but it may surface as we go through your lists. Also, I would like you to complete this brief questionnaire about some characteristics in your present situation. If it fits with your schedule, we can meet again in three days instead of waiting for a week to continue with our work.

Summary of Client-Counselor Interaction: Sudden Widowhood. The most significant aspect of the session was the client's refusal to discuss any emotions. The therapist was aware of the client's avoidance to address his feelings, but decided to accept the client's decision for the time being. The reasons were twofold. The therapist's respect for the client's wishes was combined with the untimeliness of producing client's resistance in the first session. The client was facing a tremendous struggle, and the therapist suspected that the client's underlying emotions might have actually impaired his decision-making skills. For the moment, it was more important to create an environment where the client could feel safe in exploring whatever issues he was willing to look at.

The client's way of responding to the counselor's attempt to consider staying with the children in their current environment as one of the options revealed the client's unwillingness to discuss this as a possible alternative. Again, nothing could be won in confronting the client with his resistance at this early stage. Instead, by assigning the client to work on the positive and negative forces inherent in any option, the counselor gave the client more time to reconsider his reasoning. The questionnaire provided by the therapist combines aspects of subjective perceptions of problems and solutions with loyalties adhered to by the individual (see Table 4.1 Cognitive style). The therapist's subtle statement that they may not have addressed all the aspects of the problem situation opened the door for the client to look at underlying issues when he felt ready for it. The counselor's

TABLE 4.1 Cognitive Style

Identify the problem:

1. *The current problem was caused by*
    - a) _____ A disastrous external event
    - b) _____ Responses to others
    - c) _____ My own decision
    - d) _____ The situation I was in

2. *I intend to solve the problem by*
    - a) _____ Accept it, make the best of it
    - b) _____ Change my approach to it
    - c) _____ Learn why it happened
    - d) _____ Move away from it, forget it

3. *To solve the problem, I have to*
    - a) _____ Support family member's feelings
    - b) _____ Allow for friends, colleague's feelings
    - c) _____ Act on how I feel about it
    - d) _____ Just do it—get it done.

4. *When I think about resolving it, I feel*
    - a) _____ Anger, resentment
    - b) _____ Guilt, shame, depressed
    - c) _____ Anxious, want to avoid it
    - d) _____ Relief, when I think it will be over.

5. *Where do the feelings come from?*
    - a) _____ When I act against family beliefs
    - b) _____ Promises I make and don't keep
    - c) _____ When others don't do as they promise
    - d) _____ When people don't care about me

6. *This problem happened because*
    - a) _____ I didn't know until it was too late
    - b) _____ It's in my genes—It's who I am
    - c) _____ I'm impulsive, can't control it
    - d) _____ It's a habit—since I was a child

Designating the Problem Areas

suggestion to change the regular weekly schedule and to meet instead after a shorter interval accommodated the urgency of the client's situation, and eliminated a time delay that might have weakened the impact of the session, with its obviously unasked and unanswered questions.

Case Study Follow-Up: Guilt Feelings From Unresolved Requests

For his next appointment the client arrived early with his list of options. He seemed eager to start.

Kent: You were right, there is something that we did not discuss. The questionnaire made me think of it. I had not intended to tell anybody, but I cannot carry the burden by myself. For now I cannot tell anyone in my family. After what you said the other day, I thought talking to you might give me some relief.

Couns: I am very glad you decided our relationship is safe enough for you to discuss something that troubles you so deeply. Does it have to do with your wife's death?

Kent: Yes, it does. In the hospital before she died, my wife was conscious for a while. I think she knew that she was dying because she asked me what I would do if I were alone with the children. I tried to avoid talking about the possibility of her dying. Although the doctors told me that she was seriously injured in the accident, I just did not want to accept the fact that she may not leave the hospital to continue living with us. It was like refusing to believe that she could stop breathing would prevent from happening what I was afraid of. So I wasted some of our precious time by trying to reassure her that she would get well. But she knew. She held out her hand to me to squeeze mine and she asked me to promise her that I would take the children back to our hometown to live there. I was so shocked that I could not answer her right away or that's what I thought. Now I don't know if I could not answer or did not want to answer faster. She died before I responded to her request.

Couns: What a tremendous burden you carried since your wife's

	death. Your instincts are probably right not to disclose this to your family now. At the end of our previous session, I had the impression that you might be punishing yourself for something. How do you feel now?
Kent:	I feel very guilty and yes, I have been punishing myself for not answering my wife, but I did not really know that I was punishing myself. Aren't you going to ask me what my answer would have been if she had not died so soon?
Couns:	No, I don't think I have any right to add to your burden. If at some time you decide to explore that question, I would be glad to be there to help if I can.
Kent:	It drives me crazy not to know what I would have said. Would I have given the promise? Would I have denied her last request? I don't have the courage to answer that question.
Couns:	You were placed in one of the most difficult situations that anybody can be in. In our culture, we seem to accept the requests of a dying person as something sacred, something that has to be honored. We usually don't consider the consequences for the person who is asked for the promise. What if the promise would change the person's life to a degree that it destroys his goals? Because one person dies, does that mean the living person loses his right to decide what to do? I am sure your wife asked for the promise because she thought that would be best for you and the children. Her request reflected her opinion, but how can another person know for certain what would be best for the other? In the years of your marriage, did you always completely agree on your decisions? No matter how close two people may be, they don't always have the same opinion about everything that goes on in their lives.
Kent:	That is true, we did not always agree on things, but we usually discussed it and arrived at a decision that seemed to be the best under the circumstances. As a matter of fact, we didn't agree on moving here. Marilyn would have liked to stay in our town and in our nice home. She was a teacher and felt comfortable with the school system. She did admit that there was not much room for expansion for me professionally, but she thought that we were at a comfortable stage in our lives. I was not ready to settle for the comfort yet and wanted to try other things. When Marilyn saw how important it was to me she settled for a

Designating the Problem Areas

	period of 5 years to try out life in the "big city." It was easy for her to get a part-time teaching job here. She was a good teacher.
Couns:	If your wife had not died, would you have stayed here for another 3 years?
Kent:	Yes, do you mean I should look at the situation from that angle?
Couns:	It seems to me that before making a decision on what to do with your family, your feelings about your wife's request need to be resolved. Your feelings will have a bearing on your decision, no matter how hard you are trying to ignore them. Before we look at your list of options, let's consider the possible consequences resulting from different responses to your wife's request. As you had indicated earlier, you felt guilty for not responding faster and giving your wife the comfort of your promise. Assuming that you can go back into the past and make that promise—how would you feel?
Kent:	If I had said yes, I know I could not break that promise. Without question, I would have to take the children and move back. How would I feel? I would not feel guilty, at least, not toward Marilyn. Giving up my current job would make me feel resentful, because I could not make the best of the opportunity to find out if I could succeed as a writer.
Couns:	Where would the feelings of resentment be directed at?
Kent:	The likely target would be my wife and, to a degree, possibly my children.
Couns:	That is a very honest, if painful, answer. Now, let's assume that you told your wife you could not make the commitment she asked for. How would you feel under those circumstances?
Kent:	Immediately I would feel guilty that I let her down.
Couns:	That would be natural, given what you told us about your thinking. Are there any other feelings that you might be aware of?
Kent:	Now that you are asking, there is some fear.
Couns:	Where does the fear come from? What is the concern of your fear?
Kent:	My children. What if they suffer? What if I don't raise them right?
Couns:	Your concerns are legitimate. Even when parents do their

	very best, they don't know how their children will turn out. You would not have had any guarantees if your wife had lived. Are there any other feelings that come to mind?
Kent:	When you mentioned that parents don't have any guarantees, I became aware of feeling lonely, of almost being abandoned. That is silly, I know Marilyn did not abandon me. It was not her choice to go. I sound like a very selfish person.
Couns:	Single parents often feel lonely or abandoned as they struggle with responsibilities that are normally shared by two people. Many single parents experience similar feelings to your own.
Kent:	When you talk about feelings, it sounds so natural. There is another feeling that I don't know what word to give to. When talking about not making the commitment to my wife, in addition to the feelings I mentioned, I also had a tiny good feeling. It was very fleeting, but I think it had to do with not giving in or keeping control over my future—if that makes any sense.
Couns:	It makes a lot of sense. You are in a complicated situation that would give rise to a wide range of feelings in most people. Some of the feelings may be in direct conflict with others, as you have already noticed. The tiny good feeling seems to have come from the thought of holding onto something important to you personally, not necessarily shared with anybody else. In addition to the parts of our lives that we share with others, such as family members and close friends, there is a part that is our very own. The part includes hopes, wishes, and ambitions for ourselves as well as feelings associated with them. This personal part also needs attention.
Kent:	Suddenly, I am very tired. I don't know that I am any closer to making a decision, but I feel now that I am not quite ready yet.
Couns:	You have worked hard in today's session; no wonder you are emotionally exhausted. You had the courage to look at what you have been secretly afraid of. You have acknowledged your feelings, even if you did not always approve of them. You are struggling with the responsibility for two young people and the decision only you can make for the well-being of all three of you. We did not get to look at your list of options. Without identifying your feelings, I

believe, you could not have made the best decisions, because you did not know how your feelings were interfering with them. In light of what we discussed today, I would like you to again go over your list of options and reasons why they would or would not work. Please make any changes that you think are appropriate now.

Summary of Client-Counselor Interaction: Guilt Feelings From Unresolved Requests.

The timing between the first two sessions had been optimal. The client had just enough time to remain concerned with the content of the first session, and not enough time to build up additional defenses or dismiss his concerns.

As the counselor had expected, there were significant reasons behind the client's refusal to consider his emotions. The questionnaire had triggered the client's thoughts about the reasons. The counselor's patience in the first session had made it possible for the client to disclose his deepest concerns and fears. Refraining from any curiosity or judgment as to what actions the client should have undertaken at the time of his wife's request for a commitment, the counselor explained the general reasons why people regard such a request with great seriousness. By adding consideration for the needs of the client, the counselor assisted the client in accepting his concerns for himself. The final decision will still have to be made by the client, but the awareness of his emotions will be more beneficial to his decision-making than the denial had been.

Despite the client's strong resistance to discussing emotions, the counselor managed to make the client more comfortable by relating that these feelings are natural and common to many people. The counselor praised the client for his courage to disclose his struggle over what the client perceived as shortcomings in himself, but the counselor did not agree with him that they are indeed shortcomings.

At the end of the session, the counselor acknowledged that they had not been able to go over the client's homework, and encouraged him to make any additional changes for the next meeting. When homework assignments cannot be explored because of time constraints or similar reasons, the therapist needs to acknowledge that. Otherwise, the client may think that the time and energy expanded on completing the assignment was not worthy of attention in the session and may take future assignments less seriously.

Case Study Follow-Up: Unexpected Options

Kent's employer had recognized Kent's difficulties in handling his responsibilities as a single parent. Kent was a valuable employee, and his boss offered to let Kent work part-time in the office and part-time at home. The offer made available the additional option of keeping the children here with him.

Couns: Which one of the options on your list would you like to discuss first?

Kent: My boss gave me the option to work part-time at the office and part-time at home, so I would be able to supervise my children's activities. I thought that was extremely understanding of him.

Couns: His offer shows that he values your work highly. How does this option influence your decision?

Kent: I feel great about his offer and how it reflects his opinion of my work. Continuing with my job is tempting, especially because I had applied at a local college to teach a course next semester.

Couns: You seem to be ambivalent about your opportunities. Is there anything else that bothers you?

Kent: Even with the help from my boss, the responsibility of raising two children by myself worries me. How do I know that I am doing the right thing by keeping them with me. How do I prepare them for life?

Couns: You are right. Raising children is a great responsibility, and most of us have little preparation for the task, other than perhaps following what our parents did with us or, if we did not like it, we may decide to do the opposite of what they did. If your wife were still here, you would not have worried as much, is that right? Are there any particular concerns on your mind?

Kent: My daughter is my main concern. She is at an age where boys will soon start looking at her. She is very pretty. I don't know how much she knows about boys and sex and things like that.

Couns: Have you asked her about what she thinks or if your wife had talked to her?

Kent: No, I did not want to draw her attention to that part of life, hoping that she would not be interested in it yet. I don't want her to end up like her mother and I. Her mother was pregnant with her before we got married. My mother-in-law knew that Marilyn was pregnant and she never forgave me for that. She has been pressuring me to have the children live with her and her husband. In her opinion, I am not responsible enough to take care of a young girl.

Couns: How do you feel about your mother-in-law's opinion?

Kent: I resent it, and yet she is right; it was my fault that Marilyn was pregnant. I felt bad about it at the time, but obviously I could not do anything to make it undone.

Couns: I can understand that you would feel some resentment and you are right, the pregnancy was the consequence of your and your wife's decisions and actions. In all those years you did not seem to have challenged your mother-in-law's opinion, instead you were ready to accept the blame and feel guilty. How much sex education did Marilyn have at the time, do you know?

Kent: I don't think she knew much of anything. She was afraid of getting pregnant because her mother had always warned her not to come home pregnant, but I doubt she told her much else.

Couns: If that is how your mother-in-law instructed your wife, what makes you think she would be more effective with your daughter? Has she changed her attitude about discussing sexual matters?

Kent: I don't think so, she seems as tight about the subject as ever. You brought up an interesting point. Are you saying that Marilyn was basically unprotected because she did not know anything about sex? Her mother should have been more open with her?

Couns: I don't know what Marilyn's mother could or should have done, and it does not take away your part of the responsibility. Your guilt feelings indicate that you basically agreed with your mother-in-law that you are blameworthy. If you did not agree and considered your mother-in-law's statements as her opinion to which she is entitled, you would not have felt guilty. You may have had a different opinion. It seems that the more knowledge we have about a certain subject, the better we are able to make decisions that are in our own best interest. Refusing to have or give sufficient information does not prevent temptation. In fact, as a man, you are in a good position to give advice to a young girl about approaches that a young man, stimulated by powerful sexual urges, might use to persuade a young girl to have sex with him. If we separate "girl talk" from "boy talk," we miss the opportunity to learn from each other.

Kent: I never thought of it that way. All these years I felt guilty and angry. I don't want my children to go through experiences like that. I would not want to tell my daughter the whole truth about her mother being pregnant prior to our wedding, but it might increase my children's trust in me if I am open about having experienced many of their urges and desires myself.

Couns: Being open about one's own sexual urges takes courage, but as you said, your children may feel more comfortable about confiding in you about sexual matters, rather than going to someone else where they may get half-truths. How much you want to disclose about the actual situation between you and Marilyn is, of course, up to you. If you want to protect your wife's image, perhaps Marilyn was not the only young girl you liked. I am sure you can think of a way to pass your knowledge on to your children. You can also enlist the services of a professional sex educator to help you with your children's preparation for that part of their lives.

Kent: Actually, there was another girl I was interested in. Marilyn's cousin Beatrice was on my mind a lot. We had dated a couple of times, but when I found out that Marilyn was pregnant, I stopped seeing Beatrice. She got married and moved away with her husband. Many years later I saw her again at one of those big family-get-togethers for someone's 75th birthday or 50th wedding anniversary. She looked happy and just as pretty as I had remembered her.

Couns: How do you feel about your options now?

Kent: This discussion has opened up a whole new way of thinking for me. When I first came here I wanted to make the best decision for my children without considering my own feelings or my wishes. I believed that I had to put my emotions aside because they would cloud my reasoning. I was ready to hand my children over to my parents-in-law or move us all back to my hometown. Little did I know that my feelings of fear, guilt, and anger had already interfered with my thinking.

Couns:	With your new way of considering your feelings as important as your thinking and acting, where do you want to go from here?
Kent:	Without having to be afraid of ruining my children's lives, I think the best decision at the moment is for all three of us to stay here. My job is important for all of us. The understanding my boss has shown me makes me feel confident about working in this company. I can be more helpful to my children in their careers in this town than going back to my old job. Certainly Heather is much better off here where she has already started on her future career goals. For Tim the most important thing is that we all stay together, even if he still misses his old friends. He and I will have more time together because his classes let out earlier than Heather's, and if I can work at home in the afternoons, I will be available to him. We can do our homework together. I will ask my mother to stay with us for the first couple of months until we have established a routine that works for us. Perhaps she can stay with us for 2 to 3 weeks and then return home for a while and come back to us again. We can be flexible about that.
Couns:	You seem comfortable with the decision. Having your mother here on a temporary basis sounds like a good way to start. Another benefit of your satisfaction with your job may be that as you are happier in your work, you will also be more sensitive to your children's wishes for fulfilling careers as they develop their future plans. How do you feel about responding to your mother-in-law's request for wanting to raise your children?
Kent:	I feel I am now better equipped to deal with the situation. First of all, it was helpful when you pointed out that, even in the most harmonious marriage, spouses do not always completely agree on every decision that needs to be made. Marilyn's death gave a sacred weight to her opinion in my mind. Now I am looking at it more the way we would have handled it if she had stayed alive. The welfare of our children would have been more important to both of us than to make a promise. I understand that now. Even though I don't have the luxury of her blessing, I will continue doing what I think is best for my family. As I had the opportunity to discuss this with you, I don't think I need to burden anybody else in the family with my secret.

| | What you said about preparing our children regarding their future sexual urges and the consequences of their actions by educating them has lifted some of the obligations arising from my guilt feelings. As I am more confident that I can do as adequate a job as my mother-in-law in preparing my children, I don't have to give her any reasons why I want to keep the children here with me. There is no sense in making her feel bad just because I felt guilty all those years. Our new life will not be easy, but it is comforting to know that help can be found when needed. |
| Couns: | You have come to an important point in your life, a point where you are willing to shoulder more responsibilities than you ever had before. You seem to look at them as challenges rather than just responsibilities or burdens. The emotional growth you have experienced is reflected in your decision not to blame anybody but to resolve the emotional aspects with yourself. |

Summary of Client-Counselor Interaction: Unexpected Options.

When the client's situation had been changed favorably by his employer's offer, the therapist interpreted the client's hesitation to indicate the existence of another underlying conflict that the client had not mentioned yet. The therapist's acknowledgment of the difficulty in knowing exactly how to raise children facilitated the client's admission of his mother-in-law's judgment of the impulsive behavior in his youth. The client had never challenged his mother-in-law's judgment of him, and seemed to be agreeing with her that he was indeed unfit to raise his daughter. The counselor's explanation of the dynamics of guilt feelings provided the client with an opportunity to re-examine the appropriateness of his emotions and see the past in a different light without removing the client's responsibility for his actions. The client's initial lack of awareness of how his feelings had already impaired his decision-making ability required further exploration. The result was increased confidence in his ability to take care of his children.

The other important issue centered on the disclosure made by the client in the previous session. Between the two sessions, the client had time to contemplate the significance and consequences of his wife's request for a promise that he had not been ready to make.

He appeared prepared to accept the fact that this was a decision the two spouses might not agree on, but their feelings for each other would not have changed. Had his wife recovered from her injuries, their marriage would not have been significantly impacted by the absence of the agreement. As the counselor pointed out, the client had demonstrated significant emotional growth. In the future, the client would be less likely to underestimate the significance of his emotions in making decisions.

Hope and Determination in the Pursuit of Goals

When a combination of hope and determination fuels the drive toward a certain goal, a positive outcome is usually expected. In Western cultures, hope has a positive connotation, as most people hope for the best—not the worst—to happen. People's ability to sustain hope in different situations varies greatly, based on the strength of the individual's conviction regarding the probability of occurrence of the wished outcome. In extreme cases, the person may become obsessed with the possession of what is denied, and will continue to direct all efforts toward the desired goal instead of redirecting energies toward a more realistic outcome (Lazarus & Lazarus, 1994). Strong personal beliefs resulting in erroneous judgment may lead to increased pain and loss of effective coping skills.

Case Study

Rhesa: Unrequited Love

The young divorced mother of two daughters came to counseling because she had been dating a man who had initially shown a strong interest in her. More recently he had become less ardent in his pursuit of her.

Couns: What would you like to have happen as a result of coming here? You mentioned that you wanted to work on relationship issues. Can you give me some details about the relationship?
Rhesa: I met this man through some friends. He is not particularly

	good-looking, but he is very intelligent. He knows so much and he is so sophisticated. I felt very flattered that he would pay attention to me. That was almost 2 years ago. We went for long walks and he told me about himself and his work. He seemed so different from most men I had met, except perhaps for my ex-husband. He is also very intelligent, and I often felt intimidated because I had not gone to college and was not as educated as my ex-husband.
Couns:	You are a very attractive young woman; it is not surprising that men would want to date you. Did you feel intimidated with your current friend, like you did with your ex-husband?
Rhesa:	Yes, I do, but I remind myself that I can use his intelligence to grow just by listening to him. Besides, I have other things to offer a man. I am a very caring person and try to help wherever I can. I am sure we would have a perfect relationship if he would only see that.
Couns:	Yes, I am sure you have many fine qualities that are important in a good relationship. You mentioned earlier that your friend has become somewhat less intense in his involvement with you. As far as you know, did anything happen that would account for the change?
Rhesa:	I think it happened gradually. I cannot pinpoint any particular event that would have lead to the change in him. For several months, we spent every second weekend together. When my daughters were visiting with their father, we spent a lot of time together; sometimes he would even stay overnight. On the other weekends, we would spend some time with my daughters. Usually, he would come over to our house and we would all play games and have meals together. The weekends and one evening during the week became like a regular schedule. We did not set any particular time, he just came over when he was ready. Then one weekend he did not show up at all. I called his house but only got the answering machine. On Monday he called me back and told me that he had been out of town to visit with his mother. It was her birthday. He thought he had told me about it.
Couns:	Did you remember later on that he told you about his mother's birthday?
Rhesa:	I remember he talked about getting a birthday gift for his mother, but he did not tell me when her birthday was.

Designating the Problem Areas

Rhesa: In fact, I had hoped he would invite me to come along and meet his mother and the rest of his family. I was really disappointed that he did not want me to go with him.

Couns: You had hoped your relationship had progressed to the point that he would want his family to meet you. It sounds like you had a double disappointment; how did you deal with that?

Rhesa: You are right, I was very disappointed, even angry, but I did not tell him that. I calmed myself down by thinking that he knows his family better than I do and he would know when the right time came for me to meet with them. I also thought he might have forgotten that he did not tell me about the actual time of his mother's birthday. I did not want to argue with him. He has a strange way of handling arguments. After he establishes that he is right, he doesn't want to listen to anything else. If the other person continues arguing, he will just take off.

Couns: How did your relationship continue? Did it go back to the previous pattern?

Rhesa: For a while, it did. But then it happened again. He just did not show up. This time it was a weekend when I had my daughters with me. They kept asking for him, so I finally called him. He was at home and said he did not feel like going out. I asked him if he wanted us to come over for a while, but he did not want that. He said that we did not really have a date anyway and hung up. From then on, he became unpredictable. He would call or visit for several weeks and then he would just stay away.

Couns: That must have been stressful for you, not being able to plan ahead. Did he ever offer an explanation for his behavior?

Rhesa: It was stressful. He never gave me an explanation and I never asked. His mood changed, too. He became more irritable and just didn't seem happy. I found out that he was experiencing financial difficulties. At first he hesitated, but then he confided in me. Some of his investments did not work out and now he was behind in his payments. I offered to help and he accepted that. Unfortunately, what I could give him was not nearly enough. He never told me how much he really needed. He did not want me to be upset that I could not give him more.

Couns: How is your relationship now?

Rhesa: It has not improved much. He is still irritable and I don't get to see him often, but he is not seeing anybody else. So there is hope that we will have a chance to make it together.

Couns: Do you have any criteria in mind for what has to happen for you to stay in or leave the relationship?

Rhesa: Well, if he were seeing another woman, I would probably break up with him. As long as that is not the case, I'll rather be with him sometimes than not at all. Do you mean, I should quit seeing him now?

Couns: Only you can decide whether or not to continue the relationship and what basic reasons you want to apply in making that decision. So far you do not seem to get your needs or wants met in the relationship, but it sounds also as if you have already thought about that. Another aspect, too, might be if your friend would be interested in working with you on goals for the future.

Summary of Client-Counselor Interaction: Unrequited Love. When Rhesa entered the counseling process, her knowledge of what she wanted was apparent. Equally apparent was that she had not been successful in attaining what she wanted. Part of the reason for not achieving her goals could have been her attraction to men who, in her opinion, were more intelligent or more sophisticated than she saw herself. Intimidation followed early excitement and adoration. The counselor was aware of those dynamics. Rather than to focus on this issue in greater detail now, the counselor decided to encourage continuation of the client's story. The information about her style of selecting significant people in her life would be useful in future sessions that were aimed at exploring her overall approach to life.

Observation of the client's approach of making decisions revealed that her main coping skill seemed to be firmly based on hope. Even when the prospects of getting her wishes met diminished, she was willing to limit or narrow the scope of what she hoped for rather than to abandon hope altogether.

Incongruities. The client's presentation in the session revealed a significant incongruity between her seemingly active determination in the pursuit of her goals and the underlying passivity and dependency reflected by her tenacious clinging to the last ray of hope. Most likely,

Designating the Problem Areas

the client would not have agreed with that description. If the therapist had confronted her with that incongruity, she would probably have responded with resistance. Instead, the counselor assured her that the decision was hers to make and gently directed the focus toward further exploration of her reasons for any decision.

SUMMARY

Entering a counseling relationship does not automatically provide information regarding the most efficient starting point. The decision where to begin the process of change is not an easy or an obvious one, as was demonstrated with the different case histories. Bill, the first client, thought he knew exactly what he needed to do to resolve his problem situation. His main interest was to obtain guidance on how best to obtain his goal of reconciliation with his wife and family. In his determination, he was not inclined to even remotely consider that his goal might have been an impossible one to accomplish. In the second case Kent, the young widower, expressed an equal degree of determination when he announced what topics or issues he did not want to explore.

Rhesa's case appears similar to Bill's insofar as Rhesa was equally certain in the knowledge of her goals. In both cases, the clients' goals seemed unattainable, or their fulfillment questionable, at best. In a way, Bill's recognition of a change in his goals was expedited by his wife's actions. In Rhesa's relationship, the other person was more ambiguous in his behavior, giving Rhesa more opportunity to hold on to her hopes and possibly unrealistic dreams. For a successful resolution of their difficulties, all three individuals sooner or later needed to modify their expectancies. The therapist's skillful guidance through a needed goal modification or redefinition is crucial to reduce or avoid unnecessary and time-consuming resistance on the client's part.

EXERCISES

1. Complete the Interpersonal Growth Scale for a current life situation to gain familiarity with the instrument and awareness

about your own priorities. Repeat ratings to indicate future goals pertaining to the selected situation, and, if appropriate, rate the dimensions of the situation in the past.
2. Suppose Kent had given the promise requested of him by his dying wife, but in his current situation he regrets having done this. How would you counsel Kent?

SUGGESTED READING

Beck, A. T. (1988). *Love is never enough.* New York: Harper & Row.
   The author explores common relationship problems. In describing his own therapeutic work, he introduces the use of background questionnaires and exercises as tools to enhance the therapy process.
Cooksey, E. C., & Fondell, M. M. (1996). Spending time with his kids: Effects of family structure on fathers' and children's lives. *Journal of Marriage and the Family, 58,* 693–707.
   The article shows the effects of shared time between fathers and children on children's welfare.
Meyer, D. R., & Garasky, S. (1993). Custodial fathers: Myths, realities, and child support policy. *Journal of Marriage and the Family, 55,* 73–89.
   The authors explored myths concerning custodial fathers. As they examined three data sets, they determined that many assumptions about custodial fathers are not true.

5

Identifying What Does Not Work

OBJECTIVES

1. To find out what problem-solving initiatives had been taken by the client.
2. To explore reasons for lack of success of previous problem-solving attempts.
3. To encourage client's continuing initiatives at resolving difficulties.
4. To find out what modifications in the attempted approach might yield the desired results.
5. To explore other options if previous approaches are not workable at all.
6. To demonstrate the lessons that can be learned from imperfect solutions and their modifications.

WHAT DOES NOT WORK

The purpose of exploring previous attempts at problem-solving is to emphasize the client's acceptance of responsibility for dealing with the situation. When working with single-parent families, one must take advantage of every opportunity to stress the client's independence. Investigation of past attempts often reveals that only a part of the client's attempts was not successful. Except for a small portion, the overall approach may have been workable. Rather than discouragement, encouragement of the client's initiative is the goal for the exploration.

This chapter focuses on problem-solving methods that people use in coping with difficult life situations. The approaches vary as widely as the types of problem clients bring with them. The resources consulted are as diverse as the personality traits of the solution-seekers. Case histories will describe a range of difficult life situations encountered by clients and will demonstrate their advice-seeking and coping behaviors.

PROBLEM-SOLVING GOAL

In most problem-solving considerations, success of the operation is the main goal. Willard Gaylin (1984) contrasted the meaning of success in fixed societies, such as European traditional rural and small-town societies, with its meaning in an open or upwardly mobile society such as the United States. An individual in a fixed society generally accepted his standing within a given social class. Ambitions were limited by the social class and the rural or small-town environment in which the individual lived. A measure of success would have been if the person had developed skills and professional competencies as good as those possessed by the person's father or teacher. In other words, individuals followed in the professional footsteps of their fathers, with the goal of becoming as good or as successful as the father had been in the same trade. In an upwardly mobile society, in contrast, *everything* theoretically is attainable, and achieving anything less than everything may be viewed as failure.

Success vs. Failure

In our success-obsessed society, we shy away from failure as if it were a contagious, crippling disease. Who has not heard the often quoted words of football coach Vince Lombardi: "Winning is not the main thing, it's the only thing"? Almost daily we hear examples of overnight instant success stories, but not everyone can be successful every single time. In focusing so exclusively on successful outcomes, we often lose sight of the valuable lessons that can be learned from failures.

Applying Problem-Solving

Whatever the person's presenting problem may be, it is safe to assume that the individual has made various efforts in problem-solving. There are different methods of problem-solving activities (Sanford, 1985). Perhaps the simplest method is a routine problem-solving approach. The person becomes aware of some difficulty to be resolved and, as the person can recognize it, a stereotyped procedure that leads to a solution may come to mind. An example would be that the person becomes aware that the gasoline gauge in the automobile reflects a near-empty condition. A routine solution to the problem of a low gasoline resource is to turn into a gas station and fill up the tank with the appropriate fuel.

When procedures leading to solutions are not readily available another technique, creative problem-solving, is required. The situation is too complex to yield to routine solutions; a path through the problem itself needs to be developed. Upon closer inspection, some parts of the path may yield to routine problem-solving activities, but the overall schema will require a mixture of both types of problem-solving methods. The complexity of real-life situations, as they are brought into the counselor's office, demands more sophisticated methods than can be achieved with routine techniques. The more knowledge a person has about a problem domain, the more likely that routine procedures will come to mind that, in turn, may be incorporated into more extensive problem-solving strategies. A person's knowledge of a problem increases with the experience of it. Even attempts that have not been completely successful expand the knowledge base about the problem situation.

Sources of Interference

Problem-solving activities can be hampered by various stumbling blocks, such as unexamined beliefs and values, myths and folklore underlying some beliefs, misperceptions of the situation, and available solutions, caused, perhaps, by overwhelming emotions. People faced with problems often turn to others for advice. The sources and the nature of this advice can by themselves create interference with solution-seeking activities. Indiscriminate application of lay advice, or syndicated media advice, can cause more harm than good, because the advice may not be congruent with the beliefs of the problem solver. People's beliefs are often unexamined until they themselves create problems.

MYTHS AND FOLKLORE

Previous problem-solving approaches may have had their basis in myths or folk sayings. Occasional successes in the past likely reinforced and strengthened the person's belief in the guiding value of myths and folklore.

Myths are as old as the human race. Our ancestors used myths to explain experiences that did not yet have logical explanations. Each mythological story gave meaning and purpose to different aspects of daily life, and thereby acquired the status of truth. Myths were used to explain experiences and perceptions and at the same time to justify their existence. Myths were also used to prescribe behaviors in various life situations. Grave consequences would fall on the individual who dared go against the wisdom of the myth. For instance, who has not heard of the saying that breaking a mirror would bring 7 years of bad luck to the person who broke it? The origin of this myth is found in the ancient attribution of mystic powers to any reflective surface because the reflection was considered to be part of the soul of the person reflected. Turkish women were busy embroidering *bursas*, clothes to protect objects. An especially important item was made to cover mirrors at night to keep away the "evil eye." The act of disturbing water—a reflective surface—into which a person was gazing, carried with it heavy taboos because shattering the image was thought to endanger the soul of the person. Connections of mirrors to death or danger to one's soul can be found in the myths of many cultural backgrounds (Walker, 1983).

In conjunction with myths, magical rituals evolved to insure the maintenance of cosmic harmony. Magical rituals also served the function of strengthening the various myths. Vehicles for cementing the importance of myths in people's minds can be seen in the use of analogies, metaphors, and symbols. Symbols constitute the predominant mode of expression in primary process thinking, a kind of unconscious thinking that is not controlled by the laws of logic (Bagarozzi & Anderson, 1989). Primary process thinking makes no distinction between what is fantasized and what is actually taking place in reality. In primary process thinking, psychic reality replaces external reality. The process of enacting a myth is by way of behavioral dramas, such as rituals. As summarized by Perry (1966), primitive man's attempts to explain the universe resulted in myths, and rituals expressed those myths. Rituals also served the functions of preserving a given social group and serving as basic source for communal action. Rituals are found in religious activities, such as prayer at specified times of the day, baptisms, wedding ceremonies, and funerals. Certain rites of passage or blowing out candles on a birthday cake constitute rituals.

On a less formal level, the unofficial culture of a group is expressed in folklore. Information and attitudes are transmitted and interpreted through folklore. Transmission occurs from individual to individual within certain groups through observation, custom, and practice. Folklore is simultaneously persistent and changing, according to the needs of a culture. Folklore is adaptable to changing technologies and, through its adaptability, remains a pervasive aspect in the background of people's lives. By its repetitive nature, folklore shapes people's behaviors and attitudes—often without the individuals' awareness. The effect of folk sayings is stronger than any number of public service announcements, and their power outweighs any other authority because it is transmitted from the collective wisdom on to a personal, individual level (Henken & Whatley, 1995).

Effects of the pervasiveness of folklore or myths were demonstrated in research involving teenage women and their beliefs about getting pregnant in certain circumstances (Zelnik & Kantner, 1979). The authors asked young girls about their reasons for not using contraception during intercourse. The following statements represented responses of more than half of the girls. Some stated that they had believed that they were too young to get pregnant. Others thought that because they had only infrequent intercourse, or because intercourse took place only at a certain time of the month, there would be no risk of pregnancy. Other reasons given were that women had to be deeply in love with the young man in order to become pregnant, or because one could not become pregnant at the very first time of intercourse.

Case Study

Rhesa: A Life Governed by Myth and Folk Sayings

Rhesa, the young divorced mother, previously encountered in Chapter 4, worked hard but unsuccessfully to attain the desired feelings and respect from her male friend. She demonstrated unusually strong persistence in the pursuit of this one-sided relationship. Rhesa's actions were grounded in traditional values, such as "Good deeds will find their rewards" and "It is a woman's duty to support her man." What was the underlying mechanism that kept her persisting in the face of repeated rejections?

Couns:	At our previous meeting you mentioned being in a relationship with a young man whom you are very fond of, but you had some question whether or not he is returning your feelings.
Rhesa:	I think he is not ready yet. I know I am good for him. I just have to try harder until he sees it!
Couns:	Today you seem sure that you will succeed in your pursuit of this young man. Do you have any signs that confirm your expectations?
Rhesa:	Where there is a will, there is a way! Everything worthwhile is worth working for, and a good relationship is certainly worth working for. I have made a commitment to this relationship.
Couns:	Your commitment in this relationship is firm, but you are not so sure about his commitment—is that what you mean? If so, what signs would help you to believe in his future commitment?
Rhesa:	As I mentioned last time, as far as I know, he is not seeing anyone else. He still sees me from time to time, so he must have an interest in me. As I said, where there is a will, there is a way. That's what my father used to say. I remember it well. It goes back to when I was in school, in the first grade, and I could not learn to write certain letters of the alphabet. I practiced writing them a lot, but I got so frustrated. My father kept encouraging me by saying "Where there is a will, there is a way! Let's assume that you really want to learn to write all the letters in the alphabet, then there is a way to do it and you just have

Identifying What Does Not Work 129

	to find that way." He would add, "If at first you don't succeed, try, try again." I believed him and kept on practicing until I could write all the letters. In fact, I excelled in penmanship in school. My father told me the story quite often, whenever he wanted me to persist in my efforts in other areas. One day he told me to write the saying in my best calligraphy skills. He had it framed for me and helped me hang it up on the wall in my room.
Couns:	That was a very strong message from your father. It seems you learned your lesson well. Have there ever been situations where you had difficulties reaching your goals, even though you diligently and persistently applied your father's words?
Rhesa:	No, I have used it ever since and it kept me going. Except the time when I was hospitalized several years ago.
Couns:	What was the reason for your hospitalization?
Rhesa:	They said I had an eating disorder. I was young and foolish then and wanted to be as skinny as my friends. No matter how hard I exercised and how little I ate, I never looked as slim as they did. I kept it up, reminding myself that if I had the will to be slim, there would be a way. Finally I got so weak, my parents took me to the doctor and he put me in the hospital. I felt ashamed about causing my parents so much trouble. But I also felt let down because I could not get what I wanted, no matter how hard I tried. My father finally explained to me that I could not change my bone structure.
Couns:	Can you see any similarity between your hospitalization and your current situation?
Rhesa:	What do you mean about similarity?
Couns:	As you said, your father had explained that you could not control your bone structure. How about your current situation—are there aspects of it that you cannot control?
Rhesa:	I don't think so. If I show my friend how much I care for him, he must realize that he can't find a more loving person. I am probably not doing enough yet; you know, "It takes two to tango!" I know he disapproves when I invite him to stay at my house with my daughters there. He reminded me that they are of very impressionable ages. His standards are so high. He probably thinks I am a bad mother. But I still have sexual longings. Not being married anymore does not mean that the sexual part of

me is dead. It's really confusing; when I was a young girl, men tried to convince me that I was a sexual being—as they called it. Now that I am single again but have children, all I am supposed to be is a mother. I still long for the intimacy and fulfillment of a sexual relationship. Men don't seem to have the same problems.

Couns: Your frustration is understandable. Just because your spouse is gone from your life, the need or wish for physical intimacy as part of a meaningful adult relationship is still there. You seem to think that your friend does not share your feelings. Do you want to talk more about this now?

Rhesa: Right now, I would rather focus on how to convince him that we can have a great relationship, if he just realized how much I care about him. I don't want to give up on what I know to be true. I am sure the sexual part will improve again later, when we know where we are headed.

Couns: Determination and perseverance are good qualities in most circumstances, but sometimes it can be dangerous to apply them indiscriminately and permanently. As with your eating disorder, you could have become seriously ill. Perhaps it would be helpful to keep a log or journal where you record your actions that are meant to convince the young man of the value of the relationship. The log would be evidence for yourself of how much effort you have extended and how much more would seem reasonable to you. Do you think that might be of help?

Rhesa: I can try, you can't lose by trying.

Summary of Client-Counselor Interaction: A Life Governed by Myths and Folk-Sayings. The therapist recognized that the client's style of thinking was deeply rooted in well-learned myths and folk-sayings. Her application of the sayings had become automatic. Without hesitation she quoted to herself and followed faithfully what she considered to be her guidelines for life. Attempts to identify her past problem-solving approaches and to integrate them into the overall situation were hampered by the client's perseverance in following the folk sayings.

The basis for Rhesa's continuing efforts was her belief that goal-directed activities were to be repeated with increased strength and persistence if they initially failed to bring the desired results. Her determined clinging to her treasured sayings prevented her from

Identifying What Does Not Work

considering alternatives to and consequences of her actions. Because of the potential danger inherent in her persistence—as demonstrated in her eating disorder—learning to identify what does not work was crucial for Rhesa. The counselor agreed with her on the general value of such characteristics as determination and perseverance, but also pointed out the risks involved in adhering to them without questioning.

The counselor recognized that Rhesa would not have agreed to discard her folk sayings, and instead introduced the use of a journal. The collected evidence of the frequency of applying her guidelines and the results of her efforts would be more convincing than anything the counselor could say. With the shift in focus, the possibility of the client's resistance to further exploration was reduced.

Case Study Follow-Up: Starting a Journal

As agreed upon, Rhesa had started with her journal. The first opportunity for entry was Rhesa's suggestion for a nice evening out with the young man.

Couns:	When you called the other day to reschedule your appointment, you mentioned that you had started on your journal. What was the event of your first entry, and how did it go?
Rhesa:	I had thought that having an evening out in a nice restaurant would be good for both of us. His current situation is so stressful and he deserves some relaxation. When I mentioned it to him he said that would be nice, but he had no money to take me out on a date. I understood and told him that I would be paying for my own dinner and would pick him up after work. My thought was that if I drove, he did not have to spend money for gasoline, but I did not say that.
Couns:	That was very considerate of you. Did he agree to the arrangement?
Rhesa:	Yes, he did, but . . .
Couns:	You sound disappointed. What happened?
Rhesa:	Actually, it started quite well. He had made reservations in my name at a nice restaurant. We got there in good time and I thought I looked really pretty in a new suit

	that I had bought some time ago, but did not have a chance to wear before. To avoid any awkwardness at the table about paying, I had given my friend the money to cover my part of the dinner while we were still in the car. The food was excellent and the service was good, at least I thought so.
Couns:	You handled the situation very tactfully. You are putting a great deal of effort and caring into the growth of this relationship.
Rhesa:	Thank you for saying this. I was proud of myself for considering all the possible trouble spots, beforehand. The evening should have worked out well, but it didn't. Shortly after the dessert my friend suggested we leave. Hoping that he wanted to be alone with me for the rest of the evening, I happily agreed. As I was driving home, my friend complained about the waiter. He seemed to be pushing us to drink more wine than we needed, and he was very obvious in his expectations for a greater tip than we gave him. The waiter's greed had ruined the whole evening for my friend, and he did not even invite me into his house when we got there.
Couns:	No wonder you were disappointed; that was a sad ending for all your efforts. How do you want to proceed now?
Rhesa:	I was disappointed when I described the evening in my journal, but perhaps I was not careful enough about his feelings. The next time when I invite him I will simply charge the cost for both meals and the tip to my credit card. Then there will be no opportunity for embarrassment about who is paying the tip and how much. He won't even know about it. Surely, he will appreciate that I care so much about him to arrange everything to go smoothly.
Couns:	To record the events of the evening in your journal seems like a painful exercise. Other people might have refused to relive the disappointment. I think you are quite courageous to keep track of what you are doing. If you get what you want, you will know how important this relationship was to you. If it does not work out, you will be assured that you spared no effort to reach your goal. As you are describing your plans for the next date, you are assuming financial responsibility for the whole evening. Can your budget accommodate this expenditure?

Rhesa:	It will be tight, but I can save money by not going out for lunch with my colleagues. Preparing my lunch at home and taking it to the office will be much cheaper. Besides, I can use the rest of my lunch hour for a walk. At least, I will get my exercise.
Couns:	That sounds like a good solution for living within a tight budget, no matter what the reason for your plans. I hope it will bring you the reward you want. Making decisions that will help you financially is always a good practice.

Summary of Client-Counselor Interaction: Starting a Journal. The session centered on the client's efforts to reach her goals in the relationship with her friend. The counselor's responses reflected acknowledgment of the client's feelings and their appropriateness to the circumstances. Reinforcement for decisions that would be generally beneficial for the client's situation was given without advice on how to do things differently. The main aspect to recognize in the interchange is that the counselor's statements were free of judgment concerning the client's actions. Where appropriate, encouragement for additional explorations was included in the therapist's responses.

It is important that the therapist remember to refrain from giving advice. What would be advantageous behavior in certain situations is often more obvious to the outsider than the person involved. Moreover, clients seem to look to the therapist or counselor for advice. The temptation to oblige in the context of helping the client is great. The counselor's role is neither advisor nor judge. The counselor's function is that of a facilitator in the client's process of growth and independence.

Case Study Follow-Up: Increasing Efforts

Due to the counselor's absence, Rhesa's next three appointments were canceled. When she saw her therapist again, the date she had anticipated and planned during her previous session had already occurred, again without the desired outcome. True to her determination, Rhesa was not yet ready to give up. Because her friend had complained about the inconvenience of going to a restaurant, Rhesa decided to prepare dinner in her friend's home. He did not have to think about going out and could just rest and relax while she was doing the cooking.

Rhesa: While you were gone, I had another date with my friend. Again it did not work out as I had expected. We don't really need to talk about it today because it's all written down in my journal. Instead, I have decided to go all out and pamper him as much as I can. I have already discussed it with him. Next weekend, when my daughters visit with their father, I will cook dinner at his house. He was agreeable, but he reminded me that his refrigerator was not stocked with a lot of food items for the feast, and he would not have time to shop. I told him that I didn't mind the shopping because I know what I need for the dinner. I have everything planned and I'll be using my own pots and utensils, so I won't ruin his special equipment. Except for the food, I have everything packed including two candles. Do you think it will work, or am I overdoing it? One of my colleagues says I am stupid for what I am doing and that my friend is just taking advantage of me. She is the only one I have told about this and, of course, you. I love doing things like cooking a good meal for the people that are important in my life. I enjoyed that in my marriage. What is wrong with showing someone that you love him?

Couns: Showing one's feelings is a very honest act, but sometimes it takes courage to do so. Of course, we hope that our feelings will be reciprocated. If the other person does not return our feelings, it does not mean that our feelings are wrong. We usually have our own reasons for loving someone and these reasons may still be valid. Because we cannot make someone love us, we need to learn to accept that and adjust to it as we go on with our lives. In your situation, if you think your colleague is right, you could cancel the date. On the other hand, you already made the arrangements. You could go ahead with your plans and enjoy what you are doing. Either way, the decision will have to be yours. The results can be anywhere from attainment of your goals to being a learning experience if things do not work out the way you hope.

Summary of Client-Counselor Interaction: Increasing Efforts. The session started with the client's brief report of another unsuccessful

Identifying What Does Not Work 135

outcome, but she did not want to dwell on the past experience. Instead, she informed the counselor of her new plans. The client appeared somewhat less confident in the session, and seemed to seek the counselor's reassurance.

Again, the counselor refrained from expressing judgments. The client's disclosure of her feelings was seen as positive in general, although the inherent risks were mentioned. Very carefully, the therapist used the opportunity to gently confront the client with the reality that we cannot control another person's feelings. Because the client had already made a commitment to her future plans, a stronger emphasis on reality did not appear indicated now. The therapist's mention of the possibilities of either canceling or going ahead with her plans reminded the client that she had choices, but ultimately, the decision was hers.

A significant aspect of the session was the therapist's focus on the future. While neither making promises regarding the outcome nor assuming the responsibility for the client's decision, the therapist directed the client to recognize her ability to cope with the outcome, regardless of her current decision. Thus, the groundwork for the process of growing and healing was laid.

Case Study Follow-Up: Another Disappointment

Prior to her next session, Rhesa had provided the therapist with copies of her journal pages that dealt with the dinner at her friend's house. She included a note stating that she wanted the counselor to know what had occurred, but did not necessarily want to talk about it in her session. The original pages must have been tearstained. Several words had letters retraced on the copies that otherwise would not have been legible. The content of the pages described the evening. Everything had gone well with her preparations. Rhesa did not forget a single item needed for the dinner, including her candles. She had brought food for breakfast along as well, and a little overnight kit with her prettiest nightgown. Surely, he would want her to stay all night after such a lovely evening.

While Rhesa was cooking, her friend watched television to relax from his job pressures. He seemed to enjoy the dinner, except for the candles. Rhesa did not know he was allergic to candles, but she blew them out as soon as she found out. Although the candlelight had provided a more romantic atmosphere, it was a small price to pay for the pleasure of his company. She was pleasantly surprised when he offered to help clear the table. At last he was acknowledging her caring behavior, Rhesa thought. As he helped carry items into the kitchen, her friend calmly suggested that she clean the dishes in her home rather than in his dishwasher. He really needed to go to bed soon to be fresh tomorrow morning for an early game of tennis with a prospective client. He even thanked her for the meal and wished her a good night as he walked her to her car. Rhesa had the rest of the weekend to record the event in her log.

Rhesa: I hope you did not mind that I brought in the part of my journal that describes my last date with my friend. After I came home that Saturday night, I cried most of the night until I finally fell asleep exhausted. On Sunday I recorded the event in my journal and cried some more. It was a real blow and I don't want to go through it again today, but I wanted you to know about it. As I was reading the entries in my journal, I could not come up with any ideas how to increase my loving behaviors. I could not think of how to try harder.

Couns: Yes, I read your notes and I am so very sorry for the pain you experienced. Your journal gave you the evidence that you had done everything possible. You seem ready to accept that now.

Rhesa: Actually, it is more than that. As I was crying and reading I came across an entry that I had made earlier. I had told my friend that I was seeing you. His response was that it was a waste of time and money. Therapists only wanted to tell their clients what to do and how to live their lives. If the clients don't follow the therapist's orders or things do not work out, it's the client's fault. I remembered that you never told me what to do, not even when I wanted you to. With that I started to doubt my friend's honesty and loyalty to me, even as a friend, if not a lover.

Couns: You are right, it is not my job to tell you what to do. My role is to guide you to make good decisions for yourself by yourself. My responsibility is to assist you in your growing process for greater independence. Reading your journal at the time of your disappointment took a lot of strength. What else did you discover?

Rhesa: I asked myself: Why did he not break off the relationship, but agreed to see me from time to time? He had not been courting me passionately, but the fact that he had allowed me to be with him had instilled hope in me that there could be a future for us. Suddenly, I realized that he was probably afraid that I would ask him to return my car if he quit seeing me. When we first met, his car had just been totaled in an accident and there was some trouble with the insurance company. I don't know the details. Not too long before that I had gotten a new car, but the dealer did not want to take my old car as a trade-in, so I kept it, thinking that I might drive it to work instead of the new car. I have to park downtown, and it is less of a risk to park an older car. When I told him about the car, he asked me if I would sell it to him. I did not know how much to charge for the car and he did not have any money anyway, so I decided to let him use it until his financial situation improved. I even replaced the old worn-out tires.

Couns: Your kindness did not bring you the deserved rewards, according to your interpretation of the situation. Some people cannot handle kindness appropriately. How will this affect your life?

Rhesa: Fortunately, I kept the title of the car, but I am not going to take the car back right away. I don't want him to know how hurt I am. I think I'll wait a couple of weeks before I act on that. Your question probably wasn't just about the car, more like what have I learned from it?

Couns: Right, there is more than the car. We can look at the car as a symbol for some of your beliefs. I think the exercise of keeping your journal has helped you gain awareness of things. For instance, you mentioned you realized that your friend had tried to discount your work in counseling, and you noticed that your actual experience here was different from what he said. From the pages you gave me to read, I could see how much emotional distress you went through. In spite of the turmoil, you had the strength to look critically at what you had written. You found the answers to some questions. What additional insights might you have gained?

Rhesa: I think I understand now what you meant by similarities between my eating disorder and the situation with my friend. Even if you had explained it to me then, I would not have accepted that there are things I cannot control. That no matter how hard and long I try, I cannot make it happen. My trust in my guiding spirit is shattered. Where can I turn for guidance now? I felt strong when I believed I could make anything happen by working hard enough.

Couns: As you said, your belief made you feel strong and you have achieved many things in your life because you worked hard for them. To make everything we want a reality requires supernatural powers. When other people are involved in what we want, it becomes even more complicated.

Rhesa: Shouldn't kindness beget kindness and love get love in return?

Couns: In general, we operate on that basis. Kindness is considered to be more likely to bring kindness in return than would meanness. But there are no guarantees. In the end, it is the other person's decision how they want to treat us. Perhaps it makes sense to consider the main reason for our own behavior to rest in our self-image. We want to act a certain way because we perceive ourselves that way, not because of what we get from others for it. Of course, there are consequences to our behavior, but they may not always be the determining reason for our actions.

Rhesa: Are you saying that I should be nice because I want to be a nice person, rather than because I want others to treat me nicely in return?

Couns: The reasons for our behaviors are complex. There is not any single force that shapes our actions. We all have certain characteristics that we may like or dislike in ourselves. We group them into what we call our personality. These characteristics are more or less stable. Then we have what we may call situation-specific behaviors. In other words, in certain situations we may attempt to estimate what particular actions will result in desired outcomes. In your situation, you are basically a kind and generous person and you like those aspects in yourself. In addition, you also assumed that if you demonstrated to your friend how deep your caring for him is, he would naturally love you for it. Your belief in the saying "Where there is a will, there is a way" made you all the more determined to continue with your efforts.

Rhesa: Should I change my personality? Or is there a way to be caring without being used?

Couns: There are ways of protecting oneself from being taken advantage of and still continue to be as nice as one wants to be. Although you may not want to develop a complicated bookkeeping system, it helps to stay connected to reality. For example, "Out of 10 dates I get to choose the place once or twice." Or "He always asks me where I want to go." "The last five times he picked me up at least one hour later than we had agreed on and he did not even call to let me know that he would be late." "In addition to taking her out for a great evening, she expected me to pay for the babysitter for her children." Comments like those reflect perception of a one-sided relationship. Once a person has become aware of being in a one-sided relationship, decisions can be made whether to continue as is or to implement changes, sometimes at the risk of losing the relationship. Several years ago I made up a quiz for a women's magazine about giving and getting in love relationships. I can give you a copy of the rating sheet. It was about the time when Robin Norwood's book *Women Who Love Too Much* was very popular.

Rhesa: I remember reading the book and thinking it was all about me. It took me until now to make the real connection. I came here to get help in making my boyfriend appreciate me, instead I found out I needed to trade in my guiding beliefs for a closer look at reality.

Summary of Client-Counselor Interaction: Another Disappointment.

Although the therapist was fully aware of the client's tremendous pain and expressed understanding for that pain, the focus in the session was directed toward the future. Pain becomes acknowledged and accepted, but it is not permitted to overwhelm or slow the overall growing process. By suggesting that the client keep a log or journal regarding her efforts, the therapist had made it possible for her to collect the necessary evidence of her own actions, but also provided her with a tool for future problem-solving activities. As the client still felt that the strength she had previously derived from clinging to myths and folk sayings had left her, she was already provided with a coping mechanism that is firmly rooted in reality. The therapist attempted to maintain a sensitive balance for the client. When one coping approach has failed to bring the desired results, it is advantageous to have another one available. The client was given a checklist to provide a framework for assessing relationships (see Table 5.1).

READILY AVAILABLE TYPES OF ADVICE

Available sources for advice cover a wide range of types, starting with friends and family members to ministers, teachers, and professionals, such as counselors and therapists. Syndicated newspaper columns, pop psychologists, and famous guests and hosts of radio and TV talk shows also function as advice sources. Indiscriminate application of lay or media advice entails risks, because the assistance found here is not specific to the person in need and the person's situation.

TABLE 5.1   Giving and Getting in Love Relations

	Give	*Get*		*Give*	*Get*
Verbal love expression	___	___	Physical love expression	___	___
Flowers and surprises	___	___	Consideration and attention	___	___
Compliments	___	___	Time together	___	___
Lovemaking and sex	___	___	Fidelity	___	___
Trust	___	___	Self-disclosure	___	___
Encouragement	___	___	Respect for opinions	___	___
Acceptance of family and friends	___	___	Personal freedom	___	___
Financial decisions	___	___	Decisions in general	___	___
Help with chores	___	___	Help with meals	___	___
			Total	___	___

Intimate relationships undergo changes over time, a process of growing together and growing apart occurs. To find out where you and your partner are along the path of growing together and growing apart, rate on a scale from 1 to 5 (1 being low and 5 high) yourself on what best represents your current feelings. Add the numbers in both the *Give* and *Get* columns. This will give you two scores. Compare the two scores; they are your appraisal of the situation. If you don't like the relationship between the two numbers, go over the scales again and rate them as you would like your love relationship to be. If you want, ask your partner to go through the same rating procedure as you did and compare your total scores.

Syndicated Newspaper Columns, Radio and TV Talk Show Hosts, and Pop Psychologists

Syndicated newspaper advice columns have long been a popular source. Such columns as "Dear Abby," "Ann Landers," "John Rosemond," and others come to mind readily. Few people may realize that this type of advice-seeking has been around for more than half a century. LaRossa and Reitzes (1993) have conducted a content analysis of advice-seeking letters written to Angelo Patri, an educator and author, who wrote a syndicated newspaper column and hosted a weekly radio broadcast in the 1920s and 1930s. About 7000 letters concerned with childrearing issues had been collected. Probably because mothers were the primary child-care givers at that time, only about 8% of the advice-seeking letters came from fathers.

In a counseling session, a young divorced mother of three related how her ex-husband had confronted her with different articles on child-raising practices from newspaper columns. Interestingly, he only used advice congruent with his own ideas. Apparently, the newspaper advice was not beneficial to the overall dynamics of the family's functioning.

Today, TV talk-show programs discuss problem areas currently encountered in society. As soon as a popular talk-show host or hostess explores a new topic, one can expect the topic to be discussed on other programs, often preceded or followed by a wave of self-help books. The advantages of public exploration of common problem areas include people's awareness of the existence of the difficulties and comfort for those who suffer with similar difficulties coming from the fact that they are not alone in their struggle. As previously mentioned, indiscriminate application of suggested solutions is a hazard.

Lay vs. Professional Advice

Watzlawick (1983) has warned about the traps of helping. The relationship between the helper and the help-seeker usually has one of two outcomes. If the given advice is not successful in alleviating the other person's difficulties, the advice-giver will become tired and will eventually withdraw. If the suggestions are instrumental in resolving the advice-seeker's difficulty, the relationship between the two individuals will change, because the person who was in need of advice no longer has the need and will withdraw. Actually, the relationship between the two individuals will undergo changes in either case. In the first scenario, negative feelings, such as resentment or guilt, are likely to develop. The advice-seeker may think the advice was not good enough to help and, therefore, may feel resentment. Feelings of guilt may result when the person believes his or her attempts have not been good enough. The situation becomes even more tense when the advice-seeker for some reason decides not to follow the advice-giver's suggestions.

Many people turn to family members or close friends for advice before seeking help from a minister or a professional counselor or therapist, at least for personal problems. Hinson and Swanson (1993) have considered help-seeking behaviors as a function of the person's willingness to self-disclose. Participants in the authors' study were 101 Midwestern university students from an introductory psychology class. The instruments used were the Jourard Self-Disclosure Questionnaire (SDQ), the Chelune Self-Disclosure Situations Survey (SDSS), and responses to questions obtained from the participants after reading a scenario describing a personal problem of either high or low severity. The results showed that willingness to seek help was associated with the perceived seriousness of the problem, with the perceived appropriateness of the problem for counseling, and with personal experience of the problem. The order of people asked for advice was established as first self, then best female friend, mother, best male friend, father, counselor, faculty adviser, and minister. The study also showed that the greatest amount of self-disclosure was directed to same-sex and opposite-sex friends, followed by parents. Counselors and strangers were ranked last. Problems considered too severe for friends and other help-givers to handle were more likely to bring the individual to a professional counselor. Participants cited as reasons for not contacting a counselor the belief that the problem was not that serious or it was too personal. When considering the guaranteed confidentiality in the counselor-counselee situation, these results are surprising and worth further exploration. The implications for counseling are that in most cases, when clients enter the counseling process, they have already approached other sources of help, and their problems have not been significantly alleviated by applying the advice they received.

In the United States, women are twice as likely as men to seek counseling services (Wills & DePaulo, 1991). The reason may be that traditional men see themselves as healthier than do women and men with nontraditional attitudes (Good, Dell, & Mintz, 1989) or that it is not manly to seek help. The determination of whether the men's self-reports of their psychological well-being are based on the truth, or on their denial of pain and discomfort, is difficult to make.

Case Study

Betty: Confusion in the Wake of Lay Advice

Betty, a mother of three, was suddenly widowed in her early forties. Although her husband's death came as a surprise at this particular time, he had been ill for several years. Knowing his illness, Betty's husband had avoided stress as much as possible. At work, he had chosen a less ambitious path than formerly, in his earlier years with the company. At home, he tried to avoid family arguments. When the children engaged in behaviors that had previously not been sanctioned by their parents, Betty reprimanded them or tried to employ consequences. Frequently, the children would complain to their father, with the result that he removed the consequences in order to keep his peace. The children learned quickly how to get what they wanted. Betty's authority with her children eroded and was steadily undermined.

The loss of her spouse placed Betty in the role of the primary disciplinarian and decision-maker, a role for which neither she nor the children were prepared. In a well-meaning attempt to distract Betty from her grief and guide her toward more future-oriented thinking, her uncle told Betty, "Now you have to be both mother and father to your children."

Following her uncle's words, Betty tried to fulfill the responsibilities for the children's education as previously planned by her husband and herself. The children, traumatized by their father's death, resisted and rebelled against her new authority. Before her husband's death, Betty had worked to supplement his income, both to provide extra money for their children's college education and for the parents' own retirement. Now she had to work to maintain the home, to be eligible for her own retirement plan, and for the family's health insurance benefits. The two older children demanded that Betty hand over to them what they perceived to be their part of their father's assets. They used their grief to blame Betty and make increased demands on her. Only her youngest daughter was still behaving like her child.

In her desperation, Betty sought assistance from her friends. Their advice ranged from suggestions to be patient and understanding and give her children time to get over their grief, to recommendations for the use of assertiveness and strict disciplinary actions. The more she tried to follow the advice, the more confused Betty became. Finally, one of her friends who had become tired of listening to Betty's complaints handed her a newspaper clipping from an advice column. The described situation was similar to Betty's, and ended with the suggestion that the advice seeker employ professional help.

Couns: You stated in your phone contact that you and your children have difficulty adjusting to your husband's death. Where would you like to begin?

Betty: Aside from being lonely for my husband, my biggest problem is how to handle my children. Due to my husband's illness, my two oldest children have not had a lot of discipline. Tracy, my oldest daughter, was away at college when her father died. Her grades during her first year had not been good. She is smart enough to make good grades, but I think she partied too much. A couple of months after my husband's funeral we got the bill for her next semester's tuition. Included was a notice that she was placed on academic probation because of her low grades. I explained to her that I would not pay for her college expenses if her grades did not improve.

Couns: How did your daughter respond?

Betty: Tracy flat-out told me that her father had promised her a college education and it was my responsibility to fulfill her father's promise. At first I was shocked, but then I remembered my uncle's words about having to be both mother and father to my children and I felt guilty.

Couns: How may your guilt feelings have influenced your actions?

Betty: I paid the tuition for the next semester, including the

	money for a class Tracy had to take over again. When I looked at our budget for the rest of the year, I knew I was in trouble. Our financial situation was extremely tight, unless I would dig into the capital. I had already asked my boss for a full-time position. When I told one of my friends about the situation, she told me to be more assertive and make the two oldest get part-time jobs to help with expenses.
Couns:	How did that work out?
Betty:	I had a difficult time with my friend's advice. I respect her opinion, but all my life I was used to think about others first. I grew up as the oldest of seven children. My father worked two jobs and my mother was ill a lot. As the oldest, I had to do most of the household chores and take care of my younger siblings. Often I was too tired to do my homework for school. Even though I loved school, I fell asleep in class sometimes. My dream was to become a teacher, but I had to go to work right after graduating from high school. College was not an option for me. I didn't date and didn't go out much. My husband and I met through one of my uncles who knew him from work. After we got married, I still had to work because we wanted to save money for a house before having children. My husband was in a promising career track and we could afford for me to stay home when the children were little. We found out about my husband's illness when the children were at an age that I could return to part-time work. My husband opted for a less ambitious position in the company, but with my salary, we could still maintain our comfortable lifestyle until he died.
Couns:	You indicated that your daughter did not seem to understand or accept the change in your financial situation. How did your other children respond to the change?
Betty:	Ron, my son, has been reacting differently. At first, he seemed angry, like his father's death was a personal insult to him. Ron is in his senior year in high school, and he is probably hurt because his father will not be there when he graduates. More recently, he appears to be withdrawing from the family. He doesn't say much although, at times, he is a bit bossy. I think it would be good to get him into counseling. My youngest daughter, Lisa, has become more clinging. When I am at home, she does not want to leave

my side. I guess she is afraid of losing another parent. I need to be patient and help her to regain her sense of security. Lisa is not the typical youngest child. She has not required special pampering in the past.

Couns: Each one of your three children seems to have responded quite differently to your husband's death. Your awareness of Lisa's needs and your patience with her in the middle of all your struggles speak well for your parenting skills. Providing counseling for Ron would be a good decision. If he makes use of it, he will have an opportunity to discuss his concerns with a neutral person, one where he does not have to worry about hurting the person's feelings. As you described it, the situation with Tracy appears to be the most troublesome right now. Your friend suggested to be more assertive with her and Ron, but then you indicated that you had difficulty with that, partly because of your past thoughts and actions. Would you like to work on reconciling currently needed behaviors with attitudes and beliefs from the past?

Betty: How would I go about doing that?

Couns: We can start by investigating your thoughts at the time when you had the discussion with Tracy about not paying for her college expenses if her performance did not improve. With the upcoming holiday next week, our next meeting will be in 2 weeks, just enough time for you to recollect your memories and make some notes of it. Of course, if you need to talk to me sooner, don't hesitate to call my office before our next appointment.

Summary of Client-Counselor Interaction: Confusion in the Wake of Lay Advice. By providing sufficient opportunity for the client to relate some of the background history regarding the current situation, the counselor was able to detect the main reason for the client's confusion. Following the advice of her trusted friends in combination with her uncle's recommendation, she put herself in an untenable position. The uncle's words were congruent with some of her earlier behaviors, but by following the direction, she would act against her own current needs. Her decisions now were dictated by the welfare of all the family members, including her own, not just her children's. Her friends' suggestions may have been appropriate for the situation according to their values, but not appropriate for the client's own beliefs, nor were the suggestions congruent with her earlier behaviors, thereby causing confusion in her children's minds.

Counselor's Role. The counselor's role was to offer reinforcement for the client's sensitivity to her children's needs in regards to her son Ron and daughter Lisa. At the same time, the counselor directed the focus to the main problem area with Tracy and the need for solution.

Intergenerational Transmission of Parenting Styles

Lay advice, as well-intended as it may be, is usually firmly grounded within the belief and value system of the advice-giver. On occasion, the belief system may be similar to that of the person seeking the advice, but more often there is significant variance between beliefs and values held by different people. When dealing with parenting styles and issues of raising children, differences are especially pronounced. Differences in parental beliefs contribute a significant proportion of the variation in parenting practices (Goodnow & Collins, 1990). Most people's parenting beliefs are influenced by the type of parenting they received in their childhoods. As parenting beliefs are transmitted across generations, parents' beliefs influence the parenting practices of their children who, in turn, will pass on similar beliefs and attitudes to their offspring. Lay advice, therefore, can be expected to include a wide variety of transgenerational influences; not all of them could be expected to coincide with the beliefs of the advice-seeker.

Simons, Beaman, Conger, and Chao (1992) explored how adolescents' beliefs regarding effective discipline and the impact of parenting upon child development are associated with the parenting beliefs and practices of their parents. From 451 two-parent families with sons and daughters attending the 7th grade in public or private schools in North Central Iowa, the investigators selected only those families who had a sibling within 4 years of the age of the 7th grader. Slightly fewer than half of the 451 families met the criterion. Of those, 78% agreed to participate. These families lived on farms or in small towns, with annual incomes ranging from 0 to $135,000, with a mean of $29,642. Parents' education ranged from 8 to 20 years for fathers and from 8 to 18 years for mothers.

The families were visited twice in their homes. During the first visit, each of the four family members in each family completed a set of questionnaires with a focus on family processes, economic circumstances, and characteristics of the individual family members. Two weeks later, during the second visit, family members were involved in different structured interaction tasks. The interactions were recorded on videotapes.

Parenting Measures. One of the measures used focused on mothers' and fathers' supportive parenting behaviors. Another measure was a nine-item Supportive Parenting Scale completed by the children. The child report and the observational measures from the videotapes were standardized and combined into a composite Supportive Parenting Index. The children also rated their parents' harsh discipline behaviors. These scores were also standardized and combined with observational ratings from the videotapes to form an index of Harsh Parenting. Mothers and fathers reported on the supportive and the harsh parenting behaviors of each of their own parents, using the same scales their children had used. These ratings provided measures of grandparents' supportive and harsh discipline parenting behaviors. Two additional measures were obtained by tapping the extent to which parents believed that parental behaviors shape a child's development (three-item Impact of Parenting Scale) and the parental beliefs concerning the most effective approach to discipline (six-item Discipline Beliefs Scale).

Findings on Parenting Transmission. The overall findings demonstrated that parents convey their beliefs to their adolescent children through their parenting practices. Over time, the children are able to recognize the principles expressed by their parents' actions.

The pattern of correlations obtained between the parenting beliefs of siblings supported the investigators' expectation that socialization of parenting beliefs varies by gender of the child. Boys seemed to be more attuned to discipline and girls more to the consequences of parental involvement. Expectations that girls obtain their beliefs about the impact of parenting from the behaviors of their mothers and that boys derive their discipline beliefs from the behaviors of their fathers were not confirmed. The discipline beliefs of adolescent boys were related to harsh disciplinary behaviors of both fathers and mothers, while the impact beliefs of girls were associated with supportive parenting behaviors from both mothers and fathers. The findings indicate that adolescent boys and girls are influenced by different aspects of their parents' roles, but when they construct their own parenting beliefs, they depend on both parents as sources of information.

Enmeshed Parent-Child Relations

Barber and Buehler (1996) found parent-child enmeshment to be positively related to youth problems. Some researchers see enmeshment as an extreme level of cohesion (Epstein, Bishop, & Baldwin, 1982; Skinner, Steinhauer, & Santa-Barbara, 1983). Others (e.g., Steinberg, 1990) regard cohesion and enmeshment as independent constructs, rather than as two different points on the same continuum.

Perosa (1996) examined the relationship between Minuchin's structural family model and Kohut's self-psychology constructs. Her subjects were 164 college women who completed different rating scales, developed to measure structural family integration, parental relations, intergenerational boundaries, and goal stability. Two factors, Proximity-Differentiation and Generational Hierarchy-Differentiation, accounted for most of the variance (90%). Analysis using the two factors as predictor variables and two scales measuring self-expression as the dependent variables indicated that women raised in families with strong cross-generational alliances are likely to display narcissistic personality traits and to have difficulty setting goals. The investigator combined different subscales, representing the factor Proximity-Differentiation to measure family members' ability to maintain a separate sense of self (Perosa & Perosa, 1990). The scale combination represented the factor Proximity-Differentiation, and suggested a family pattern in which the young woman develops a clear sense of self and functions autonomously if her parents (especially her mother) are not overly involved with her and take responsibility for meeting their own emotional needs.

Another combination of subscales represented the factor of Generational Hierarchy-Differentiation, reflecting a family system composed of clear intergenerational boundaries, where the parents support each other and do not depend on the child to meet their emotional needs. In this study, the two factor scores (Proximity-Differentiation and Generational Hierarchy-Differentiation) made up the predictor set of linear composites. The criterion set of linear composites was formed by the two measures (Superiority and Goal Instability) of Kohut's self-psychology constructs. The implications were that young women raised in homes with parental conflict and parents' dependence on their daughter for fulfilling their emotional needs are likely to have difficulty setting goals for themselves. The young women are also likely to feel confused and unable to complete their projects. They may display a tendency to unrealistically appraise themselves, to seek admiration, and to exhibit narcissistic personality traits.

On the basis of her findings Perosa concluded that, in general, Minuchin's structural family model is congruent with Kohut's psychoanalytic theorizing about the self. A major limitation of this study is the fact that the investigator relied solely on the subjects' self-reports through the use of the various scales. No measures were obtained from the parents of the young women regarding their perceptions of the relationships. Another limitation is the lack of male subjects in the study. One can only speculate what the results would have shown for the adjustment of young men with these measures. Struggles to separate from parents may be particularly difficult for men, resulting in engulfment anxiety (Quintana & Kerr, 1993) as men are socialized into demonstrating greater independence from parents.

According to Kohut (1984), narcissistic needs develop along the two lines of grandiosity and idealization. The grandiose part of the self perceives itself as the powerful and entitled center of the universe. The adolescent experiencing narcissistic injury in the grandiose part of the self may entertain aggressive fantasies of power, or act out arrogantly in interactions with others. The adolescent may also indulge in drug and alcohol abuse or delinquency. Thomas et al. (1996) studied the effect of single-mother families and nonresident father's involvement in these families on delinquency, alcohol, and drug abuse in Black and White adolescents. In their sample of over 600 households, the investigators found the highest rate of problem behavior among White male adolescents in single-mother families without the support of a nonresident father. As in previous studies (e.g.,

Hagan, Simpson, & Gillis, 1988), daughters were not found to display the same risky behaviors and delinquency as did sons.

For optimal development in adolescence, clear boundaries distinguishing between parents' and children's status, power, and roles are necessary (Minuchin, 1974). In enmeshed, or cross-generationally overly involved family situations, the boundaries are ill-defined and fluctuating, interfering with the normal separation-individuation process of adolescence. Adolescents growing up in a family with weak cross-generational boundaries are often confused about their own roles and identities. Enmeshed family systems are particularly vulnerable to ineffectual parental discipline. In order to be effective, parents need to set standards for their children, they need to monitor the children's behaviors, and they need to be consistent in enforcing rules (Maccoby & Martin, 1983).

Research (Bank et al., 1993) has shown that monitoring relative to discipline was especially important with children advancing into preadolescence and beyond, but less important with younger children. To carry through on effectual discipline, a certain emotional distance or neutrality between parent and child is necessary. The enmeshed family system is not conducive to objectivity, a basic requirement for effectual parental discipline.

Case Study

Laura: Enmeshed Parenting Style

Laura, an attractive mother of a 15-year-old girl, had followed the advice of friends and colleagues when attempting to institute needed discipline and structure into their lives. Laura and her former husband had been childless and decided to adopt a baby. Their first opportunity at parenthood was Gina, whose mother gave her up for adoption a few days after birth. Gina was a beautiful little girl who seemed to fit well into the family. Marital problems developed over time and Laura and her husband divorced when Gina was about 11 years old.

Laura's expectations for parenthood were based on her own childhood. She patterned her parenting skills after what she remembered from her parents. Simons, Beaman, Conger, and Chao (1993) and coworkers have hypothesized that parents who themselves had been raised by supportive parents will most likely repeat their parents' supportive style. Laura's memories of her childhood were rather idyllic. Her parents did not need to discipline her much. She was a cheerful girl who liked to please her parents and others around her. Her school grades were good and there were no behavior problems. Her teachers and peers liked her. Her parents often told her how lucky they were in raising her. During her college years, Laura applied herself diligently in a field that was traditionally occupied by men, and in due time she found a promising job in her chosen career.

After the divorce, Laura's husband moved to another state, leaving the sole responsibility for raising their daughter to Laura. Laura's liberal parenting style was not counterbalanced anymore by her husband's more authoritarian approach. According to past research (Maccoby & Martin, 1983), effective parenting includes setting standards, monitoring children's behavior, consistency in enforcing rules, and eschewing punishments. Laura's parenting style could not be described in those terms. The result was a degree of freedom for Gina that the teen was not ready to handle. As minor difficulties developed, Laura still believed that trust and acceptance were the best techniques to raise a well-adjusted child. She did not insist on a curfew for Gina because she wanted her to develop responsibilities on her own.

When Laura started to date again, she confided some of her experiences to Gina. The boundaries between parent and child became vague and blurry. Gina became more of a friend and confidant to her mother than a daughter. Their enmeshed relationship became psychologically and emotionally intrusive. Gina felt entitled to the privileges of adulthood. Laura's parenting style proved to be ineffective, and she sought the advice of friends and co-workers. Attempts to integrate the advice into her own practices escalated the situation into crisis proportions. Finally, Laura was encouraged by the court system to seek professional help.

Couns: I am glad both of you could come, so we can all start together to work on the situation. Laura, how do you feel right now? Are you ready to fill me in on the events that brought you here?

Laura: I feel terrible about my failure as a mother. Perhaps her

	father was right, I am too lenient with her. I believed that the way my parents raised me was right and I tried to raise Gina the same way. When the trouble started, I asked my friends for advice and even with that help I did not succeed. Gina is rebelling against me. At times, I am afraid of her, like I am not in control.
Couns:	What was the help or advice that you received from your friends?
Laura:	Lately, Gina had been skipping school and did not tell me about it. One day the teacher called me at work, asking me about Gina's illness that made her miss so many days. It turned out that Gina had typed her own excuses and forged my signature on them. Naturally, I was shocked. Before confronting Gina, I talked to some of my colleagues about it. They suggested I take disciplinary action and ground Gina for the times she had skipped school. They also recommended I set a strict curfew for Gina.
Couns:	How did that work out?
Laura:	It made everything worse, Gina did not come home when I told her to and she skipped school even more. Gina was suspended from school when I told the teacher about the forged signature. The worst thing was when she brought those savages into our home who vandalized the place. After that I grounded her indefinitely. My friends agreed I had to put down the law.
Couns:	How did Gina respond to that?
Laura:	I hate to admit this, Gina actually threatened me with physical retaliation if I grounded her.
Couns:	Is that what you meant earlier when you said you felt afraid of your daughter?
Laura:	Yes, that is true. One day I tried to keep her from leaving and she pushed me aside, saying that if I laid a hand on her, she would report me for child abuse.
Couns:	How did you deal with that?
Gina:	(interrupting) She locked me in, just like an animal in a cage!
Laura:	Yes, I did lock her in. After her threat, I knew I could not physically restrain her by holding her. I had to go to work. I did not know what else to do. There was nobody to share this burden with. I tried calling her father for help. He was out of town on vacation with his family. Being worried about Gina, I called home several times, but she never

	answered. Finally I left work earlier than usual. When I came home I saw a window had been broken out and Gina had escaped that way. That's when I called the police and reported her missing.
Couns:	How did you feel during that time?
Laura:	It was the hardest thing I ever did in my life. Even going through a divorce was not as bad as this. I felt utterly alone and helpless. I felt guilty and ashamed for calling the police on my own daughter, but I was even more worried about what could happen to her when I did not know where she was. I asked my parents if they would let Gina stay with them if she was willing. I knew I had lost and I was ready to let Gina go away if it would help us.
Couns:	Gina, how do you see the situation?
Gina:	I don't know, everything was fine until Mom flipped.
Couns:	What do you mean by everything was fine? And how did your mom flip?
Gina:	It was just normal, you know, Mom went to work, I went to school and had fun with my friends. Mom did not fuss much about what time I had to be home and didn't get bent out of shape when I did not clean my room as often as she wanted it. We didn't have big arguments over things like that. I thought she trusted me. She told me about her boyfriends and asked my advice what to wear. Mom told me about the men she dated because, as she said, she wanted me to know with whom she went out. She did not tell me details about what they did, except maybe about the restaurants they went to. She often asked me what I thought looked good on her and how to do her hair, things like that.
Couns:	So you thought you were more like friends than mother and daughter?
Gina:	Yes, like confidants. I felt really betrayed when she pulled this stunt on me!
Couns:	You sound angry. What stunt are you referring to?
Gina:	Of course I am angry, wouldn't you? All of a sudden, she grounds me and doesn't want to give me my allowance.
Couns:	What led up to that?
Gina:	I had my friends over to the house, the ones she called 'savages'. They got a bit out of line. One of them smoked and must have burned a hole in the carpet. Another one

> apparently left a big scratch in Mom's rosewood coffee table that she bought in China. He must have put his keys down on the table. There were lipstick marks on one of the pillows on the sofa. Mom just threw a fit when she came home. She told me I could not go out anymore, could not bring home any friends, and I had to pay for the damage with my allowance. That's not fair, it wasn't my fault. I did not know what my friends would do. How can she blame me for that? It's just like the other counselor said, it's Mom's fault.

Couns: What counselor was that?

Gina: Oh, that's Tim, the counselor Mom took me to after I was suspended from school. I had signed Mom's name on the notes, so she would not be bothered by it. I don't have to go to school every day. I am smart enough to know what's going on, even if I miss a class here and there.

Couns: Yes, you seem quite intelligent. What do you want to do after you graduate from high school?

Gina: I am going to be a veterinarian.

Laura: Ever since she was a little girl Gina has been talking about becoming a veterinarian. She is very good with animals. She always had pets and she takes care of them. The animals just take to her and follow her. I think she would be good as a veterinarian and she is bright enough to make it through school if she applies herself.

Couns: You have given me enough background information, so we can start working on what you want to have changed as a result of coming here. The next time I would like to meet with each of you individually. Please make a list of things that you would like to be different and indicate what you would be willing to do to make it so. In other words, look at yourself for what you can do as well as what you would like the other person to do.

Summary of Client-Counselor Interaction: Enmeshed Parenting Style.

Whenever possible in working with families, starting with conjoint sessions is good practice. If the therapy process starts with one person and later involves another family member, the risk is great that the second person feels that an alignment between the counselor and the first person has already been established. Children may think the counselor is siding with the parents, if for no other reason than that the counselor is another adult.

Without taking sides, the therapist provided equal opportunity for the clients to express their opinions and feelings in the session. Realizing that probably neither one had been given a chance to explain their feelings calmly and clearly, the counselor set the stage for the mother to report in her daughter's presence what considerations had prompted her actions. Similarly, Gina was encouraged to express her side of the events that had led to the current situation.

When Gina mentioned another counselor, the therapist decided against detailed explorations at the moment. Most likely, a discussion of previous counseling would have further undermined the mother's already shaky sense of control. Normally, the name of the previous counselor would have been included in the intake forms and consent to obtain information from that source could be obtained when appropriate. By inquiring about Gina's plans, the therapist directed the focus to the future. The moment was enhanced by her mother's praise of Gina's talents. Both mother and daughter drew together in a moment of agreement, giving a calm and promising ending to the first session.

Case Study Follow-Up: Following Friends' Advice.
Laura's sense of defeat dictated the focus of her individual counseling sessions. Her attempts to raise her daughter in a loving and trusting atmosphere had failed. Implementation of advice from others had worsened the situation. Everyone else seemed to know how to bring up children, but she had failed. Her self-confidence was badly shaken.

Couns:	Our first session was difficult for you, Laura. I was impressed by the way you handled your side of the interaction. Although you admitted being afraid of your daughter and not approving of her behavior, you did not blame Gina for the way your relationship developed.
Laura:	I am the parent! Sometimes I get angry with Gina. As a parent I should know better, but I could not even handle the situation with my friends' advice.
Couns:	You seem to blame yourself for not doing better with your friends' advice regarding the difficulties with Gina. When you think back on it, were your friends' recommendations congruent with your own ideas about raising children?

Laura:	No, as I mentioned the other day, I tried to raise Gina the way my parents raised me. They gave me a lot of freedom to develop my interests. They would never have done what I did to Gina, locking her up!
Couns:	You just made an important point about wanting to bring your child up the way you were raised. Many parents are influenced by their own experiences in growing up. Some people pattern their parenting style on what they remember their parents did, while others may want to adopt a completely different parenting style because they think that their parents did not do a good job. Then there are those who use some of their parents' ideas as a basis and add skills from various other childraising philosophies. The advice from your friends and colleagues came out of their own frameworks and, apparently, their opinions did not fit well with your philosophy. The result was a tremendous clash of directions that was confusing to Gina and impossible for you to continue to implement. By changing your practices so completely to what your friends recommended, you acted as if your own philosophy had been worthless.
Laura:	Yes, that must have been confusing to Gina. I did not feel comfortable in punishing her the way I did, but I thought I needed to do something fast to put a stop to what was happening. There is something else. I did not want to bring it up in front of Gina, but I think it has some influence on our situation. Gina's father has remarried and he and his new wife have a little son. From what Gina told me, she felt neglected at her last summer vacation with her father. She said she was just a live-in babysitter. She started cutting her classes after she came back from her father's. I think she feels deserted by her father and she did not like it that I called him for help. It probably made things worse because she may think that I am giving up on her, too. Being an adopted child, she is probably more sensitive to rejection than other children are. I don't want to blame all the difficulty on her father. Most of it must have come out of our life together.
Couns:	Did Gina's adoption make you more protective of her than if she had been your birth child?
Laura:	It's strange you would say that. I always felt that adopting a child puts a greater responsibility on a parent than

raising a child you have given birth to. I thought I had to prove myself as a parent. When you give birth to a child, you are automatically that child's parent. Perhaps that is the reason why I was so eager to follow the advice of others; I wanted to make sure I did everything right. The day Gina was suspended from school I asked the school counselor for a recommendation of a counselor for us. She referred me to Tim, the counselor Gina mentioned.

Couns: Is he no longer available to you?

Laura: He is still here, but I felt uncomfortable with him. I thought he blamed me for all the trouble. At first, I was glad that he was quite young because I thought Gina would trust him more than she would an older person. Initially we saw him together, just like you started out with us. Then he saw Gina a couple of times by herself. After about four or five sessions with Gina, he asked us both to come in together. I was surprised that this was supposed to be the last session. Tim said that there was basically nothing wrong with Gina; she was just a typical teenager. He added that the two of us had been too close. He used the word "enmeshed." The way he explained it, it sounded as if I had taken over too much of Gina's life and she was rebelling against it. I felt he thought I was a bad mother, but he did not tell me how to be a better one.

Couns: That must have been painful for you. Gina seemed to have understood the counselor's statements in much the same way you did, judging by what she said last time. In enmeshed families, the lines between parent and child tend to become blurry. At times, the parent may confide in the child more than the child is capable of handling. The child feels special and more mature than its peers, and often encourages the parent to continue in the relationship. Difficulties arise when the child assumes privileges that are part of adulthood. The poorly defined boundaries between parent and child in enmeshed relationships also cause problems when the parent sees a need for disciplinary actions. The child considers herself an equal rather than a child, and regards discipline as unfair or unjustified.

Laura: The way you are explaining the enmeshed family system, I can see some similarities in our relationship, and can

Identifying What Does Not Work

	understand why my use of the recommended discipline backfired so badly. I wished I had a better understanding of it before. What can I do to recover?
Couns:	You can start by examining your beliefs. From what you said before, you wanted to give your child all the opportunities to grow and unfold into her own personality, as you had been able to do. Not everybody can handle the same amount of freedom; some children need more guidance than others, and we don't know exactly why. You can interpret the parent's responsibility as observing the child's growth and adjustment to the environment. The child's unlimited explorations can be dangerous. A parent who does not adhere to a punishing parenting style may want to gently but clearly make the child aware of consequences connected to certain actions. The parent needs to be prepared to apply the consequences, because most children will attempt to find out whether or not the consequences will indeed occur. In some ways, the more liberal the parenting style is, the more consistency is required from the parent's behaviors.
Laura:	It sounds like I need to make major revisions in my parenting. I would like to stay within my original belief system and give Gina freedom to choose her own lifestyle, but I need to teach her that freedom brings with it responsibilities—is that what you meant by consequences?
Couns:	That is an excellent way of describing it. The privileges of adulthood include responsibility and appropriate judgment. As a parent you can allow her as much freedom as she appears able to handle by assuming the responsibilities for that level of freedom. When you consider the situation where Gina invited her friends without asking your permission, she may have thought that she was your equal and you have invited your friends without asking her. The privilege of adulthood here includes the judgment for what friends to invite and the responsibility for their behaviors while in your home.
Laura:	I'll try to explain this to Gina. I want her to know my plans to improve our relationship. She may not agree with my ideas, but at least she knows them and can express her opinion. I have learned that I cannot change my position completely from what I believe in. I hope that

	Gina and I have a chance to build a new relationship for ourselves with your guidance.
Couns:	I will be happy to assist you in whatever way I can. Gina will be coming in for her individual session tomorrow. After that we can have another conjoint session and go from there.

Summary of Client-Counselor Interaction: Following Friends' Advice. The counselor began by acknowledging the client's difficulty in her relationship with her daughter, but immediately gave her reassurance by praising her way of handling herself in the confrontation of the previous session. When the client mentioned the previous counselor, the time was opportune to obtain more details about the past counseling experience. As the counselor had perceived the experience to have been painful for Laura, an explanation of what the previous counselor may have meant by the word "enmeshed" was appropriate. The counselor's explanation removed any need for defensiveness from the client and, in fact, made her more open to contemplating changes. The fact of Gina's adoption was used by the counselor to further help Laura understand how her egalitarian and enmeshed parenting style, combined with her conscientiousness and sensitivity about being an adoptive mother, contributed to her sudden strict adherence to her friends' suggestions and Gina's confusion and rebellion.

SUMMARY

Clients' previous problem-solving attempts are explored. Some attempts may have worked well, but not necessarily perfectly. Other approaches may have been largely unsuccessful. For the single parent, maintaining self-confidence and initiative are important characteristics that need repeated emphasis. By finding out what part of the approach did not work to the client's satisfaction, the client gains not only more knowledge about the problem situation, but also feels more confident when some aspects of the attempt appeared promising for a solution. In exploring some of the reasons why a particular attempt did not work out, the individual gains self-awareness into underlying beliefs and values that may be incongruent with the person's actions in the problem-solving approach. In avoiding consideration or acceptance of any failures, the person becomes deprived of the benefits of the learning experiences inherent in less-than-perfect solutions.

EXERCISES

1. Complete Table 5.1, *Giving and getting in love relationships* (Maass, 1986).
2. Imagine yourself as the parent of a teenage child. In the recent past, you have noticed changes in your child's behaviors. The child seems to be avoiding your presence and you have noticed that the child is associating with a different group of friends. Your child frequently does not adhere to the specified curfew and seems to spend significantly less time at home and with studies. When you question your child, the child gives ambiguous answers.

    You ask a friend for advice. The friend recommends strict measures. The child should be made to stay at home after school, do homework and chores. For every minute the child is breaking the curfew, one hour of the child's time is forfeited.

    Examine your own beliefs about parenting; are they in agreement with your friend's recommendations? Is your parenting style different for sons and daughters?

    Assume that you followed your friend's advice. You tell your child in no uncertain terms what is expected of the child. Two days later, on Friday, you hear your child sneak into the house after midnight. You confront the child and announce that the child will not be allowed to leave the house during the whole weekend. The next morning you find the child's room empty. The next time you hear from the child is through a telephone call from the police station.

    What are the reasons for failure of the earlier intervention? Was your discipline approach too weak? Too harsh? Did it not work because your own beliefs of parenting were not congruent with the actions suggested by your friend? What might you have learned from this chain of events? What steps would you want to consider next? Again, would there be a difference in your actions according to the gender of your child? If you were an advice-giving friend, what course of actions would you recommend? How would your recommendations be similar to or different from what your own parents may have done? If the parent had come to your office, as a counselor, how would you have proceeded in this case?

The scenario is sufficiently vague to yield several different stories, according to the way readers supply the details.

SUGGESTED READING

Bagarozzi, D. A., & Anderson, S. A. (1989). *Personal, marital, and family myths: Theoretical formulations and clinical strategies.* New York: Norton.
The authors trace how personal myths mesh to form conjugal and family myths, influencing individual development and coloring family life in ways that lead to predictable behaviors and relationship patterns.

Simons, R. L., Beaman, J., Conger, R. D., & Chao, W. (1992). Gender differences in the intergenerational transmission of parenting beliefs. *Journal of Marriage and the Family, 54,* 823–836.
The study describes how the authors tested several hypotheses regarding how adolescents' beliefs concerning effective discipline and the impact of parenting upon child development are associated with the parenting beliefs and practices of their parents.

6

Introducing the Idea of Choices

OBJECTIVES

1. To facilitate client's awareness of the existence of choices.
2. To uncover hidden stumbling blocks in accepting choices and options.
3. To resolve stumbling blocks and stressors that may impact the decision-making process.
4. To help client accept the possibility that a certain decision may not be the perfect solution.
5. To demonstrate that readiness to explore options brings with it increased control and self-sufficiency.
6. To help client gain awareness of the impact of values and beliefs on the perception of choices.

CHOICES

Discussing characteristics of determinism and purposivism, Prescott Lecky (1969) considered the psychological function of the two concepts to be the same, as far as the principle of cause and effect is concerned. Both are attempts to give meaning to sequences of events. Differences between determinism and teleology are seen in the sources giving rise to and maintaining the action of an event. Teleologists maintain that action results from a "pull" of the goal as the organism engages in purposeful behaviors toward the goal, while determinists view the sequence of events as originating from the "push" of the cause and moving toward the consequence or result. In addition to the perceived cause of a given sequence of events, a more subtle difference in the temporal aspects of the events is evident. Determinists considering the push of the cause as the origin are focusing on the past, whereas teleologists are looking to the future (the goal). In Lecky's opinion, both views are attempting to construct a line that has only one end.

Current thoughts about human actions have turned away from the idea that behavior is predetermined. The concepts of intention, choice, and purpose have received a more prominent place in studying human behavior. William Glasser (1998) recommends replacing theories that emphasize external control with Choice Theory, a theory based on the premise that we choose everything we do and feel, including our own unhappiness. Other psychologists expressed similar concepts some time ago. When formulating his list of irrational ideas causing and sustaining people's emotional disturbances, Albert Ellis in 1962 introduced the idea that people erroneously believe in external causes for their misery and lack of control over their sorrows. Even if biological and environmental factors determine human behavior to a degree, people still have choices about how to feel and act in given situations (Ellis, 1979).

Factors Involved in Decision-Making Behaviors

In order to advance knowledge about people's decision-making behaviors, research work in the field would benefit from considerations regarding the decision maker's subjective view of uncertainty about the given situation, as well as the objective characteristics of the situation. Some explorations have focused on various factors operating in decision-making processes.

Subjective Uncertainty vs. Environmental Uncertainty.

Sniezek and Buckley (1993) distinguished between subjective uncertainty, the individual's personal experience of not knowing what outcomes to expect in a given situation, and environmental uncertainty, the reflection of objective reality and its predictive probability for certain events to occur. Several factors contribute to subjective uncertainty. The person may not have access to all available information; the person's knowledge of the availability of information may be incomplete; or any combination of the two factors may interfere with the person's possession of a complete set of knowledge around a specific event.

A need for change was expressed by Cannon-Bowers, Salas, and Pruitt (1996) when they discussed establishing boundaries of a paradigm for decision-making research. The authors recognized the limitations inherent in classical decision-making research that focused mainly on sterile, contrived situations with outcomes that had little significance for the decision makers in the real world. To improve human decision-making ability, the authors proposed naturalistic decision-making perspectives that focus on decision-making needs in complex, real-world environments. Factors to consider in the research include among others uncertain, dynamic environments; multiple-event feedback systems; meaningful consequences; multiple or ill-defined goals; and time constraints.

Characteristics of the Decision-Maker. Characteristics of real-world decision situations are important, but even more consequential are the characteristics of the decision makers themselves. The level of confidence that decision makers have in their own abilities to make sound decisions varies greatly, from extreme confidence to serious underestimation. Another characteristic is reflected on a continuum from people who like to take risks and seem to thrive on the excitement of "living on the edge," to those who demand guarantees before moving in any direction. Some individuals may be predominantly overconfident or underconfident in appraising their own decision-making capabilities, for most people, levels of confidence change as a function of decision quality over time and situations.

Rather than focus on absolute levels of confidence for a given situation, Sniezeck and Buckley (1993) proposed a confidence-accuracy space type of approach that emphasizes the examination of differences between confidence levels over conditions. Events of zero decision quality or complete failure to select the best alternatives can occur at the extreme ends of the confidence continuum. Individuals who are continuously convinced of having selected the best alternative, and those who are completely certain of having failed to do so, occupy the extreme positions at the confidence continuum. In the real world, events of zero decision quality are rare. Environments characterized by randomness will reward even completely ignorant decision makers with an occasional correct decision, just by chance alone. Thus, individuals who are unwilling or unable to make decisions in their own best interest are at times reinforced for their passivity by experiencing satisfying outcomes without exerting the effort.

Stumbling Blocks in Facing Choices

People may not be aware of the fact that they have choices; others may even resist the very idea of alternative ways of feeling and behaving. Awareness of the existence of choices brings with it an invitation to decide, to choose among options. Improvement of decision-making skills can be achieved through a learning process.

The Stress of Making Decisions

The act of making a decision is often accompanied by stress resulting in anxiety in the individual about to choose (Langs, 1991). The decision stress has at least two reasons. Irvin Yalom (1980) has defined decision as the bridge between wishing and acting. Therefore, deciding implies a commitment to a specific path. By choosing or selecting one alternative, the individual rejects or loses the other options (Assagioli, 1973). The other source for the decision stress is the individual's demand that the decision be the correct decision. Accepting responsibility for possibly having chosen the wrong option leaves many individuals paralyzed and unable to move in any direction. They either try to ignore the existence of options, or attempt to manipulate others to make the decision for them. They go to any length to avoid experiencing post-decisional regret.

Self-Imposed Helplessness

Individuals who firmly believe that they have no choices in a given situation, or who resist considering alternative actions, place themselves in a condition of helplessness that most often is not imposed on them by environmental forces but is self-imposed. Repeated failures to reach a desired goal may lead to a conviction of hopelessness and to capitulation, a condition of learned helplessness, according to Martin Seligman (1975). In failing to think their way through to satisfying choices, some people may give up thinking altogether, and instead act on their emotions. Inadequate thinking skills can increase reliance on affect, and uncontrolled affect can further undermine good thinking (Fischhoff & Downs, 1997).

Case Study

Becky and Ruth: Two for the Price of One

Becky and Ruth, two single mothers—one a widow, the other a divorcée—made their first counseling appointment. They requested to be seen together.

Couns: The telephone intake notes mentioned that you want to be seen in conjoint sessions. Does that mean you have the same or similar problems you want to discuss?

Ruth: Yes, we have basically the same problem. We are stuck, we are broke, and we have no future where we are now. The reason for wanting to be seen together is that we cannot afford individual sessions, even at the sliding fee scale. The only way for us to come here is when Becky can borrow the car from her parents-in-law. We have to scrape the money together for gasoline and for a babysitter if her mother-in-law is too sick to watch our children. Our problems are similar and we thought if we could share sessions, we could see you more often than if we had to pay for individual sessions. We could learn together.

Couns: I appreciate your openness and your initiative. Conjoint sessions sound reasonable in your situation. You know that by coming in together, the confidentiality for what is discussed here will be in both your hands. As is the case with group therapy, the therapist cannot guarantee confidentiality, but can only stress the importance of it to all participants. Becky, would you tell me more about what you and Ruth hope to achieve?

Becky: It was really Ruth's idea about coming here together, but she is right, we could not afford it otherwise. As Ruth said, we are poor and we don't know how to get out of it. There are no jobs in our town that we could do. The biggest employer is the foundry and they hire mostly men because it is physically hard work. My husband used to work there. The only other place is the little cafe. Ruth and I share the waitress job there. It does not amount to more than one full-time job. We come in as needed and have no health insurance or other benefits. We have tried to do some cleaning and babysitting for extra money, but that is not working out either. We just don't know where to turn anymore.

Couns: You seem to have already explored your resources. I am not sure I know how to help you.

Ruth: Becky has told you the situation as we see it now. We thought we might be able to get a house-cleaning and babysitting service that the two of us could handle. I am doing some typing and office work for our church without pay; just to keep my typing skills up. We mentioned our plans to the owner of the cafe. He suggested that we offer our services for free initially. Then if people liked our work, they may agree to pay us and we could start a small business that way. We have been doing this for almost a year, but nobody wants to pay us. Whenever we carefully bring up the question of money, they tell us they can't afford to pay. The best they can do is to return a favor from time to time. Sometimes they let us have some of the leftover cleaning materials for our own homes.

Couns: In your opinion, are the people in your town really unable to pay you?

Becky: Some are, but they are not even the ones who ask us that often to help them. Several of the people who ask us could afford to pay if they wanted to. The real trouble now is, we can't even stop working for free. People get upset when we turn them down and give us smaller or no tips at the cafe. At first we did not believe that was the reason for our shrinking tips, but Ruth kept track of the people whose tips got smaller. They were mostly the people we had tried not to work for free anymore. The suggestion sounded like a good idea. Our boss could not know it would backfire and we don't want to complain. He

Introducing the Idea of Choices

	meant well.
Couns:	What a disappointing turn of events. You both seem to be trying very hard to help yourselves. Becky, you mentioned that your husband had worked at the foundry, where is he now?
Becky:	My husband died two years ago in an accident and Ruth is divorced and is raising her two children by herself. Between the two of us, we have three children to take care of. We have become very close friends through all of that. It's a long story; it would take hours to tell you.
Couns:	Let me make a suggestion to you. You came here together to reduce the expenses for each of you. Instead of telling me your background histories during our session, I would like each of you to write down your own story as you see it and bring it with you the next time or mail it to me if you want to. I am also giving you each a short questionnaire to complete about how you see your situation. Our time in the sessions will be devoted to working on what you want to accomplish now or for the future, although I am still unsure about your expectations of me.
Ruth:	I like your suggestion. You have an understanding for our difficulties. In my opinion, we don't have a chance to get out of poverty while staying in our hometown. We need to make decisions and to take some risks, but we are scared. We talked about leaving town, but where would we go with three children? What would we do? We think we would be better off doing things together rather than each of us alone. We need a completely neutral person to listen to our ideas and to help us figure out if a certain plan makes sense. Our families and neighbors are ready with advice, but it does not seem to work out in our best interest. While we are considering possibilities on how to get out of our situation, there are also some difficulties with our families that we need to work on. For instance, I have a terrible relationship with my mother. You will probably see that when you read my story. Becky is totally dependent on her in-laws. They are really nice people, but Becky cannot make a move without their blessings.
Couns:	When you said you are stuck, that did not appear to be an exaggeration. You seem to have some hope of getting "unstuck" or you would not be here. Also, what I thought you mentioned was that you wanted to explore opportuni-

ties of leaving or changing your situation while at the same time working on ways of coping differently with the current situation. Our work will then proceed on two different levels. In addition to completing the questionnaire and writing your background stories, I would like you to write down ideas you may have had about changing your future. Then please mention the relationship you want to start working on first.

Summary of Clients-Counselor Interaction: Two for the Price of One. The initial interview was quite different from most expected counseling sessions. From the clients' descriptions, they had followed advice from others, as other clients had done in the previous chapter. Now their situation seemed almost hopeless. The counselor did not hesitate to admit that the counselor's function in the scenario appeared vague. The clients described troublesome life situations, but they seemed unable to envision options for change. Because of the clients' determination, the counselor agreed to work as efficiently as possible with them, but left no doubt that they had to do their share of work by immediately assigning them substantial homework.

The therapist's plan was to help the clients to explore their financial situation, to keep the responsibility for their goals placed firmly with the clients, and to see how determined the two young women really were. Although initially the clients were not very eloquent in defining their expectations about the therapist's function, with patience and gentle guidance, the therapist managed to direct the clients' focus onto two areas that they all could agree to work on.

Case Study Follow-Up: Autobiographies

Prior to their next session Becky and Ruth mailed their background histories to the therapist. Both women had grown up in the same town, but their childhood experiences had been quite different.

Becky's Story

> My childhood was a happy time, even though I lost my parents at a very young age. I hardly remember them, and what actual memories I may have of them blends in with the stories my grandparents told

me about them. My grandparents raised me in a very gentle, loving way. I do not remember ever being punished. When people in town mentioned how pretty I was, my grandmother said to me that it was my responsibility to be as pretty on the inside as God had made me on the outside. Early on my grandmother taught me to cook and bake, to sew, crochet, knit, and do other crafts. She also taught me to make my own patterns when I was old enough to learn that. I remember having many ice cream or tea parties for my friends. My grandmother saw to it that I was doing a lot of the work, such as baking cookies, making the lemonade or tea, and setting the table, as well as cleaning up afterward. Setting the table used to be my favorite activity because I could make it look so pretty. I wanted to have parties every day, but grandmother said if people had parties all the time, they would not be special anymore.

My grandmother made most of my clothes. She told me it was fun for her to sew pretty dresses, skirts, and blouses for me, but she also bought jeans and other things for me. I think she wanted me to have some clothing similar to what other children wore, probably to protect me from being teased. She was such a wise woman. I am sorry I did not realize that at the time.

School was a rather unremarkable experience. I had many friends and was a cheerleader in high school. My grades were average, with the exception of art. I was doing very well in drawing and other art projects. In my senior year I started dating Greg, the most popular boy in town, the best player on the high school ball team. An outstanding memory from that time is that my grandmother made my gown for the prom. It was a real surprise to me when she gave me a beautiful strand of pearls that had been hers for as long as I could remember. As I was waiting for my date to pick me up, my grandfather took me aside and told me the story about the pearls. They had been his gift to my grandmother when she had given birth to their only child, my mother. While working on my prom dress, grandmother kept thinking about the pearls and how beautiful they would look on me. She had planned to save them for my wedding, but she told grandfather that the prom would be a good occasion to give me the pearls. My grandfather did not agree with her at first and suggested she loan the pearls to me to wear to the prom. Grandmother firmly stated that in her opinion I should not wear anything borrowed. My grandfather gave in and remarked that perhaps grandmother could borrow the pearls from me if she wanted to wear them. I think my grandfather told me the story to let me know the depth of my grandmother's love and the meaningfulness of the gift.

Soon after graduation from high school, Greg and I got married. I was so much in love with him and my life seemed like a fairy tale then. Grandmother made my wedding gown, but she invited me to participate in the choice of the material and the design of the style. Life seemed perfect when I became pregnant with our daughter. Soon after I found out about my pregnancy, my grandfather suffered a heart attack. He never got his strength back and died a few months later, having another heart attack. One day, perhaps a week before his death, I went over to their house to visit. The door was open as usual, but I could not find my grandmother in the kitchen or the living room downstairs. I went upstairs and realized my grandmother was in the bedroom, sitting next to my grandfather's side of the bed. They talked in low voices and had not been aware of my presence. Just as I tried to quietly go back downstairs, I heard my grandfather thank my grandmother for giving him back the daughter that had been taken from them by death. He was talking about me and the way my grandmother had raised me. At that moment I had a glimpse of the deep love, trust, and devotion my grandparents had for each other.

Soon after my daughter's birth, my grandmother died. I missed her a lot. She had given me a little camera to take pictures of my daughter as she was growing up. Her last gift to me seemed to say that time is passing by fast and we need to make our own memories. My marriage did not remain happy. Greg soon became bored with spending his evenings and weekends with a wife and baby. He stayed out in the evenings, drinking with friends. At times he came home drunk and pushed me around. There were even rumors that he was seeing other women. Shortly before our daughter's third birthday, he was killed in a motor vehicle accident. Because of his blood alcohol level he was declared to have been at fault. After the insurance company paid for the injuries and damages sustained by the other driver, there was no money left over to replace our car. Greg had never taken out life insurance. We had to move in with my parents-in-law. My mother-in-law is in failing health and my responsibility is to keep the household going in exchange for room and board for my daughter and myself. I am allowed to use their car for shopping, running errands, and occasional drives for my own needs. I guess, I am lucky to have a roof over my head and to be able to make a little extra money working at the cafe. I don't feel lucky, though; there is no future. How can I prepare my daughter for a more independent life when I am dependent on others for everything? What example am I setting for her?

Ruth's Story

What a task to recount my misery! Some girls, growing up with only brothers as siblings, are treated like little princesses. I was the stepchild in my family. My mother focused all her attention on my two brothers. I was just good enough to do the household chores. When I brought home good grades from school she did not praise or encourage me. To her my good grades were unimportant because there would be no money to send me to college. Any money invested in education was earmarked for my two brothers. Thinking back on it now, it seems as if my mother kept me busy with chores, so that I would not have much time to study. Doing the household chores did not earn me any praise either. Mother made me feel I was just barely getting by with the quality of my work. When I was old enough I had to work in the cafe during the summers. The money I earned was taken away from me to help pay for my older brother's college expenses. My father was not mean to me. In his own way he loved me, but he never stood up to my mother, certainly not on my behalf.

The only person paying attention to me was a young man who came into the cafe on his way through town. He was a truck driver from another state. He tried to talk to me when I served him his coffee. I felt embarrassed and angry at the same time about the tips he gave me. I was embarrassed because I thought he wanted to pay me to talk to him, and I was angry because I knew my mother would make me turn over the money for my brother. The young man tried to date me, but my mother would not let me go out. He persisted in coming through our town from time to time, always stopping at the cafe for coffee or a snack. Finally, he asked me to marry him. I had just turned 18. When I told my mother, she showed no interest in him. She simply disapproved of the idea of my getting married. The timing was not good; my older brother had just dropped out of college in the middle of his second year, My mother was disappointed about that. Not only had the money for his tuition been wasted, but college money would soon be needed for my younger brother.

The thought of getting married was tempting to me, because I would be able to leave my mother's house. For the first time, I rebelled against her when I told her I would get married whether or not she approved. My mother responded by saying I might as well elope with the young man, because she did not intend to spend a penny on a wedding she did not approve of. At the time, I believed my mother was against the marriage because she would not get any more money through my work. In addition to being angry, I felt too ashamed to get married in our hometown with everybody knowing that my parents would not even provide for the smallest wedding. There was nothing left but to follow my mother's suggestion. After we returned from our short honeymoon, we rented a small house, and I continued to work at the cafe because my husband was on the road so much. We did not have much in common, but I was busy taking care of my two children, a girl and a little boy. After the birth of my son, my husband did not return home from one of his trips. I found out he had changed employers without telling me about it. He did not send any money for us to live on, and I finally divorced him. I never saw him again. The money I made at the cafe was not enough for us to live on and I had to apply for public assistance. My mother never let me forget how embarrassing it was to have a "welfare mother" as a daughter. Although our relationship never improved after my husband's desertion, my mother offered to let me work at home cleaning and cooking for her at holidays in exchange for leftover food to take home to my children. I am too afraid to rebel now because of my children. In addition, I am afraid to make decisions. The only time I ever decided anything on my own was to get married against my mother's will. Look what that got me! I feel incompetent in making decisions and helpless in changing my situation. My mother is in control of my life more than ever before and I don't know how much longer I can take it.

Couns: Both of you have done excellent work in telling me your background histories. Your situations appear quite difficult. From what you said last time, you both have a relatively safe place to live, but you cannot get a handle on increasing your finances or get started in any kind of business in your town. That seemed to be the main concern in your decision to see me. Before we get started with this issue, I would like to check out another point. Ruth, when I read your story I was concerned about the amount of anger and bitterness it reflected, and the urgency in the way you feel about your relationship with your mother right now. A lot of strong negative feelings seem to be bottled up in you.

Ruth: It's been a troublesome situation for many years, but you are right, recently my negative feelings have become much stronger. I told you in my report about the food packages my mother would give me after I did most of the cooking and cleaning for her on holidays. Well, when I noticed that she also packed food for my two brothers to take

Introducing the Idea of Choices

	home with them and they had not done anything to help, I really became angry. Sometimes I feel almost unable to keep myself from throwing the food packages in her face. My relationship with my brothers was never very close because of my mother's favoritism, but now it's getting worse. I find myself making sharp remarks to them when it's not really their fault.
Couns:	What do you think has kept you so far from rejecting the food packages?
Ruth:	Mainly thinking about my children. I feel I should not jeopardize anything I can get for them. My parents are the only grandparents they have. Partly that is my fault for marrying their father. My father tries to be kind to them, but he is no match for my mother. With what little attention my mother pays to my children compared to my brothers' children, she is showing the same differential treatment to my children as she did to me and my brothers. She pays some attention to my son, but my little girl might as well not exist. It really infuriates me.
Couns:	It must be painful for you to see your mother repeat that differential treatment with your children. It is like going again through the unhappiness of your own childhood. But tell me, what is the effect of the extra food on your family's life?
Ruth:	It makes my food budget last longer, and sometimes there is a little extra money that I can use for a special treat for my children.
Couns:	I can see the good feelings you have about your children. When you talk about them you have a special smile on your face. They must know how important they are in your life. The way you are raising them makes them feel special in their own ways. Your daughter will be spared the unhappiness you experienced when growing up and are still experiencing today. What would be a realistic estimate of the value of those food packages that your mother gives you for helping her with the chores?
Ruth:	Thank you for saying what you did about my children and myself. I do take comfort in the way I show my love to them and how they respond to me. They are great children and I am proud of them. In answer to your question I would say that the leftovers are worth between $15 and $20 on big holidays, such as Christmas, Easter, and Thanksgiving. On smaller holidays, such as anniversa-

	ries and birthdays, it may be more between $8 and $10.
Couns:	If you did not have the food packages, could your family survive on the money you get from your sources of income?
Ruth:	We would have to; yes, we could—but without special treats. Are you saying I should not take the leftovers, so I would not have to be angry about it? I am glad you brought this up today. With Thanksgiving coming up, I have felt more angry than usual.
Couns:	I cannot and will not tell you what to do. My job is to help you explore and find out what is best for you and how to make your decisions based on your own beliefs and values. You are right, one way of reducing your anger may be to reject the food packages. How long the state of reduced anger would last, I don't know. For the moment, let's look at anger itself, removed from your particular situation. We will come back to it later. If we talk about anger in general terms, it lends itself more to a learning experience that can be applied to many other situations and may be meaningful for Becky, too.
Ruth:	Becky, I am sorry, I did not mean to monopolize the session.
Couns:	We know you didn't. Anger is a powerful emotion, where does it come from? Usually we experience anger when things are not going our way. Perhaps our rights are being violated. Perceived helplessness plays a significant role in the development and maintenance of anger. The greater the degree of perceived helplessness, the angrier the person feels until the anger either turns to rage and acting-out behaviors or to depression and eventual withdrawal from action. People respond differently to anger; some say it makes them feel strong. The feeling of strength may be a result of overcompensation for the degree of helplessness they experience. If the person can do something to correct an unsatisfactory situation or make it acceptable, instead of feeling angry, the person would feel good about being able to make constructive changes. Ruth, can you see how this may apply to your situation with your mother?
Ruth:	When I saw my brothers leave my parents' house with food packages similar to my own I felt this overwhelming anger come up in me, almost a rage. That's when I came close to throwing my food package in my mother's face.

Introducing the Idea of Choices

	What saved me was my children's tiredness; they wanted to go home. In retrospect, it would have been a moment's satisfaction, but I would have regretted it later. And it is true, I felt absolutely helpless watching my brothers and their families walk away smiling. What can I do about this year's Thanksgiving?
Becky:	You and the children could come over to us for Thanksgiving. You know you are welcome, my parents-in-law like you. The children could play together and we could talk. I would pick you up and drive you home, so you would not have to walk home.
Ruth:	Thank you very much, Becky, for being such a good friend. We would have a good time together and maybe we will do that some day. But right now it would be like running away. I think there may be another lesson in today's session, right? (*turning to the counselor*)
Couns:	The two of you have a wonderful friendship, something that makes you both stronger. Observing the way you feel about each other gives me great pleasure, but you are correct, there is another lesson. By not spending the holidays at your parents' house you may be able to avoid the angry feelings. From your description, your mother would probably not like to prepare for the holidays without your help. She may even ask you to help before and after the holiday. In that case you would not have to see what your brothers get, but how much would you get?
Ruth:	Probably a lot less. The best thing for me would be if I were not even around to be told to help and then see the differential treatment. I have no place to go to be out of town with my children for almost a week. I have no car and no money. I am stuck. Is there a way I can handle myself without running away and without feeling so angry or helpless?
Couns:	You said earlier that on big holidays the food you get from your mother for helping her can be as much as $20 in value. You also said that you could live without that if necessary. How would it be if you stretched the food items for as many meals for your family to save that amount of money out of your food budget? Instead of spending the money on small treats for your children, act as if it did not exist and put it away for some future project that can help you in your search for independence. Although we don't know yet what your and Becky's projects will be,

	certainly you will need some funds. Saving the money and making decisions on how to use it for your own good may make you feel less helpless than if you let the money disappear in your overall household expenses. You can't do anything about the food your brothers get and what they do with it. If they feed it to the dogs, you could not change that.
Ruth:	How did you know? My younger brother always asks for extra bones for his dog.
Couns:	Without knowing about your brother's dog, I meant to show that you have no influence on what others do, but you can decide how you want to invest what you get. When you separate the food items from comparing yourself to your brothers and the negative feelings associated with that comparison, you are in a better position to evaluate if the food can be useful to you in your overall long-range planning or if it is too insignificant to bother with.
Ruth:	My mother would still be in control of me.
Couns:	Only to the degree of what she gives you for your work. What you do with the food and how you feel about it are the aspects of the situation that are in your control, not hers. If you decide to help your mother this Thanksgiving or Christmas as you did in the past, you could remind yourself that you will decide on how to invest whatever goods you earn. You can even congratulate yourself on how wisely you are putting the food to good use toward your future rather than feeding it to the dogs like your brother, but that is still his decision.
Ruth:	I think I am slowly getting the picture: My anger may cause me to lose what little extra resources are available to me. This is a whole new way of thinking and it is not easy. I guess I'll have a chance to test the new thinking pretty soon.
Couns:	You are quite right, Ruth, maintaining your new thinking within an environment that is filled with mental and emotional cues from the past will be difficult indeed. Perhaps you can prepare yourself with the aid of imagery and behavior rehearsals, something we will talk about in another session.
Becky:	As you were talking, I wondered if this kind of thinking would apply to our situation with the people in town. When we started cleaning and babysitting for some members of our community with the hope of getting paid for

our services in the future, we often got some cleaning items or leftover yarns I could use in making my afghans. Now that we told them that we can't work for free anymore, we not only don't get these things, we also find a reduction in our tips at the cafe. Should we have handled that situation differently?

Couns: That is a good point, Becky. You are correct, there are many areas of application to what we talked about. It's great that you noticed the similarity in the situations. Of course, each situation has specific aspects that need to be considered. Both you and Ruth could investigate how much or how little you may have gained from your past activities for the community. Sometimes the efforts are not worth the returns, and sometimes they are. The two of you need to decide what is worth your while.

Your observation makes one point quite clear. By sharing your sessions you can both learn from the same situation. You made a very wise decision. I congratulate you on your good judgment. Now before ending today's session, I would like to give you another homework assignment. I would like each of you to make three individual lists of activities. One list should include all the activities that you know you can perform. Another list would be made up of activities that you are not so sure you can do well, but you have an idea that you might be able to perform them. The third list is the fun list. Here you can dream and write down activities that in your wildest imagination you would have liked to do if you had the opportunity. On this list, please don't worry about whether or not you could actually perform the activities. The purpose for developing the three lists is to see if there are activities on the different lists that overlap and may be combined to guide you toward future endeavors.

Summary of Clients-Counselor Interaction: Autobiographies.

The clients' goals had not been well defined in the first session, and the counselor decided to focus on the current feelings of one of the clients. The therapist did not dictate the focus of the session, but checked out the clients' agreement before starting in the changed direction. As the session developed, the client revealed how her strong negative feelings interfered with making sound decisions for herself. The counselor offered support for the client's emotional distress and then directed the attention toward the reasons for her emotions. As both clients were interested in gaining greater individual independence, the explanations of underlying forces in the development and maintenance of anger were especially appropriate. Without making decisions for the clients, the therapist outlined where the clients were not in control and where they could exercise control if they were aware of the dynamics in different situations.

Because much of the attention was centered around one client's feelings and actions (Ruth), the therapist was aware of the need to keep the other client (Becky) equally involved in the session. Normally the counselor would not speak for the client (Becky), but at the time the counselor had a double agenda. One client needed to be reassured that she had not unduly taken advantage of the time spent in the session. The therapist attempted to set that client's mind at ease, while at the same time including the other into the interaction. The counselor also recognized and emphasized the importance of the clients' friendship as a source of strength for both of them.

One of the clients correctly generalized onto another situation the lesson learned using her friend's current situation. Her observation demonstrated that she had been actively involved in the session and that they could indeed learn twice as much by sharing their learning experiences. The therapist confirmed the clients' good judgment in deciding to share their sessions. With the assignment of new homework (see Figures 6.1 and 6.2) the therapist returned the focus to the clients' initial goal.

Things I know I can do	*Things I hope I can do*	*Things I wished I could do*
cleaning, organizing space, reading, typing, comparison-shop	learning more about photography, traveling, participating in group discussions	writing book reports for journals, studying history, archeology, literature; going to college, teaching

FIGURE 6.1 Ruth's list of activities.

Introducing the Idea of Choices

Things I know I can do	Things I hope I can do	Things I wished I could do
cooking, baking, knitting, sewing, crocheting, drawing, arts & crafts projects, gardening, reading, making patterns	dancing, playing an instrument, singing, learn budgeting, learn to talk in front of groups of people	planning big parties, teaching arts & crafts, decorating professionally, buying art objects for others, learning and teaching color-coordinating

FIGURE 6.2 Becky's list of activities.

Case Study Follow-Up: Activities Lists

For their next session, Ruth and Becky had worked on their lists of activities. Both stated that their lists were not completed yet, but it was a good beginning.

Couns: I see you have done a lot of thinking about your homework assignment. Your lists are impressive. Becky, your interests seem to cluster strongly around creative and feminine activities. As you can see, some of the items on the list where you know how to do things, such as cooking and doing arts and crafts, certainly could be correlated with things on your "wildest dreams" list. When you say that you would like to plan big parties, I assume that you mean that professionally now. I remember reading about it in your story. Many of your skills could be useful. Your talents in cooking, drawing, and decorating would certainly find application in planning parties, so would knowledge of music and dancing for the entertainment part. Where did the idea of planning parties come from?

Becky: When I grew up, I never had big ambitions. I really just wanted to be a good wife and mother. When I dreamed about my future family life, I always thought it would be nice if I could turn every day of our lives into a party. Hearing my grandmother say that having parties every day would take the specialness away, I was disappointed. Later I thought, perhaps I could do it for different families and different people each day of the week. I had forgotten about that until you gave us the homework assignment, and I thought I might as well write it down.

Couns: I am glad you did. It is an excellent example of how some of our ideas stay with us even if we are not always conscious of them. The ideas may lead us toward certain activities, but we don't know that for sure. When we take the time to look at ourselves, as you just did with the exercise, many parts of our lives are more logically connected than what we give ourselves credit for. Perhaps you would enjoy working in the catering business, planning and organizing festivities for special occasions. That is only one possibility. I am sure as we study your lists in more detail, other ideas will come to mind. Ruth, have you thought of how some of your activities could combine into a possible career path?

Ruth: I could probably do some report writing for people to make a little money, if I had a typewriter or word processor. When I look at the different interests that I wrote down, it seems to me that they are all connected to my dream of going to college. Perhaps I wanted so badly to go to college because I wasn't allowed to while my brothers were given the opportunity. Every time I thought about college, I was afraid that my obsession was rooted in envy. Writing down the things I am interested in, at least, gave me the idea it wasn't just envy. For most of the things I would like to do, I would have to go to college to study them, or obtain a degree to be teaching them. In that respect, the exercise was valuable, but I still am not any closer to a goal.

Couns: You seem to think that college is absolutely impossible for you. Have you made any inquiries about possible financial aid that might be available to you? Had you ever taken the Scholastic Aptitude Test when you were in high school?

Ruth: No, there seemed to be no sense in doing it, as my parents would not support me financially. Also, I would have had to leave home, because there is no way of commuting to any college from our town without a car. So I never even took the test. I guess, I just gave up. Now it is too late;

Introducing the Idea of Choices

Couns:	with two small children it would be even more difficult. Certainly, going to school with two young children at home would not be easy even if the college were in the town you live in. Have you ever wondered how you would have done on the SAT? You seem quite intelligent. It might have been interesting to find out.
Ruth:	Do you think I could still take the test, even though I am not in school anymore?
Couns:	I don't see why not. The test is given at different times and in different locations. People can sign up for it whether they are in school or not. Your local school, library, or a learning center would have more details on that. They and bookstores probably have books on how to practice for the test. What kinds of feelings did you experience while you were writing your lists?
Ruth:	I did not like the assignment, but I did it because you considered it to be important and because Becky did it. She did not seem to mind, but I felt very sad as I continued with it.
Couns:	Where do you think the sadness came from?
Ruth:	I know this sounds silly. I felt like I was dying all over again and I haven't even died the first time. How can I explain it?
Couns:	I think I understand what you mean. The first time you realized that your parents would not support your wishes, you may have felt as if something died in you. Your hope, your aspirations, your spark for the future, all appeared to be lost. When you worked on the homework assignment, you may have gone through the same process of feelings again as you did in the past. From what you said earlier today, you seem to think it is as hopeless now as it was then. No wonder you felt sad. The assignment was not easy for you and it took courage on your part to continue with it. Perhaps not everything is dead yet. Remember, you said earlier that you believe it is too late to go to college. Your feelings of sadness would be a natural consequence of that belief. The question is, how realistic is that belief? We will talk more about beliefs later on. Let's see how Becky felt when she worked on her assignment.
Becky:	I agree with Ruth, my feelings were strange, too. In fact, I cried when I remembered what my grandmother had said. I don't know whether I cried because I miss her, or

whether it was because of the disappointment that having parties every day would not be good. When I stopped crying I felt sad too, but not the way Ruth described it. With me it was more a sadness that I had lost, or rather misplaced something and I needed to find it again. Afterwards I thought some more about it and I decided to make more party days for my daughter and myself. Probably my husband's parents would like a bit of joy around the house. It may not lead to anything big or anything I can make money with, but I want to use what talents I have to make our lives happier. Who knows, with more practice I may get to be real good at it. I decided to buy some seeds and grow flowers next year to put them in all the rooms of the house. Starting with seeds is a lot cheaper than buying the plants. With the remnants I still have I can make some coasters or placemats and combine them with the flowers into gifts for friends for their birthdays or to make a special day for them.

Couns: Becky, that is wonderful. You have used the exercise to bring your spirits up again. I am sure, as you go along with your plans, more exciting and creative thoughts will come to you. In addition, you will be in control of your own feelings and to a degree of those around you. By making it a special day for your friends, you are practicing your creative skills and your activities will be different from those when you gave your services away for free.

Ruth: Becky is right, we need to do what we can to keep our spirits up. I wished I had her talents. She can make so many beautiful things. I enjoy looking at them. For myself, I have decided to give it a try looking at my mother differently. What you said last time made a lot of sense, although it is hard to keep my mind on it. If I can concentrate on using mother's food packages for my work as a means to save up some money for future plans, instead of comparing what I get with what my brothers get for not doing anything, I would probably feel better about it. I also thought it would be easier if I had a plan how to apply any money that I can save, but I could not come up with a goal where the small amounts would be an incentive. With the two big holidays, Thanksgiving and Christmas, coming up, changing my attitude would be helpful. As Becky was talking, I thought about investing

> some of the money in materials for Becky's art work. Perhaps we could invest in Becky's talents to produce decorative things that people would buy. We would have to go to another town and look for a store that might take her work on consignment. The process would be slow with our limited funds. If we cannot sell the items, we would have enough birthday and Christmas presents for years to come.
>
> Couns: You have come to a good start. Both of you already seem to be more hopeful and future-oriented in your thinking. How would it be if you kept a record of your ideas? Write everything down for a week or so and then prioritize your ideas. You probably want to get started soon to make use of the momentum of your hopeful spirits. When you keep a record of your ideas, you can always go back to another idea if the first one does not work out for some reason. Besides, having more than one plan on paper may give you new ideas on how to combine some of them for a more effective approach. This can be your homework assignment for the next session. Keeping a realistic eye on your limited funds, how many different ways could you invest them for a reasonable return without risking more than you can afford?

Summary of Clients-Counselor Interaction: Activities Lists. The previous homework assignment facilitated both clients' focus on the future. In completing the assignment, both clients had experienced very strong but different feelings. In bringing the emotions to the surface, the counselor helped the clients to realize how important their past dreams and goals had really been to them. Neither one had been aware of the impact of their emotional losses when they discarded their goals out of necessity. As they felt some of their past emotions surface again, a ray of hope emerged that lead them to consider possibilities for the future. Surprisingly, Becky, the less directive of the two young women, was expressing stronger feelings of hope than Ruth, who usually appeared more active than her friend; but for both, the focus shifted to more promising issues about their future.

Toward the end of the session, the therapist prevented the clients from making hasty decisions that would be cast in stone. Their excitement about planning a new approach seemed to lead them to accept the first solution that came to mind. While the proposed approach was not an impossible one, it may have been somewhat unrealistic, insofar as Ruth was willing to invest all her funds in Becky's work. Becky's talents may have been a good basis for the investment, but the difficulty Ruth expressed about working for her mother's food packages indicated that in order to reduce the resentment, Ruth needed to feel some added benefit for herself personally. By suggesting a period of contemplation and further exploration of possibilities, the counselor prevented a premature decision that could have required more delayed gratification than Ruth could handle now, and could have resulted in disappointment.

Forced Choices Due to Sudden Singleness

Single parents are often placed in a position of sole decision-maker quite suddenly, through divorce from or death of a spouse. In the normal process of maturation, individuals gradually develop decision-making skills. When sharing substantial parts of one's life with another person, many significant decisions become joint ventures rather than individual selections. Over periods of time, considerations of others' opinions have become stable habits in situations requiring decisions. The sudden removal of the other person frequently leaves the single parent facing a task that up to now had been handled by two people. Betty, the widowed mother of three children, who was introduced in the previous chapter, faced just such a crisis situation.

Case Study

Betty: Decisions and Choices Forced by Widowhood

Betty started her next session by asking the therapist's permission to pay her co-payments for the counseling sessions for several months ahead. The counselor, surprised about this unusual request, explored her reason.

> Betty: I am at the end of my rope. I had to cancel my credit cards, at least, those that my oldest daughter Tracy had

been allowed to use. In order to pay the amounts Tracy had charged, and the tremendous telephone bill from her long-distance calls, along with payments for the mortgage, car insurance, and the high food costs, I will have to sell a piece of property that my husband and I had bought for our retirement. Closing the deal on the property will take some time, but I have been able to get an agreement with the phone company and the credit card companies to pay the debts off in installments. Any money coming in from my job I have to use for food, gasoline, and utilities. Even with the sale of the property I will have to cut corners in our spending for a long time to come. With what I am going through now and not knowing what to do next, I cannot afford to have no money for my sessions. Just the thought of not being able to come in for my sessions raises my anxiety level sky-high.

Couns: I can see the tremendous shock you must have experienced when you found out about the debts. In spite of it you have already made decisions on how to deal with some parts of the situations that require immediate attention and you have taken steps to act on those decisions. Your approach has worked well and your debtors were probably impressed with your sincerity in handling your responsibility. You had to sacrifice some of your property; I hope you can salvage a part of it for your own retirement. How are your children responding to this?

Betty: That is the most difficult thing to handle. When I confronted Tracy about the debts she had incurred for the family, she just told me to file bankruptcy. My son, being the only male in the family, seems to see himself as the head of the household. He stated that was a great idea and would certainly take care of the financial burden. He seemed more concerned with being able to get his own car for a graduation present as my husband had promised him. I told them that bankruptcy was not an option. I have to come up with ways to keep our living expenses down, but I don't see what else I can do.

Couns: You rejected the idea of filing bankruptcy but, as you said, you need to spend less money on a daily basis. As you continue to think about it, what possible strategies come to mind?

Betty: The easiest way would be if Tracy moved out. She is old

	enough to be on her own at 20 years. She could get a job and support herself. I don't think she has any intentions of doing that, though, and I cannot bring myself to throw her out. If she had no place to live, she would probably get even more involved with the people she used to run around with. She could get into trouble and I would feel too guilty that I had driven her to that.
Couns:	So you don't want to force her to leave home. Can you think of any other way to control your finances? A way, that would not lead to guilt feelings?
Betty:	With a little money, I could find a used or a small new refrigerator that I could lock and keep in my bedroom. Then I could keep the expensive food items that I need for dinner in there and leave other foods for snacks in the big refrigerator in the kitchen. But it would be too horrible to keep food locked away from my children! What kind of a mother would I be!
Couns:	How are your other two children behaving in this situation?
Betty:	They are generally pretty good in following my suggestions, although my son has been disregarding some of my notes on the foods lately. Lisa, my youngest, does not seem to eat much now. She complained of pains in her stomach and having bad dreams. I found out that she is worried we may have to leave our home.
Couns:	You have made some changes to cope with an essentially difficult situation. You have taken steps to increase the safety of your family and you have developed some plans on how to operate within your financial boundaries. Some of your plans have been successful, while others apparently have not worked so well. You could see those that did not work out as failures. In reality, though, you have learned more about the particular problem situations by finding out what does not work. Once you acknowledge that, you can direct your energies toward other possible solutions—as you already did.
Betty:	You mean the lockable refrigerator? I can't go through with that. Tracy would probably tell everybody that I am keeping the food locked away from my kids. What would people think!
Couns:	Being a single parent often puts you in a lonely position. You have to make decisions to the best of your knowledge

Introducing the Idea of Choices

and ability without the luxury of having the support of a spouse. Some of your decisions will not meet with your friends' applause. No matter how popular some of your decisions may be in the eyes of others, only you know how much struggle and pain went into making them and how justified they are when considering the whole situation. You know how you have considered different options and the likely consequences resulting from them.

Betty: I think I understand what you mean. I know that financially we cannot continue to live the way we do now. Implementing changes is not my children's responsibility, although it would be nice if they showed more understanding. When I weigh the possible consequences of having Tracy leave home and compare those with the consequences of locking up some of the food, I think my daughter's safety is more important than her approval of my decision. She may think I don't love her and that will be painful to me. I have a chance to work overtime, starting next week. At first I thought of using that money to take the family on a short trip to one of my sisters' place. It is too far to drive and I thought of flying out there. That would have been nice but I think I better use the money to pay for my unpopular decision.

Couns: You have made a difficult decision, one that may be unpopular in the eyes of others. In the view of your own values and beliefs, you have considered various possibilities and their consequences. When you started out seeking the advice of others in your difficult situation, you had not been aware that some of the advice would not fit in with your values or your past behaviors, as we had discussed previously. The incongruence led to confusion. Now you have learned that in order to feel comfortable with your decisions, they have to be congruent with your values. Actually, you are following some of your friends' advice, you are more assertive, but you are tempering your assertiveness with characteristics that are not in conflict with your values. When you accepted the loneliness of your current decision-making position within your family, you were able to focus your energy on possible solutions that are within your reach.

Betty: I did follow my friends' advice. Linda, my friend who gave me the newspaper clipping, has actually given me the best advice. Without the newspaper clipping I would not be here.

Summary of Client-Counselor Interaction: Decisions and Choices Forced by Widowhood. The previous session reflected the client's struggle in weighing the consequences of decisions she had to make for the safety of her family. The counselor was well aware of and acknowledged the tremendous emotional pain the client experienced. Rather than encouraging prolonged focus on the pain, the counselor decided on facilitating the client's goal-directed thinking. The client needed to use what little time she had to explore solutions, consider their consequences, decide on a course of action, and start implementing her decisions. Her financial situation demanded swift action. Although she had made some decisions to resolve parts of her problematic situation, regarding other parts, she initially saw herself as helpless and unable to find a solution.

Responsibility Developing. Later on, the client's willingness to shoulder the burden of responsibility for some harsh-appearing decisions was reinforced by the counselor's supporting statements. When explaining the reasons for the client's earlier confusion, the counselor emphasized that considering other people's advice in and of itself was not a mistake, but following the advice indiscriminately without regard to her own values and philosophy of life created the stumbling block that prevented the desired outcome.

Effects of Values and Beliefs on the Perception of Choices and on Decision Making

In considering possible choices, our judgment about the feasibility or practicality of the choices may be clouded by conflicts of underlying values (Knaus, 1983). Not only may conflicting values operate within ourselves, but our values may also be in conflict with those held by significant others around us. In order to arrive at decisions that are in our best interest, awareness of the values that guide or determine our actions is important. As demonstrated in Betty's case, when she followed others' recommendations regarding solutions to problematic situations, part of the failure to achieve the desired outcome was

Introducing the Idea of Choices 191

due to actions that were incongruent with her underlying values. Even when decisions and actions are congruent with the values and beliefs held by the person, the outcome may not be in the person's best interest because some beliefs may be based on experiences that are incomplete or incorrect.

Case Study

Earl: Conflicting Values: Marriage, Fidelity, Parenthood

Earl, a young, still-married father of two daughters, originally entered counseling to work on improving his marriage. He had felt emotionally rejected by his wife for some time. If he initiated sexual activities, the best he could hope for was passive compliance from his wife. She never showed any passion that would lead him to feel loved or desired by her. If he tried to hug or kiss her, she pulled away.

Couns:	You stated your presenting problem as wanting to improve your marriage—how does your wife feel about this? Is she going to join us?
Earl:	My wife doesn't know that I am here because I am not sure that the marriage can be saved.
Couns:	It sounds like you are not quite sure whether you want to improve or leave your marriage.
Earl:	That is true. LaTonya, my wife, has been cold to me for several years. I don't know why she even married me. She almost called off our engagement, but finally went through with the wedding. For a while it was not so bad, but after the birth of our younger daughter she seemed to turn away from me. I thought perhaps she was afraid of becoming pregnant again. We had talked about not having more than two children. LaTonya had a tubal ligation, but her attitude toward me did not change. A couple of years ago she found herself a part-time job and with her new friends from work she started to go out at night to concerts or movies. She has been coming home quite late, saying that she and her friends had stopped at a restaurant after the concert. More recently there were some weekends that she did not come back until Sunday morning. Her excuse was she stayed with one of her

friends after the concert rather than come home by herself at night. The last time she came home on a Sunday morning she had a black eye. She said she had fallen in the dark coming out of the restaurant and her friend had taken her home. She went straight to bed with a headache.

Couns: How did you respond to that? Did she ever invite you to come along?

Earl: No, she didn't. In fact, I once asked her if she wanted me to go with her, but she said that her friends would think that I didn't trust her. After all, it was only once or twice a month that they have their girls' night out. She is right; I don't trust her now.

Couns: You seem troubled and suspicious, what are your fears?

Earl: Yes, I am suspicious—who wouldn't be? I don't know if she is always with her friends as she says. I don't know whether she is having an affair with another man, but it looks to me as if she is at least contemplating it.

Couns: What are your expectations of me, how can I help you?

Earl: First I have to find out what LaTonya is really doing. If she does not have an affair, I want us both to come in for marriage counseling. If she has been seeing another man, I need your help in getting through the divorce and perhaps help my daughters to adjust to it.

Couns: It seems your decisions are already made, depending on what you find out. What are your feelings for your wife?

Earl: I don't really know. My love is not the same as when we first met. For so long I have felt lonely, nobody to hold me or really care about me. Perhaps I have done something to hurt LaTonya and am not aware of it. If there is a chance for us, I am willing to work to change in myself what is necessary to make us happy. But if she has been with another man, there is no chance I can ever forget that. The marriage would be over.

Couns: You seem determined to proceed in either of two ways as you explained. What are your plans about your daughters?

Earl: That's where I need your help if I have to divorce LaTonya. She has been a good mother to our daughters. She is doing a great job with them. I will miss them terribly.

Couns: You have already decided that in case of a divorce your daughters will continue to live with their mother, even though you love them as much as a father can.

Earl: The girls are my only happiness; I spend a lot of time with them in the evenings and on weekends. They come

	to me for help with their homework, and I am glad they do. We are really close, but they have to live with their mother. I firmly believe children need their mother, especially girls. They should not be separated from their mother while growing up. I would never take them away from LaTonya, no matter how much she may have hurt me.
Couns:	Ideally, children should have both a mother and a father. There is no doubt that children need a mother, but there is also no reason why fathers would not be as good a parent as mothers. Evidence has shown that in general mothers and fathers can function equally well as primary parents. In your individual case, however, you and your wife will make that decision based on your beliefs and values. How would you like to proceed for the immediate future?
Earl:	My next step is to find out whether or not LaTonya has betrayed me. The future of my family and my actions depend on that. I would like to make another appointment as soon as I have that information—if that is agreeable with you.
Couns:	Yes; that is agreeable. If you and your wife decide on marriage counseling, you would want to consider her schedule too in setting up the next appointment.

Summary of Client-Counselor Interaction: Conflicting Values—Marriage and Fidelity. During this initial session, the counselor realized how the client's strong beliefs influenced his decision-making. While the client was strongly committed to his marriage, he valued marital fidelity even more. He made it quite clear that he would not consider one without the other. An equally strong value was reflected in his decision that if the marriage ended, his daughters would live with their mother. Beyond the statement that both men and women have the ability to be effective primary parents, the counselor did not attempt to lead the client to consider other options at this point. In the face of the client's strong convictions, such action would only have alienated the client. Moreover, as the client expressed his suspicions regarding his wife's infidelity, he also seemed to look for someone to trust. By his decision, the counselor would be the person to trust for assistance with his future actions. The therapist responded to that need.

Case Study Follow-Up: Conflicting Values—Parenthood

At his next session, Earl reported that LaTonya had indeed been involved with at least one other man. Earl had initiated divorce proceedings and moved out of his home, leaving the house for his daughters and their mother. Although his attorney had recommended that Earl sue for custody of his daughters, Earl had declined the recommendation because he remained firmly convinced that his daughters needed their mother full-time. In the few remaining counseling sessions Earl mainly tried to adjust to the emotional pain of not having his children with him.

About 2 years later the counselor received an urgent call from Earl. He wanted to be seen as soon as possible.

Couns: Your call sounded urgent. We have not met for quite a while, so I assume that you are faced with a crisis situation. Please fill me in on what has happened to bring you back.

Earl: Thank you for seeing me so soon. Something terrible has happened and it's all my fault. I received a phone call from the Child Protective Services about my older daughter Revena. They think she may have been sexually abused by my ex-wife's boyfriend. I knew that her boyfriend was staying overnight on the weekends that my daughters spent with me. Perhaps you remember I told you that LaTonya had come home with a black eye from one of her concerts when we were still married. Well, it seems that her boyfriend can be quite nasty, especially when he had something to drink. At times, I had seen bruises on LaTonya's arms and face when I picked up or dropped off my daughters. The girls told me there had been arguments. Sometimes they did not want to go back home. I wished I had listened to them.

Couns: I remember you told me about LaTonya's black eye when we first worked together. Now you are blaming yourself for something. Did your daughters tell you what went on in their home?

Earl: Not exactly, they just did not want to go back sometimes. I probably should have asked more questions, but I did not want to interfere with their and their mother's life. I always trusted LaTonya to be a good mother. She would never let the children be hurt knowingly. I still believe

Introducing the Idea of Choices 195

	that. As far as I can sort out the situation, LaTonya had been drinking with her boyfriend. She passed out and that's when he went into my daughter's room and molested her. Later on he threatened her that if she told anyone, he would hurt her mother and her little sister. The Child Protection Services asked me if I could have the girls live with me. How can the girls trust me again after I left them unprotected? If I had followed my attorney's advice, perhaps I would have been awarded custody and this tragedy would not have happened.
Couns:	When you first decided to divorce LaTonya you firmly believed that children belong with their mothers. That belief may have come from your parents or what people in general say. In the case of strongly held beliefs, we act as if our beliefs are true. When we believe that something is true, we don't even think of questioning it. We simply act on the belief without considering other options. At the time, you decided what you thought would be best for your children, even though you missed their presence. You were willing to sacrifice having them with you every day for what you thought would be in their best interest.
Earl:	That is true, I was convinced that I was doing the right thing. I remember my mother saying that children always belonged with their mother. Nobody else can know what they need. The relationship between a mother and her children is a sacred one. My mother would have given her life for every one of us if necessary. How can something so strong be wrong?
Couns:	With your own mother as a model, you had good reasons to believe as you did and, as I said earlier, we usually do not question strongly held beliefs. Your experiences were incomplete; you did not know how other mothers behaved and you did not know that a man can be as effective a parent as a woman.
Earl:	I think you tried to tell me that when I decided to divorce LaTonya, but I would not listen. You could not have convinced me to think differently, just as my attorney could not change my mind. Where can I go from here? How can I know whether or not my beliefs are true?
Couns:	First you could try to find out the basis for a given belief; where did it come from? In this case your belief came from your mother, but you could ask yourself if that means

that all mothers are good mothers, or if you have heard of some that are not as good. Similarly, are there fathers who are great parents in the absence of a mother? Evidence for answers to these two questions is available. Another useful question would be: What are the consequences if I act on my belief? One of the consequences would be that other options will not be considered. In the case with your children, another consequence would be that you are limiting your own control over your children's welfare while at the same time reducing your responsibility for them. Evaluating the effects of possible consequences will be a step in the overall decision-making process.

Earl: What you are saying sounds terribly complicated and time-consuming. Who has the time to go through all those steps before making a decision?

Couns: You are right, questioning the basis for our beliefs and considering consequences that may result from our actions takes time, especially in the beginning. As with many other things, practice makes proficient. The more frequently we activate the challenging process, the more efficient we will become at the whole process. Usually, the significance of the decision to be made will justify the time spent, not only because of the different aspects of life that will be impacted, but also because of the emotions that accompany the outcomes of the decisions.

Earl: If I had known what would happen, I would have listened to my attorney and to you. Certainly I feel bad about what happened to Revena, and I will try to obtain full custody for my daughters. Having them live with me full-time will be difficult because of my job. Perhaps my mother can help me take care of the girls while I am at work. Also, I have started dating again. I wonder how my new friend will respond to having my daughters around all the time. I feel a bit better now after talking to you. The Child Protective Services recommended counseling for the girls and have already referred them to a counselor. They also suggested I join the girls in their sessions even though I told them I was seeing you, as my attorney recommended.

Couns: If I can be of help, I will be available to you and your family. In the meantime you can discuss with your lawyer and the Child Protective Services what would be the best course of action.

Summary of Client-Counselor Interaction: Conflicting Values—Parenthood. When the client returned due to a crisis situation, the reason for his return was not quite clear. At first, the client appeared devastated about the abuse of his daughter. He also seemed to want to know what impact his decision had in the development of the crisis. The therapist attempted to explain that most people make decisions based on what they think is best, according to their beliefs and values. Sincerely held beliefs often do not require questioning in the mind of the person, and a certain path of action will be pursued without exploring other possibilities.

At this point, the interaction between the client and the counselor changed direction. The client seemed to have little interest in becoming involved in a cumbersome decision-making process. He admitted that in the past he had not listened to his attorney nor to the counselor, indicating that at the time he had been aware of the attempts to assist him in considering different options. His current concerns seemed to center around the impact the new living situation would have upon his daily life. Although concerns like that would be natural under the circumstances, the therapist did not perceive any expressed willingness or readiness for continuing work on the issues.

Perhaps the reason for the client's return was his statement to the Child Protective Services about seeing a counselor and he did not want to be lying. The therapist was aware that the time was not ripe for embarking on a more meaningful counseling process, but left the door open for future work if the client felt a need. Had the counselor pushed for more involvement, the client would not have made any commitments. He also would have felt too uncomfortable to return in the future, even if he wanted to.

SUMMARY

As the different case histories demonstrated, consideration of options is not always a natural step in the decision-making situations many clients face. Choosing between several options can be overwhelming, depending upon the attitude surrounding the choices. Selecting one option over others means rejecting the others. What if one of the other options would have resulted in a better outcome than the one chosen? The responsibility for selecting the correct or the best option renders many people paralyzed. Unless they can have a guarantee for making the absolute best choice, they are unwilling to move in any direction. Sometimes, as in the case with Ruth and Becky, options are not as apparent to them and they see themselves stuck in a hopeless situation. When forced with the necessity of making decisions, the most efficient choice may be an unpopular one that meets with no support from others, as happened in Betty's case. Finally, clinging to deeply entrenched beliefs and values prevents clients from exploring alternatives that may work but are incongruent with their values. In other instances, decisions that are incompatible with the person's values may dictate actions that the individual feels uncomfortable with. Those actions are usually doomed to failure.

The exploration and selection of choices is a complicated process that requires patience, willingness to take reasonable risks, and courage to accept responsibility for the outcomes—positive or negative. In the safety of the counseling session, the client is encouraged to explore different solutions with consideration of how well a given approach fits with the client's overall lifestyle and beliefs. The counselor's role is to guide the client in the search for decisions and to select those that are not leading to more conflict but rather are congruent with the client's life. Without the client's willingness to actively participate in the process, significant changes in the client's unhappiness cannot be expected.

EXERCISES

1. Following the counselor's instructions for Ruth and Becky, construct your own three lists of activities.
2. Recall from your memory a situation where you had to make a choice among several available options. Was the situation stressful for you? Where did the stress come from? When you made your choice, was it congruent with your values and beliefs?

SUGGESTED READING

Ellis, A. (1994b). *Reason and emotion in psychotherapy* (Rev. ed.). New York: Birch Lane Press.

The author describes the theory and practice of rational-emotive therapy, demonstrating how emotional reactions can be traced to exclamatory sentences stated by clients. Rational-emotive treatment is compared with other popular therapeutic methods.

Glasser, W. (1998). *Choice theory: A new psychology of personal freedom.* New York: Harper-Collins.

The author states that people choose everything they do, even their own misery. Taking more effective control means making better choices as people relate to those around them. The focus of the book is on major relationships that are in obvious need of improvement.

Sniezek, J. A., & Buckley, T. (1993). Becoming more or less uncertain. In N. J. Castellan, Jr. (Ed.), *Individual and group decision-making* (pp. 87–108). Hillsdale, NJ: Erlbaum.

The chapter explores the roles of subjective uncertainty or confidence in decision making. Factors associated with changes in confidence about the quality of decisions are identified and implications are addressed.

7

Starting and Proceeding Along the Chosen Path

OBJECTIVES

1. To help client focus on a particular approach for problem resolution.
2. To explore skills and techniques that aid in achievement of the desired outcome.
3. To increase awareness of possible stumbling blocks along the path.
4. To resolve stumbling blocks if they have surfaced.
5. To guide client in behavior rehearsals that are appropriate for the client and the situation.
6. To guide client in refining and modifying skills during repeated practice or rehearsals.

PROCEEDING ALONG THE CHOSEN PATH

The preliminary work done in previous phases, such as deciding on the problem area and selecting a particular approach to employ for resolution, has prepared the client for the actions required for the achievement of the desired goals. Various skills and techniques are explored. As in all the other phases, opportunities exist to enhance actions and occasions arise to uncover stumbling blocks that had been unknown up to then.

UNRESOLVED EMOTIONS

The existence of interfering underlying unresolved emotions can be discovered in any phase of the counseling process, but appears particularly frequently when the client is actually seriously contemplating, imaging, and practicing new behaviors. The concomitant emotions and contemplated new behaviors must be explored.

Case Study

Becky and Ruth: Revisited

Ruth and Becky, introduced in an earlier chapter, were ready to contemplate behavioral changes, especially because Ruth felt she needed preparation for the upcoming holidays.

Couns: You both look very happy today, as if you discovered something pleasant.
Ruth: I think it is working.
Couns: What do you mean, Ruth, what is working?
Ruth: What we are learning here is working. This year, before my mother even asked me to help her with the cleaning, I had made up my mind to think about what the food packages could do for our plans for the future, just as we had discussed in our session. I tried to program my mind every morning, imagining myself in my mother's house cleaning and thinking that the important thing was to earn whatever I could. After my mother called me, I arrived at her house in a good mood and started right in on the cleaning.
Couns: Very good, you actually got a head start on your imagery skills and you seem pleased with your success.
Ruth: Yes, I really was off to a good start! After I had done some of the rooms, my mother talked about the lack of space in the hall closet. She complained that people were wearing heavy coats in the winter and there was not enough space for the guests' coats. When I looked into the closet I saw quite a few of her own clothes hanging in there. I suggested to take them out to make room for the guests' coats. She thought that would be a good idea, except that

her own closet was already overflowing. I offered to help her organizing her own closet. We went up into her bedroom and got everything out of the closet. In one corner of the closet I saw two big boxes with yarns, remnants, and old materials. When I pulled them out I could see that we could make two levels in that space where she could hang blouses, jackets, and other short items in the top row and possibly hang skirts or put shelves for shoes and handbags on the lower level. I put all the dresses and longer items to one side and coordinated them nicely according to seasonal use with handy little dividers between them to separate different sections. We had a nice space left for the two-level arrangements.

Couns: You really worked hard and quite creative in the way you reorganized the space.

Ruth: Yes, for once, my mother was pleased with what I did, but then she did not know what to do with the boxes of remnants. Some of the materials were pieces left over from drapes that she had taken down a long time ago. There were half-completed sweaters that she had started to knit years ago and never finished. Mother seemed a bit embarrassed when she saw her unfinished projects, and said that the things would probably be too small now for the persons she had intended to make them for, but it would be a sin to throw them away. As calmly as I could, I suggested that perhaps Becky could put the items to good use for her daughter.

I know my mother likes Becky. She always talks about how Becky is taking such good care of her parents-in-law. No matter what her husband was like, Becky being a widow is so much more respectable than her own divorced daughter living on welfare. I was afraid if I asked for the materials for myself, my mother would find a reason why she did not want to give them away. But if she gave them to Becky, that would be a good deed.

Mother hesitated a bit but said asking Becky might be a good idea. I also thought my mother would not be unhappy to get rid of these reminders gracefully and quickly, so I just mentioned that Becky was watching my children and would come by later to pick me up after we finished the cleaning for the day. I carried the boxes out to the door and let my mother enjoy her newly organized closet. At the end of the day when Becky came over to take me home, my mother asked her if she could use the materials. Becky was surprised, but she thanked my mother and we quickly carried the boxes to Becky's car. We enjoyed looking at the remnants and thinking about how Becky would turn them into beautiful and useful things. The boxes were like a treasure to us.

Couns: It sounds like you had a wonderful opportunity to obtain an inventory for starting on your future business. You said that you knew your mother would not give the materials to you, but she would be more inclined to give them to Becky. How did you feel at that moment?

Ruth: Oh, it hurt. I was not happy thinking about it and I felt some anger come up in me, but then I reminded myself of the promise I made to myself before I started on this year's Thanksgiving cleaning. I was able to say to myself that it was more important that we take advantage of all possible resources than to get angry with my mother to the point that neither one of us would get the materials. That is what I meant earlier when I said "it works." Preparing myself in my mind for the situation really helped.

Couns: Congratulations, *you* made it work! You felt the pain over the lack of approval from your mother, but as you rose above the hurt, your thinking became logical and goal-directed. You were able to decide what would be in your best interest. A lot of strength and courage went into realizing and accepting the probability that your mother would be more likely to give the materials to Becky than to you. That kind of strength will serve you well. What a tremendous victory for you! Your mental preparation paid off. Can you think of additional ways to remind yourself to keep your goal-directed attitude in the face of painful situations?

Ruth: Yes, Becky and I talked about it. Whenever either one of us gets stuck in a situation, or does not know what to do next, we ask ourselves "What would our counselor say in this case?" Becky came up with the idea of a reminder for me. She is aware that I need help because of all my stored-up anger. Becky knows how to make braided buttons and matching pins as well as earrings. She is making a set for me and I am going to put the pin on whatever garment I wear when I go over to my mother's house.

	When I feel myself getting angry, I will look at my pin and remember what it stands for, the improvement of our lives.
Couns:	The two of you are amazing in how you have given directions to your life in such a short time. You make a great team. You seem to learn a lot from each other and with each other. You have truly started on your chosen path for improving your situation.
Becky:	Yes, we did and we had a great time with it. We went through the boxes of materials and discussed what we could do with them. We made some plans and worked on some designs. I had not realized what Ruth went through to get the remnants for us.
Ruth:	As you had suggested, we discussed in more detail some of our possible plans. Another, more selfish, thought came to my mind. Instead of grieving over not having been able to go to college, I could find out if I am intelligent enough to get in. With some of the money that I can save from the food packages, I could sign up for the test. I would not want my mother to know because she would just say that it is a waste of money. For that reason I may have to go to the next town to take the test if Becky drives me. When I mentioned it to Becky, she was all for it.
Becky:	I think it is important for Ruth to know if she could get into college. Perhaps there would be a way to obtain financial aid. If she can't get in, at least she would know once and for all and could turn her attention to other goals.
Couns:	You have a point, Becky. If Ruth could resolve her question of whether or not she can become accepted at a college, she would have another decision point to address.
Ruth:	After Becky and I discussed our plans, I did some research about colleges because if I take the test, they send my scores to one or two colleges for free, so I would need to apply to them. I found some college catalogues in the library. One school has a recently established scholarship for a single mother from our state who has the academic potential to better her own position in life and to work on improving the quality of family life in our state. The studies should lead toward a legal or political career or as a service provider in the field of family life.

Couns:	You sound excited about your research. The scholarship appears promising.
Ruth:	I am excited, but unfortunately, this college is at the other end of the state. I would not be able to commute, even if I had a car. Another interesting point is that the college started a pilot program for running a day-care center on campus. Students and staff are allowed to bring their children for daytime childcare. Staff members have to pay a fee, while students can use the service free of charge, but they have to work a certain number of hours per week in the childcare center to help with the children and to keep the costs down. It sounded like a real neat idea. I feel this would be tailor-made for me if I could get the scholarship. Without a scholarship, I could not even think of going to college. I know, there are loans available, but with two young children I could not go into debt for that much money. I took some books home from the library to brush up on my math. I am going to try my very best on the test.
Couns:	You have done your homework well and you seem determined to give it your best effort. Whatever the outcome, you will have more information about yourself and your capabilities. Obtaining that information takes great courage. In a way, it is like diving into a pool, not knowing whether the water will be warm or cold. Before we end for today, I would like to encourage you to continue with your planning as well as with your mental imagery and behavior rehearsal for difficult situations in the future. You have put your skills to good use already and there may be further opportunities for application.

Summary of Clients-Counselor Interaction: Revisited. The counselor observed the smiles on the clients' faces and opened the session with an encouragement for them to report on the reasons for their happy attitude. As Ruth described how she had prepared herself for working at her mother's house without the usual anger and resentment, the counselor took the opportunity to emphasize that it was Ruth's achievement to make the new approach work. It did not just happen; Ruth decided how she wanted to act. While praising her for assuming control in the situation, the counselor did not neglect to explore

Starting Along the Chosen Path

Ruth's feelings when she realized that her own mother would be kinder to Ruth's friend than to Ruth herself. Obviously, the acknowledgment caused her pain. Aware of the struggle within her, the counselor took great care to emphasize how Ruth had risen above her hurt and had grown so much stronger through the experience.

The counselor also applauded Ruth and Becky for the additional planning they had done toward implementing changes in their lives. Because Ruth's attempts at mental imagery as a tool for her attitude change had worked well for her, the counselor reminded and encouraged her to continue with the practice.

Case Study Follow-Up: Additional Unresolved Feelings

After the initial successes experienced by Becky and Ruth in their next session following the Thanksgiving holiday, Ruth appeared discouraged. The counselor began by acknowledging the non-verbally expressed affect.

Couns: I am glad to see you both and hear about your most recent experiences. Ruth, you look troubled. Did anything happen to disappoint you?

Becky: Yes, Ruth, you were so quiet on the way over here. I thought I might be talking too much.

Ruth: I had thought I was doing so well, preparing myself to face my mother and the holidays, especially after I did not let my anger interfere with getting the materials for us when I helped my mother with the cleaning. But on Thanksgiving Day itself I felt awful. All my good intentions and the imagery practice seemed to have left me.

Couns: Please, tell us what happened if you are ready to talk about it.

Ruth: Actually, it started out pretty good. I dressed up the children and put on my pin that Becky had made for me just in time. The children behaved well and my mother had no need to complain about them. As we finished the cooking, set the table, and got everything ready for the meal I was still in a good mood and felt confident that I would handle the situation as well as I had done with the house cleaning before. Then my mother told me to serve

	the food to everybody at the table. All of a sudden I felt this wave of really bad feelings come over me.
Couns:	How would you describe your feelings? Try to give them a name.
Ruth:	There was anger, I am able to recognize that feeling pretty well now; but there was something else. I think it was more like shame.
Couns:	You think it may have been a combination of anger and shame. Do you remember what you were thinking as you served the food?
Ruth:	My sister-in-law was holding up her plate requesting to exchange the piece of turkey I had given her. She complained that there was too much skin on it. She is pregnant with their third child, probably another boy, and she makes such a fuss over having the proper nutrition. She never helps much when she and my brother come over to my mother's house, but now that she is pregnant again, she just sits there.
Couns:	Is that what went through your mind, or can you remember any other thoughts?
Ruth:	Well, yes, that would just explain the anger part. There was more. I remember thinking that I don't amount to more than my mother's servant and I was worried that my daughter might be embarrassed for me.
Couns:	Those are painful thoughts, no wonder you felt bad. How would you describe your relationship to your sister-in-law?
Ruth:	We were never close. In school she always acted like she was somebody special. I did not pay much attention to her then, but when she married my brother I had to accept her as part of our family. My mother seems to be almost a bit intimidated by her, probably because her family is financially better off than our family.
Couns:	It sounds like there is quite a bit of tension between the two of you. Your sister-in-law constitutes a more or less permanent part of your environment, therefore, this would be a good area to practice your coping and imagery skills. What did you mean by your daughter might be embarrassed?
Ruth:	I wanted my daughter to grow up differently, with more options for her own life. I didn't want her to think she is less capable or less worthy than other children. But if she sees her mother being a servant in her grandmother's

	house instead of an equal to her brothers and their families, I wonder how that might affect her. I considered not taking her along anymore. She might be better off with Becky.
Becky:	We would be happy to have her with us but, Ruth, wouldn't she wonder why she can't be with her own family, her mother and brother?
Couns:	Considering the effects of your behaviors upon your children shows what a good mother you are, Ruth. Not taking your daughter to your mother's house on family holidays is an option to keep her from feeling bad about you. As Becky pointed out, your attempt to protect your daughter may backfire. She may misinterpret why she can't be with you. Perhaps you can turn this into a learning experience to show your daughter how important it is for her to work hard for her own independence by learning well in school and looking for small jobs she can do after school. She may also understand better why you are not using money saved from the food packages for little treats. In addition, your daughter may be able to help you in little ways at your mother's, or keep an eye on her brother. Seeing the visits at your mother's house as a team effort might serve to bond the three of you closer together. Becky's observation makes sense and shows a lot of insight and consideration for your and your daughter's feelings.
Ruth:	You are so right. Becky knows my daughter well; she would probably be hurt or confused if I left her behind on holidays. She is a sensitive child and she always wants to help. Letting her know the facts of our life may turn out to be a valuable learning experience. I better set myself down and write another script on how to interact with my sister-in-law. If I can do it with my mother, I can do it with other people. I need time to rehearse: Christmas is coming.
Becky:	What do you think of starting a new tradition? We will have a party after each of the holidays. I'll fix the food and little homemade treats. We will play games serving each other. We can draw lots who will serve whom. Serving can be fun among people who love one another.
Couns:	That's an excellent idea! Your children will learn that at times we do things because they are necessary. At other times, we can enjoy the same activities because we are

doing them with or for people we love. Again, the two of you have turned a painful situation into a successful learning experience. You both have so much going for yourselves and are working so diligently on improving the quality of your lives. It is a pleasure to observe your growth.

Summary of Clients-Counselor Interaction: Additional Unresolved Feelings. At the beginning of the session, the counselor noticed Ruth's sad affect and immediately directed the focus to the underlying circumstances. Even if the counselor has prepared an agenda for a particular session, clients' mental and emotional states take precedence and need to be attended to as soon as possible. As Ruth described what she had considered a setback, the counselor helped her to identify her feelings and connect them to what might have gone on in her mind at the time of her unpleasant emotions. Recognizing this client's tendency to easily get caught up in anger, the counselor redirected her attention to the other, less frequently experienced, emotion.

Responding to both clients at the same time, the therapist praised Ruth for her sensitivity to her daughter's feelings and Becky for her caring and insightful comments. Acknowledging the clients' resourcefulness and hard work that once again had helped them to succeed in converting a painful situation to an experience they could learn from, the counselor expressed the pleasure felt over the clients' continuing growth.

Unexpected Emotions Likely to Surface in Connection With Behavior Rehearsals

As seen in the above case study, feelings of guilt, shame, anger, or self-doubt are commonly expected to reappear, but, other less frequently expected emotions, such as anxiety and relief, are equally likely to surface in connection with imagery and behavior rehearsals.

Richard and Bernice Lazarus (1994) consider relief an emotion that does not need to be discussed in detail because it is associated with positive outcomes following an unpleasant situation. The authors consider relief to be an emotion with two stages, a negative and a positive one. An emotional situation starts with some type of distress and is thought to end with termination of the distress when the dreaded event does not materialize. On a personal level, according to the authors, relief signals to the person that everything is all right and that further coping with a threatening situation is no longer necessary. The main significance of relief is considered to be the fact that it occurs so frequently in people's lives and it sets the stage for coping behaviors to be initiated.

Thinking of relief as a simple emotion that does not need further attention appears to be a gross oversight when considering the role it seems to play in the development and, more importantly, the maintenance of phobias. A comparison of treatment outcomes in clients presenting with phobias and episodes of extreme anxiety failed to identify predicting variables. Criteria such as age of client, precipitating event, client's age at onset, or duration of illness did not appear to be predictor factors regarding positive or negative outcome of treatment or necessary duration of treatment (Maass, 1979). One predictor about improvement in the client's condition seemed to be related to the feelings that the client experienced immediately following termination of the feared situation. Whether termination of the threatening situation occurred after having lived through the situation, or simply through avoidance, did not seem to matter as much as did the experienced emotions.

Some clients reported feeling relieved after the feared experience and, as mentioned by Lazarus (1994), the greater the fear had been, the more intense was the feeling of relief. Other clients identified their responses as embarrassment, shame, or even guilt. Clients who felt relief in general had a more difficult time overcoming their strong fears than those who experienced embarrassment or shame. The experience of relief apparently worked to reinforce the clients' perception that there was something inherently dangerous or threatening in the situation. While the fear was not appropriate to the actual situation, it was appropriate to the clients' strong beliefs that they were indeed caught in a dangerous situation. In experiencing relief, the clients validated beliefs that were not appropriate to the real situation.

In addition, the intense feelings of relief have a rewarding effect, and after having so narrowly escaped the imagined disaster, individuals do not see any great need to take the essential step in the process of change: that of challenging their misperceptions and faulty beliefs. Strong avoidance tendencies usually continue.

Lazarus (1994) saw the main psychological interest of the relief dynamics in the period prior to the relief when the individual is trying to evaluate and cope with the anticipated danger, hoping that it will not actually occur. If the disaster does not strike, the felt relief will not only reinforce the original faulty perception of the situation, but also will validate importance of hope over actual coping behaviors. In the pursuit of treatment, the main psychological interest would be more beneficially directed toward the moment directly following the relief.

Case Study

Lynn: Fear of Going to Church

Lynn, a young divorced mother of two sons, believed that she had made an adequate adjustment to her recent divorce. After experiencing difficulties in continuing with her regular Sunday church attendance, she decided to seek professional help with the situation that she had tried to resolve unsuccessfully by herself.

Couns: You stated as your presenting problem attending church. What about going to church is difficult for you? Is this a difficulty of long standing?

Lynn: The whole idea of going to church suddenly frightens me. It started after my divorce. While preparing my sons and myself for church on Sunday, I started to feel anxious as if something awful was going to happen. My heart was racing, my hands became clammy with cold sweat, and I had difficulty breathing. My oldest son saw me tremble and asked me if I was sick. I thought that perhaps I was coming down with something, so we decided not to go to church. After a while I began to feel better. By that time it was too late to go to church, but we went over to my sister's family in the afternoon.

Couns: You were not really ill then? What happened the next Sunday?

Lynn: The same thing, I felt shaky and sweaty again. For a couple of weeks I made excuses that I was too busy to go to church and my sister took my sons with her. Finally, I decided I was not going to give into this weakness. I wanted to fight it, but it got worse. Even though I felt shaky again and close to suffocating or fainting, I forced myself to go to church. I decided to sit in the back, so people would not notice me. After the sermon was over, I quickly collected my sons from the children's group and went straight home.

Couns: How did you feel when you got to your car?

Lynn: I felt much better, like I could breathe again.

Couns: You felt better—in what way? Could you be more specific? If you had to name a feeling, what would it be?

Lynn: I would say it felt like relief, like my ordeal was finally over.

Couns: You used the word "ordeal"; that sounds pretty painful—almost like a threatening or even dangerous situation. Is that how you felt at the time?

Lynn: Yes; that's exactly it. I felt like I was in a very threatening situation and I was scared. How silly of me to feel scared in a church!

Couns: The church in itself probably did not arouse your fears. More likely you were afraid of what you thought would be the consequences of your being in that church at that time, just as a person who suffers from claustrophobia is not frightened by the small room itself, but by the visualization of the consequences of being trapped in the room. People are afraid of the consequences, such as being unable to get out, or not having enough air to breathe, and finally suffocating. In your case, where did the threat come from? Do you remember?

Lynn: I don't really want to think about it, it was too awful. I am getting to feel shaky again. Can't we quit instead of bringing up bad memories?

Couns: I realize this is very painful. You are in a safe place here. I will help you calm down. Please take a deep breath in, as deeply as you can. Now exhale slowly, slowly and hold your breath. We'll try to go for 10 seconds. Now inhale again deeply, exhale slowly, and hold again. Let's do it again, breathe in deeply, slowly exhale, and hold. Do you feel better now? You can learn to use this breathing exercise as one tool to help you cope with anxiety. You

	might want to do the breathing exercises for a longer time. About 10 minutes would be a good time, but sometimes it takes even longer, depending on the intensity of the anxiety. Do you think you could go on now with finding out where the threat or danger as you perceived the ordeal might have come from?
Lynn:	I'll try, I do feel a little bit better now. I felt that I would be exposed or accused of having committed a crime and everybody would point the finger at me.
Couns:	What crime did you think you had committed that would lead people to chastise you?
Lynn:	The thing that comes to mind is that I am depriving my sons of having their father living with us. Perhaps if I had tried harder, I could have prevented the divorce. Perhaps I was concerned too much with my own hurt feelings and not enough with my sons' happiness.
Couns:	From what you say I get the impression that you are blaming yourself for the break-up of the marriage. When you think back about your reasons for the divorce, how does that agree with what you just said?
Lynn:	It does not agree at all. When I filed for the divorce, I did not think there was any way to save the marriage. Actually, my husband did not really spend much time with the boys or with me. He came to church with us only occasionally and preferred to be with his girlfriend.
Couns:	When we look at what you are saying now, would that have led to your feelings of guilt and fear you described earlier?
Lynn:	No; that's a good question. Are you saying I had no reason to be afraid?
Couns:	I think your fear was probably warranted by something. It may not have been warranted by the actual situation, but your feelings of fear and anxiety were appropriate to your thoughts as you described them. Did anybody ever blame you for your sons' deprivation?
Lynn:	Nobody actually blamed me, but my sister has made some statements about how sad it is that my sons don't have a role model on a daily basis. She thinks that at their current ages they need a male role model for their mental and emotional development.
Couns:	Let's summarize the situation: When you went to church you felt uncomfortable or afraid because you thought that

	the people in the congregation would chastise you for being divorced. Your thought was mainly based on your interpretation of what your sister said, not on what the people in church actually did. Is that correct?
Lynn:	Yes, the way you describe it; that seems accurate.
Couns:	Now, let's look for a moment at the feelings you experienced when the situation was over and you were safely sitting in your car. Your feeling of relief again seemed to be logical or appropriate to your thoughts, based on your sister's statements rather than on the actual situation. But your relief may have confirmed your idea that this was indeed a dangerous situation. You may have felt that you just narrowly escaped a grave danger. By confirming the perceived dangerousness, your feeling of relief also reinforced your perception of danger and increased your fears and anxiety every time you considered approaching the situation again. Can you see how this circular action exacerbated your anxiety?
Lynn:	The way you describe it, it sounds all so logical, but also a bit ridiculous. I feel embarrassed to have scared myself silly over nothing.
Couns:	It is logical in a way because our feelings are logical to our thoughts, beliefs, and perceptions. There may be more factors contributing to your anxiety. So far, we have only focused on your thoughts generated by your interpretation of your sister's statements. Was there anything in the behavior of the people at church that may have strengthened your perception of danger?
Lynn:	I had not been consciously aware of it, but now that you mention it, at some time I remembered the people's reaction when a male member, a father of two little girls, became widowed. His wife had died of cancer and the whole congregation rallied to his side, especially the women. They all wanted to help and comfort him and invited him for dinner. I too felt sorry for him at the time. After my divorce, nobody seemed to want to comfort me. Do you think I interpreted that to mean they were against me? Just as I interpreted my sister's statements to mean that I had neglected my children's welfare?
Couns:	It is possible, but only you can answer this question by going back into your memory and exploring what your actual thoughts were at the time. If you can't clearly re-

	member, you can ask yourself "I felt and responded in the situation as if I thought what?" In fact, you seemed to have done that in a way when you asked your question.
Lynn:	What can I do to overcome this fear?
Couns:	First of all, you can practice the deep breathing exercises that I introduced you to earlier. I will give you a handout that describes the exercise in more detail. The next thing is to be willing to accept a bit of discomfort. By now you may have become afraid of becoming afraid of the feared situation. Then you can remind yourself that you have done the best you could regarding your marriage and divorce. It is highly unlikely that anyone in church will openly chastise you. You don't know what other people are thinking, but you can control your own thoughts. As you have used your fantasy skills to imagine the terrible things that might befall you in church, you can use those same imagery skills to keep yourself focused on reality and how to challenge your fear-producing thoughts. We can continue to work on this aspect at our next meeting.

Summary of Client-Counselor Interaction: Fear of Going to Church. In this first session the counselor expediently checked about the client's feelings following the end of the dreaded event in order to plan the approach for the remaining work. The counselor was cognizant of the fact that the client had attempted to fight her weakness by deliberately exposing herself to the uncomfortable situation. The fact that the client was not able to overcome her fear in this manner came as no surprise to the counselor. Although Implosion Therapy as developed by Stampfl (Rychlak, 1973) has been successful in some cases by immersing the client in the feared stimulus situation, experiencing the feared situation is not necessarily sufficient to eliminate the exaggerated fear or the powerful avoidance tendencies (Beck, 1976).

When the client started to feel anxious in the session, the therapist seized the opportunity to introduce a coping technique to be used immediately, such as the deep breathing exercises developed by Maxie Maultsby (1975). The therapist did not agree to let the client discontinue with the exploration. If the counselor had stopped with the exploration, the client's perception of having been in great danger at church would have been confirmed again. Instead, the counselor reassured the client that she was safe and would be helped. When the client had recovered sufficiently, the counselor directed the focus toward possible underlying thoughts or beliefs that may have contributed to the fear. Once some of the thoughts surfaced, the counselor helped the client question those thoughts as to their congruence with reality.

The counselor demonstrated how the client's feelings logically followed her thoughts; first when she anticipated the feared event, then being in the situation, and finally after she had emerged from the dreaded event. All the while, the client's feelings served to confirm her perceptions regarding the danger of the situation and strengthened her beliefs about it, thus reinforcing and intensifying the phobia.

As the client understood how the process worked, she expressed embarrassment. The counselor did not agree or disagree about the significance of the embarrassment at this time, but took it as a sign of progress, and decided to continue with the exploration of the client's perceptions to uncover additional fear-producing or fear-confirming aspects of the event.

Although the client's reactions of fear and anxiety appeared to be responses to an external stimulus situation—the church—the anxiety reaction follows an inner drama—the imagined devastating consequences of being trapped in the situation. Despite the fact that the client dreads the consequences rather than the situation itself, the client usually describes the discomfort in terms of the situation where the anxiety is experienced. Therapists may be misled by the client's statements; exploring in detail characteristics inherent in the situation, instead of tuning in to the drama transpiring in the client's fantasy (Maass, 1979).

Physiological or Psychological Cause. In the past, several investigators (Danaher & Thoresen, 1972; Davis, McLemore, & London, 1970; Rehm, 1973) have reported difficulties in attempting to correlate imagery and behavioral measures in systematic desensitization. The difficulties may have been based in part in the misinterpretation of the client's reports. According to cognitive (Schachter & Singer, 1962) and cognitive behavioral (Beck, 1976; Ellis, 1962) models, the client's images and covert verbalizations mediate emotional and physiological arousal. Beamish and coworkers (1996) in their literature review came to the conclusion that, according to cognitive theory, the catastrophic misinterpretation of the bodily sensations results in or escalates panic attacks. Krech, Crutchfield, and Livson (1969, p. 611) contrasted the Cannon-Bard theory—that the emotions and the body reactions occur simultaneously—with the James-Lange theory, that physiological changes precede the emotions and the perception of the bodily changes leads to the emotional feeling. Thus, the question remains: Does the individual's misinterpretation of the consequences of being in the situation lead to the physiological responses of anxiety, or does the misinterpretation of the physiological symptoms bring on the anxiety? From the senior writer's clinical experience, it appears that the cognitive assessment of the consequences of being in the situation leads to the physiological responses that, in turn, serve to reinforce or validate the experience of the perceived danger.

More recently, review of the literature has shown that the use of progressive relaxation as a specific technique has not been as effective as cognitive restructuring. Moreover, it is not as effective as combinations of cognitive-behavioral techniques (Beamish et al., 1996).

Helpful Techniques for the Attainment of Behavioral Changes

Behavioral changes do not occur automatically. The decision to adopt different behaviors in a given situation is usually made when the individual realizes that previously used activities have not brought the desired results. While progressing along the chosen path, the client has a choice between several techniques that can be used in planning and rehearsing new behavioral approaches. During the planning and rehearsing stages, the identified goal is ever present in the individual's mind as the different parts of the road map are being explored, considered, altered, defined, and adopted. Most situations involve interactions with others, and here the anticipation of their possible actions and responses constitutes another significant part of the process. Changed behaviors demonstrated by the client will most likely bring about changes in the responses of those around the client. As the client develops new behavioral plans, the responses of others need to be considered in the planning as best as can be anticipated by the client. The client's activities in the planning and rehearsing stage can be likened to that of a writer who is developing the script and then the actor who is delivering the script. Clients frequently argue against the use of behavioral scripts and rehearsals because they think that their actions should come about spontaneously. Not to diminish the importance of spontaneity, in important situations the value of preparation is often reflected in the outcome.

When Roberto Assagioli (1973) discussed his notion of the "skillful will," he described an interesting scenario between the will and other psychological forces, such as drives, emotions and imagination. If the will is in opposition to these strong psychological forces, it can be overpowered. People who conceive of will as a force may attempt to push themselves toward a designated goal. An example would be a person using all her willpower to remain compliant with a certain diet. In an emotionally charged situation that may give rise to feelings of sadness, disappointment, or depression, the person may convince herself that a piece of cake or a dish of ice cream would really help restore the emotional balance. After having indulged in consumption of the dessert, the person typically would chastise herself for being weak and having no willpower at all and possibly abandon the use of will in the future. A more effective way of using the will is to develop a strategy where the will can stimulate and direct the other psychological forces toward the goal. The skillful will functions in combination with, rather than in opposition to, the other psychological forces.

The skillful will can be a useful concept when planning, programming, and executing important actions. In combination with imaging and rehearsing techniques, it constitutes a powerful and effective strategy for preparation in decision-making and for successful behavior patterns in general.

Case Study

Kent: Preparation for Family Conference

The widowed father of two children, encountered in Chapter 4, contacted the counselor again. He had run into an obstruction in proceeding along his chosen path.

Couns: How have you done with your family since we last met?
Kent: Actually, we are all doing quite well. I accepted my employ-

er's offer to work part-time at home. Usually, the children and I leave home together. When they go to school, I go to the office and do my work there. With this schedule, we can all have breakfast together and discuss what needs to be done that afternoon or evening. I think it is important to start the day together. At first the children wanted to run off without breakfast, and it took me a while to convince them of the benefits of having this opportunity to check out the rest of the day while at the same time having a nourishing meal.

Couns: You are taking your responsibilities as a parent very seriously. Your children are in good hands.

Kent: I am glad you said that. It goes right to my reason for being here today. When I thought I did not need to give specific reasons for my decision to stay in the city with the children, I had underestimated my mother-in-law. She has not accepted the fact that I am raising the children here by myself. She has used my son's initial disappointment about not returning to our hometown to influence her husband and her brother and his family. She even enlisted the help of my mother who had stayed with us for a short time. My mother is not against our living here, but she said we should at least discuss the situation with the whole family. Before I was aware of what my mother-in-law had been up to, I had agreed to go back home with my children to spend the Christmas holidays there. The publishing company is traditionally closed between Christmas and New Year's and so are the schools. Taking the children back to spend some time with their grandparents seemed like a good idea, but now my mother-in-law has planned this big family conference to discuss my children's welfare. I know, legally she cannot take the children away from me unless there is neglect on my part. I could cancel our visit, but that would look like I am afraid of my parents-in law. They are still my children's grandparents, and my children are entitled to a good relationship with them.

Couns: As we had just mentioned, you are a very conscientious parent and neglect would certainly not be an issue that your mother-in-law could use. You are also right in considering the importance of your children's relationship with their grandparents. Are you planning to participate in the

	family conference, or is there a way to convince your mother-in-law individually not to push the issue? I remember you had some hesitation in making it known that your wife had been pregnant prior to your wedding.
Kent:	I am glad you remember that, so I don't have to go into all the details now. What you said in the past about sex education made a lot of sense to me. I have talked some with the children about it and also mentioned the possibility of seeing a sex educator if they wanted to. They responded favorably to the whole issue and we are going to proceed with further explorations as needed. If my mother-in-law persists discussing Marilyn's pregnancy in front of the whole family, I will use the concept of sex education as an argument and I will also tell my children about their mother's condition before the rest of the family finds out. Even if I can convince my mother-in-law not to bring up the pregnancy issue to discredit me, there will still be some type of family conference because she has already announced it.
Couns:	You have done a lot of thinking about the family conference and you seem ready to stand your ground. Is there any way you can prepare yourself?
Kent:	That's why I am here. I thought it would be a good idea to prepare myself and, hopefully, you would be my mentor.
Couns:	It seems there are two possible paths for the situation: If you can convince your mother-in-law to be considerate of her daughter's image, then the encounter with the whole family will likely be less emotionally charged and you can give them your reasons for staying here. If she is willing to have the whole background disclosed, the situation can become much more tense and volatile. This situation would require a more intense type of preparation. Of course, the first encounter with your mother-in-law in this matter can also be expected to be volatile. In summary, within the two possible paths, you have three different interactions to consider.
Kent:	That's true, I had not really sorted it out as clearly as you just did. The other day I found the lists of pros and cons that you had assigned me to do regarding my decision of where to live at the time. I think the lists will be quite helpful now because they are still valid in how they led me to the decision I made then and would make again.

Couns: Great! With that past homework assignment you are now a step ahead in the current process of preparing yourself. You have a lot to do between now and Christmas. How do you want to approach the preparation now that you have a rough outline of the different possibilities?

Kent: As I remember, in the past I did not do well when I neglected to consider my feelings. I want to make sure that I consider not only my own feelings, but those of the other family members.

Couns: You have learned well from your past experience and you will be doing well considering the feelings of others as they impact the discussion and resulting decisions. The most difficult and most important interaction will probably with your mother-in-law. Usually people who want to prepare themselves for such an event find it beneficial to work on a script. The script would focus on what and how they want to communicate to make their points. Then, if at all possible, it helps to be able to predict the responses of the other person or persons. If we also know from experience how they would most likely respond emotionally, we could use that to refrain in our own expressions from using statements that will trigger unwanted emotions in the other person. For instance, many people are more difficult to interact with if they feel attacked or accused. Instead of listening to an otherwise sound argument, they will direct all their energies to defend themselves and to show that the perceived accuser is wrong.

Kent: That makes a lot of sense. I never thought about it in that way. Writing those scripts will take a lot of time, but I can see where it may work.

Couns: Another important aspect is to keep track of your own emotions as they become part of your communications and as they may arise in you from the other persons' responses. In your scripts, you may want to include statements to yourself as to how you want to feel during the interactions and then rehearse the scripts out loud, to see what feelings are elicited in you. We don't always know how another person will respond, but the more we know about the person, the better we are able to guess or predict. Sometimes it is helpful to go back in your memory and look at past interactions that the person may have had with you or with others as you witnessed.

Kent:	This sounds like writing a play. How elaborate do I have to be?
Couns:	As much as you think the situation warrants. Yes, it is like writing a play and in addition to being the playwright, you are also the actor and director. You can use your imagery skills to find out how comfortable you are with your scripts. Then you can continue to rehearse and see yourself in the actual situation behaving and feeling the way you want to. Most likely, the more you rehearse and imagine yourself in the situation, the more comfortable you will feel. Repeated practice may actually make your muscles move to express your learned behaviors as if the behaviors had been a natural part of your behavioral repertoire all along.
Kent:	I never thought of myself as an actor, let alone a director, but the writing part should come a little easier for me. I can't help but think this is faking it or, even worse, am I playing with peoples' minds and feelings?
Couns:	That is a good question and I am glad you brought it up. On the surface one could certainly consider the kind of preparation you are planning as an act of manipulation. You are not doing this to gain an unfair advantage. As you said, legally you are entitled to make decisions about your living arrangements and those of your children. I understand that your purpose for this event is to communicate the reasons for your decisions in such a way that the bonds between your children and their mother's family will remain intact and healthy. Furthermore, if indeed you come to the conclusion that your chosen behavior or communication pattern is generally effective, you may want to incorporate it into other parts of your life. Rather than playing with peoples' minds, it becomes a learning experience, resulting in some lasting cognitive as well as behavioral changes.
Kent:	I see, you mean it would become a permanent part of my overall life, not just something to gain an advantage for the moment. I like that aspect.
Couns:	Yes, I am glad you understand this process to be more than superficial manipulation of others. If you want to start working on your scripts, we can go over them at our next appointment.
Kent:	I can see I will be busy. I am almost getting excited about

being able to direct the interactions rather than just to respond to them helplessly. Oh, I thought you might be interested to know that I am not worrying anymore about what I would have done if Marilyn had lived a few minutes longer. I think it's more important to focus on what I do with our future lives.

Couns: Thank you for telling me about it. You sound like you have reached a point of peaceful acceptance of what happened in the past.

Summary of Client-Counselor Interaction: Preparation for Family Conference. During his return visit to counseling, the client demonstrated that the past sessions had been helpful to him in making his decisions and that he had gained more awareness and understanding about the importance of his feelings. The counselor acknowledged the client's good work in taking on the responsibilities of a primary parent to his children. The acknowledgment served as a smooth transition to the client's current concerns. In exploring the parameters of the current problem situation, the therapist facilitated the formation of an action plan for the client. As the upcoming meeting with the family was an important event in the client's mind, the therapist encouraged him to prepare himself for it as best as he could. Emphasis was placed on the significance of considering the other persons' emotions and their influence on the direction of the communication. Detailed instructions on writing scripts, being aware of surfacing feelings, and using imaging skills for behavior rehearsals completed the initial phase of the preparatory process.

Ethical Concerns. The therapist responded in detail to the client's concerns regarding the ethical basis for his plans, pointing out that the client mainly wanted to communicate his side of the issue in such a way that it would not endanger his children's relationship with their grandparents. The considered preparation process was not merely an instance of play-acting, but an opportunity for additional learning.

SUMMARY

Once a given aspect of the client's life has been agreed upon for problem resolution, the time has come to outline the various steps leading to the defined goal. In this phase, necessary skills and techniques are explored and undiscovered hurdles may surface.

In the case of Ruth and Becky, the clients had made good progress toward their goals. Ruth, in particular, had been pleased with the success of her preparation for difficult situations until unresolved emotions interfered with her planned behaviors.

Other opportunities for unresolved emotions to appear are during the practice of imagery and mental rehearsal. As clients experience the emotions, their immediate exploration will often lead to uncovering of the underlying reasons, as demonstrated in the case of Lynn.

Finally, a major portion of this counseling phase is devoted to introducing skills and techniques that can be applied in the attainment of desired outcomes. The case of Kent is a good example here.

EXERCISES

The reader is encouraged to think of a past experience that resulted in mental or emotional discomfort. If the situation were to recur, how would imagery and mental rehearsal techniques be helpful? What script would the reader write for him or herself? What other unresolved feelings may surface? What signals may they reflect?

SUGGESTED READING

Ellis, A. (1962). *Reason and emotion in psychotherapy.* New York: Lyle Stuart. (Revised 1994 edition; New York: Birch Lane Press.)
  The book is a comprehensive work on the theory and practice of REBT. The revised edition describes its differences from other psychotherapeutic approaches.
Lazarus, R. S., & Lazarus, B. N. (1994). *Passion and reason: Making sense of our emotions.* New York: Oxford University Press.
  The authors explain how emotions are aroused and maintained, and how they impact our perceptions of ourselves and our environment.
Maultsby, M. C., Jr. (1975). *Help yourself to happiness.* Boston: Esplanade Books, Marlborough House.
  The author demonstrates how emotions work and how to make desirable emotional changes by practicing rational self-analysis.

8

Reevaluating Progress

OBJECTIVES

1. To provide an opportunity for clients to express their overall satisfaction with progress.
2. To explore changes in clients' functioning regarding gains or losses experienced through counseling.
3. To reinforce clients' efforts and application for new learning.
4. To increase awareness of clients' potential for competence and independence.
5. To uncover possible additional stumbling blocks, such as conflicting values.
6. To emphasize the importance for repeated application of newly learned skills.

REEVALUATING

Clinicians decide upon and implement clients' chosen treatment strategies that they believe will be appropriate and effective for the clients' circumstances. Clinicians also would want to find out how close the actual treatment results are to their expectations. If the treatment did not produce the desired impact on the client's condition, decisions on whether to discontinue treatment or employ different strategies are indicated (Barrios, 1988).

In addition, most professionals in the helping disciplines are faced with the public's increasing expectations for accountability of practitioners' treatment approaches and the need for development of standards of care and assessment procedures. Among the most frequently considered measures of quality in client care are client satisfaction and treatment outcomes (Steenbarger & Smith, 1996). A basic underlying element to treatment outcome is the idea of change. It is assumed that clients' level of functioning will show beneficial changes as the result of interaction with the counselor (Lambert, Ogles, & Masters, 1992).

TREATMENT OUTCOME CRITERIA: CLIENT SATISFACTION, CLIENT CHANGE

Various instruments to assess satisfaction and outcomes have been developed over time, but the measurement of therapy or counseling outcomes is a complex task that has not yielded to simple dissection (Schacht & Henry, 1992). The difficulties inherent in therapy outcome research are reflected in a comment addressing Seligman's 1995 analysis of a *Consumer Reports* study of psychotherapy effectiveness and the flaws observed in the analysis (see Brock, Green, & Reich, 1998). That is, regardless of the complexity and difficulties connected with evaluating counseling or therapy processes, successful outcomes for clients involved in the process are not only the goals of the therapist, but the assumption and expectations of the general public. To meet the goals and expectations, standards of care are based on various factors. One of the factors will most likely be the structure of the counseling process itself (Granello & Witmer, 1998).

Evaluation as Integral Part of the Counseling Process

Independent of, but congruent with, the developments surrounding the quality-of-care issue, therapists are well advised to incorporate a phase of reevaluation into the overall therapy process. The planned check on progress made so far affords a better understanding of the client's abilities and gives an opportunity for encouragement to continue with the work. Even if there have been setbacks or a success smaller than desired, exploration of underlying reasons is important. At the same time, the benefits of considering smaller successes as building blocks for greater future achievements can be emphasized.

Case Study

Becky and Ruth: Two for the Price of One Reevaluation

The two young single mothers encountered in previous chapters appeared ready for a closer look at the gains or losses experienced in counseling up to the present. The current session reflects a reevaluation of their progress.

Couns: Both of you have worked efficiently on modifying some of your attitudes and your outlook on the future. How would you describe what you learned so far?

Ruth: For me, the most surprising part is that even when a situation appears hopeless, there can still be choices if we look deep enough. Nothing in our situation has really changed dramatically from when we first came to see you.

Couns: You are absolutely correct, Ruth; your and Betty's circumstances have not changed at all. Whatever paths you embark upon from here for a resolution of your problems have been with you all along. Being so firmly engrossed in a situation often does not afford us an accurate view of the overall circumstances. By coming here you have been able to step outside a bit and turn yourselves into more objective observers.

Becky: I was just thinking about that yesterday. Any change would be easier to see in Ruth's case because she may actually leave town and start over in a different place. With me, on the outside it does not look much different. I will be staying here at least for now and will continue to live with my in-laws. My resources are much the same as before. The scraps of materials and yarns, the skills my grandmother taught me, and my imagination or talents are the same, but my focus is different. Before I made little things to make our immediate surroundings more cheerful. As I ran out of places to put little doilies, my imagination seemed to have turned inward and shriveled up until I was not doing much beyond mending and making clothes for my daughter and myself because we needed them. When I made the pin and buttons for Ruth to remind her of her goals when working for her mother, I realized I was in need of reminders myself.

Couns: Both of you have made extremely important discoveries when you became aware that you had skills and tools for change within yourselves. You were not necessarily dependent on changes from the outside. Becky, you seem to be saying that as you saturated your immediate environment with your talents, you actually stunted further growth of them because you did not see an opening beyond your home and your town. Now you are directing your talents beyond daily needs and you are looking to the outside world as a possible marketplace for your creations.

Becky: That is so true. My first step outside was to look at bookstores on college campuses to get an idea what students would like. I have made a few things, such as book covers, bookmarks, pillows, and even a few T-shirts. The camera my grandmother gave me at my daughter's birth is coming in handy now. In addition to recording my daughter's development on film, I am taking pictures of my products to make kind of a portfolio that I can show to prospective buyers.

Couns: That is a great initiative! In addition to finding out that most solutions to our problems are available within us, what other discoveries did you make so far?

Ruth: My biggest discovery was how much my anger really paralyzed me. Looking back now, it seems that the anger was so overpowering, I could not think of much else. When you told us that anger is closely associated with helplessness, that really hit me! I hate feeling helpless. Somehow the anger seemed to emphasize the helplessness, building up even more anger and finally, when I felt worn out physically and mentally, I was ready to give up and feel hopeless.

Couns: You described the anger cycles very well, Ruth. Anger is a very powerful emotion and can take a lot of energy out of us. The sooner we are able to recognize it, the better off we are. We don't want to push anger out of our awareness as some people do by denying its existence within them. To regard anger as a signal that things are not the way we want them to be can be a tremendous asset in developing plans for action. Just as you did with your imagery and behavior rehearsals, preparing yourself for doing the cleaning, cooking and serving for your mother on holidays, you recognized the anger you still felt toward

Becky: your sister-in-law. Usually anger is more pervasive than we realize. Feelings of anger are not confined to just one or two people or situations in our lives. Anger has a way of spreading as our overall dissatisfaction increases. Becky, is there anything you would like to add?

Becky: I noticed that my in-laws are treating me differently ever since I decided to put more pleasure into our lives. The other day my mother-in-law said that I didn't have to ask permission to use the car unless I want to be gone for most of the day or two. She wanted me to feel more independent and she added that the way I take care of them and the house is much more valuable than the room and board for my daughter and myself. Without us their life would have been very sad and lonely after their son's death. She wanted me to consider the house our home and told me that she and her husband had made changes in their wills. All their belongings are to come to me and my daughter, even if I were to remarry. My mother-in-law also admitted that she had been aware of my husband's drinking and that she had been afraid that I would leave him. As a favor, she asked me not to discuss Greg's drinking with his father because his father could not bear hearing anything bad about his only son. I feel a lot closer to my mother-in-law now. I think she is trying to be a real mother to me, something that I appreciate, especially after my grandmother's death.

Couns: Both of you have made significant gains since we started working together. You have taken the initiative to put into practice what you learned. If you like the results you have achieved so far, you may want to think of other areas where you can apply your new way of thinking. The more you practice your new skills, the faster they become habits that will feel familiar and comfortable to you.

Summary of Client-Counselor Interaction: Reevaluation. At the opportune time, the counselor invited the clients to take stock of the results their efforts had brought them so far. Although nothing basic had been added to their original circumstances, options had emerged or been brought into their awareness. The fact that the clients realized that the options had all been within their domains was praised and emphasized by the counselor to strengthen the connection between the clients' initiatives and the results. While underlining the clients' increasing independence, the focus on their discovery also served to build up their self-confidence. Another important facet emphasized by the counselor was that continued practice would be beneficial in turning new skills into elements of well-established behavioral repertoires. Additional practice would also come from applying new learning to other life situations, as was pointed out by the counselor in a transitional step to the next counseling phase.

The skillful therapist will make the most use of the reevaluation phase by reinforcing the clients' new learning and coping skills, as well as their attempts at gaining self-confidence and independence. Minor setbacks can be used to point out what part of the strategy worked while directing the focus to other aspects that may need more practice. By the time clients enter into the reevaluation phase, most of them will have had ample opportunity to become aware of, challenge or dispute, and replace self-defeating beliefs with more effective and self-enhancing beliefs.

Procedures for Reevaluating. The processes of disputing clients' self-defeating or irrational beliefs are considered a main element of the Rational-Emotive Therapy process. Extensive disputation strategies for challenging beliefs have been described by Kopec, Beal, and DiGiuseppe (1994). The disputing or challenging activity may involve up to 90% of the therapeutic process. It is not sufficient to demonstrate to the client that a given belief is dysfunctional and that as long as the client holds on to the self-defeating belief, the client will experience negative emotional and behavioral consequences and negative outcomes. The existence and availability of a more effective alternative presents another requirement for the client's successful relinquishing of a faulty belief.

Another process of reevaluation can be considered to occur when clients renew their contacts with the counselor some time after having left the therapy process. The reasons for reentering counseling can be of a wide variety. Previous problems may not have been resolved as completely as believed, or new problem areas may have arisen. Whatever the reason, the client's returning to the previous therapist constitutes an act of evaluation of the client's past experience. In general, it can be assumed that the client's return reflects a level of satisfaction with earlier work.

Case Study

Bill: Reluctant Divorcé

Bill had first sought counseling when his marriage had deteriorated to the point where his wife insisted on a divorce. His request of the counselor was to help him get his wife back. As described in an earlier chapter, the request was ill-fated.

Couns:	It has been a long time since we last met. I assume that you adjusted somewhat to your divorce. How are your sons doing? I remember you were quite concerned about having to leave them.
Bill:	A lot has happened since then. When I first saw you, you helped me sort out things. I did not want to accept the possibility of a divorce then, but you helped me realize that the marriage had not been as good as I had wanted to believe. Now I am at another point where sorting out is needed.
Couns:	I am glad that you think we can face another hurdle together. Please fill me in on some of the events that you consider necessary for me to know before we go on.
Bill:	As you may remember, at the time of the separation and through the divorce I was living with my parents. Of course, that was only a temporary situation. I knew they were ready to retire to a warmer climate. Before deciding on where to live, I had a lot of thinking to do and I did not know what my financial circumstances would be. As I wrote down some of the needs and wants for my new situation, I came to the conclusion that I did not want to travel that far to my job each day. My job was my stability and security and I like my boss and the people I work with.
Couns:	I remember how satisfied and secure you felt with your work and the people you work with. Your job was a point of stability during all the turmoil you went through.
Bill:	I don't know what I would have done without my work. Finally, I made the decision not to return to the small town where my sons were still living. The decision was difficult to make because I wanted to be close to my sons. I looked around in the area where my sister is living with

her family. They live in a very nice, stable neighborhood on the south side of town. With my sons visiting every other weekend, I knew they did not want to spend all their time with me, but needed companionship with children their own age. My sister's children are about the same ages as my sons. Also, if I could find a home closer to my sister, we could help each other out, taking care of our children. She and her husband need time to themselves to keep their marriage alive. What I learned the hard way, I can use to protect her from having similar experiences.

My sister kept her eyes open for me. A small, two-bedroom house with a family room and a nice yard became available. It meant that my sons had to share a bedroom during their visits, but with the child support I had to pay, I could not afford a larger house. The family room was a bonus because it could double as a bedroom for my sister's children when I kept them overnight.

Couns: You have done a lot of exploring options and have selected a workable solution for your situation. Your efforts in planning have paid off. How do your sons like your new home?

Bill: After they got over the initial shock that I was not going to return to our little town, they seemed to enjoy the new neighborhood and especially the company of their cousins. That part worked out well, but Linda, my ex-wife, ran into some trouble. The young man she had met at the restaurant seemed to get tired of the fact that Linda had our two sons to take care of and could not get out as often in the evenings as she did when I was still living with her. He did not want to spend his time in the house with Linda and the boys. He also thought getting a babysitter was Linda's responsibility, not his. She asked me for more money, but I did not think that was justified and refused to pay more. Apparently, arguments with the young man became more frequent, leading Linda to become depressed. One evening after a particularly nasty argument she made a suicide attempt by taking an overdose of the medication prescribed for her by her family physician. While Linda was in the hospital, I took care of the boys until her discharge. Fortunately, it was during the boys' summer vacation, so I didn't have to worry about

	getting them to school. My sister helped me a lot during that time.
Couns:	Your careful planning certainly showed the benefits that you had considered from the beginning, although for different reasons. How is Linda now, has she recovered?
Bill:	That brings me to the reason for my being here today. After her suicide attempt Linda's lover ended the relationship. He was not willing to burden his life with such complications. Linda's depression increased and, unknown to me, she had started to abuse alcohol. After a while Linda approached me for reconciliation of our relationship. I almost called you then. Less than a year ago, I thought that was what I wanted most, but now I did not feel right in going back. I remembered the rating scales you had me complete when I first came to you. I still have them and I looked at them again and realized that we could not pick up where we had left off. The marriage had deteriorated too much for that.
Couns:	Your past efforts paid off. You had gained more knowledge about yourself and the marriage that helped you with the current decision.
Bill:	I am glad to have worked through that before Linda's offer. I did suggest she seek counseling to help her over the disappointment with her lover and to find a future for herself. When I mentioned your name she became upset because, as she said, you made it too easy for me to get over the divorce. I thought that was a rather strange remark, but I did not press her. Perhaps I should have.
Couns:	Are you blaming yourself for something that happened to Linda?
Bill:	Maybe I am and I hope you will help me with resolving that if I need it. As I said, I didn't know Linda was drinking too much. She continued to work in the restaurant on the weekends I had the boys, but could not work as many evenings as before when I was there to supervise them. The boys complained that Linda was moody and irritable. They wanted to spend more time with me. Because the court order gave me visitation rights for every other weekend and some holidays, I did not think I could do anything to change that. Well, to make a long story short: Linda's drinking increased, she had a couple of court-ordered inpatient treatments due to driving while under the influ-

	ence, and another suicide attempt. My attorney recommended that I sue for full custody of our sons because, as he said, two suicide attempts render Linda automatically an unfit mother. In addition, he mentioned that Linda's parents could request custody for their grandsons. If they were successful, the children would be moved out of state. I don't know if my attorney is correct, but I also don't want to involve my sons in a court battle.
Couns:	What an unhappy development for you and your family. Your reluctance to have your sons subjected to the legal hassles is certainly understandable. Your attorney is the legal expert and you trusted him before when you engaged his services for the divorce. Do you have any reason to change your mind about him? If so, you could probably obtain additional information from your local bar association.
Bill:	I trust him; he has been quite open and straightforward during the divorce proceedings.
Couns:	Has your lawyer advised you as to what might happen if you don't sue for full custody and leave everything as is?
Bill:	Yes, he said it would not look good for me if I did not do anything about my sons because I know about Linda's problems. According to him, there is a good chance that Linda's parents will sue for custody to protect Linda and if I haven't done anything about the situation before that, the judge may hold it against me, interpreting my lack of action as lack of interest in my children's well-being.
Couns:	I think your concern about your children has been well documented, but if it comes to a legal matter, your attorney is the one to listen to. I am certainly glad you have someone you trust. Let's look at the reasons for your reluctance to go to court. One reason you already mentioned is to protect your sons from legal procedures, such as painful court hearings. Are there any other reasons for your hesitance?
Bill:	Trying to take the children away from Linda may really push her over the edge. The children are all she has left after a failed marriage and being deserted by her lover. Also, how would I be able to take care of the boys full-time without giving up my job?
Couns:	Let's look at one issue at a time. Are you concerned that Linda would attempt to kill herself again and this time would succeed?

Bill: Yes, and it would be my fault. If I had not rejected her attempts at reconciliation, she might never have tried it in the first place. I could have saved her and the children from that.

Couns: Do you believe that if Linda committed suicide, it would be your fault?

Bill: It would seem that way, everybody would think so.

Couns: To your knowledge, is Linda still abusing alcohol? And if she is, is that your fault too?

Bill: Yes, she is still drinking. That's why my attorney recommended that I take action. But I don't think I caused her drinking. She did that when things with her lover went sour.

Couns: Didn't you tell me that Linda's first suicide attempt occurred while she was still in the relationship with this young man, quite some time before she wanted you to come back again?

Bill: Oh, okay. She did swallow those pills after an argument with him. She may have tried to scare him into coming back to her. But she tried again later after he had already left her.

Couns: If you believe that you are to blame if Linda makes another suicide attempt, what do you see as the basis for the belief?

Bill: She was not happy with our marriage. I neglected her by working so hard.

Couns: Perhaps so, but did she try to kill herself then because of her unhappiness?

Bill: No, she found another way to be happy without me. But when you get married don't you take on responsibility for that other person?

Couns: In some ways we do, but it depends a lot on the individuals within that marriage. Did they get married because they thought they could not live without the other person, or did they get married because they wanted to share part of their lives with the other?

Bill: I am not sure I understand what you mean by that. When we are in love, don't we usually think we cannot live without the other person?

Couns: Dependency is a concept with a wide range. Persons with various degrees of dependency needs fall all along the continuum. Some people feel safer with an extreme degree of dependency, where they do not engage in any activity without the other person by their side. Others can live very well by themselves and have many activities that they enjoy individually in addition to the activities enjoyed by both. Although they know they can live independently, they have decided to share their lives with another person. In a relationship like that, both contribute and the lives of both are enriched. Their living together is more like a privilege that they earn than a need to be fulfilled in order to make it through life. The danger with extreme dependency is that feelings of love can change into fear and resentment, as relationships change from a partnership of equals to that of master and slave connection.

Bill: Some of what you are saying seems to apply to me in the past. Although I was the one who went to work every day to make a living for the family, when Linda told me about divorcing me, I was scared. I didn't think I could go on without her. Looking back on it and being honest, it was not all love that made me feel so desperate then. Probably, my love for my sons was stronger than my love for Linda. I am shocked and a bit ashamed to admit that.

Couns: Those are natural reactions to what you discovered about yourself. Please remember that your fear was temporary and that you learned to become independent and self-sufficient again emotionally as well as financially. How does our discussion tie in with the belief that you are to blame if Linda makes another suicide attempt and that you can prevent it by going back to her?

Bill: Looking at relationships, the way you just described it, is scary. Believing that I can prevent Linda's suicide attempts would place the responsibility for her whole life on my shoulders. How can anybody work all day and worry about his wife's suicide all day? I know, I am exaggerating, but it feels like I would be the slave afraid to make a mistake. Suicide attempts could be the whip to keep me in line. I would not like to live that way!

Couns: We have had a long session today and have done a lot of work. As you continue to think about the different aspects of the belief we discussed, I would like you to spend additional time on considering consequences that would most likely result if you acted on that belief. You have already mentioned one, but I would like you to include your sons in the scenario and how their lives may be affected. This can be your homework for the next session.

Summary of Client-Counselor Interaction: Reluctant Divorcé. The client who had been seen previously in connection with his upcoming divorce returned to counseling as new developments required significant decisions impacting on his life and those of his sons. The counselor acknowledged the client's success in structuring his living situation following the divorce. After the client had given an account of the events that had transpired in his life since his latest counseling session, the counselor was careful to explore the client's feelings with him, especially as they related to the described events.

When one of the client's self-defeating beliefs surfaced, the counselor guided the client toward exploration for the basis of the particular belief. Additional feelings surfaced, and the counselor reassured the client about the naturalness of his emotions. The counselor's educational attempt to discuss relationships served to validate the client's emotions and to lead him to consider consequences of acting on his belief. Knowing that the client after the session would be concerned again about the fate of his sons, the counselor included the likely consequences affecting the sons in the homework assignment for the client. Throughout the session, the counselor was cognizant of the legal implications of the client's current circumstances, and repeatedly encouraged the client to follow his attorney's recommendations because the client seemed to trust his attorney's advice. The counselor carefully avoided involvement in an interaction that the counselor is not qualified for, namely giving legal advice.

Reevaluation by Previous Clients. Clients who return to counseling after having worked on some problems in the past can be seen as initiating the reevaluation process. In many cases, clients have experienced some degree of success in their areas of concern, and may be in a plateau phase where they feel capable of handling their circumstances more or less independently. The reason for returning may be that a new problem area has developed or that the client decided to continue and bring the previous solution to a more elegant completion. Smaller successes are often encouraging in working toward even bigger accomplishments. In the rare case where the client up to that point has not experienced any success as a consequence of counseling, explorations similar to those used in the phase of "identifying what does not work" can be employed to uncover some as yet hidden stumbling blocks. Such persistent stumbling blocks strongly indicate the presence of firmly held beliefs that have not yielded to the challenging process.

Case Study

Earl: Conflicting Values

Earl, who was first introduced in Chapter 6, had not been ready to involve himself in counseling on a regular basis beyond the requirements of the Child Protective Services involving the custody and care for his two daughters. Several months had gone by when he called in for another appointment.

Couns: The last time I saw you, you and your daughters had started in family counseling, as recommended by the Child Protective Service because of the possibility of child sexual abuse by your ex-wife's boyfriend. I hope that the counseling was helpful. Are your daughters still living with you?

Earl: You have a good memory. Yes, my girls are still with me. The counseling was really more for my daughters than for me, and they have adjusted well to that painful event. Today, I came back for myself, although when I first came to you, it wasn't really much help. The situation with my wife had already deteriorated too far, and divorce seemed to be the only solution.

Couns: Yes, I remember you thought your wife had been involved in an extramarital affair and you could not forgive her for that. Have you changed your mind about that?

Earl: No, I still feel the same way about LaTonya. But I wonder if I missed some things you tried to tell me then.

Couns: Perhaps we can relate to that when you tell me what is troubling you now.

Earl: At the time when I had to take full custody of my daughters, I had just met another woman whom I really liked. She had been divorced some time ago and was still quite hesitant about dating. Taking care of my two daughters

	in addition to a full-time job did not leave me much time for dating, but I really liked her. I had told her that I had undergone a vasectomy recently. On her birthday I took her out to a nice restaurant and we had a wonderful evening that ended with a bit of champagne in her place. Thinking that I had a vasectomy, she did not use any birth control methods. I had forgotten to tell her that my urologist had not cleared me yet. I still had to submit another sample. When Lucille told me about being pregnant she was quite upset. She wanted to discuss the possibility of having an abortion. I told her that was a crime. Preventing conception is one thing, but once a child is conceived, abortion would be murder. I could not agree to that and told her we would get married as soon as possible. My daughters would probably be happy about the baby.
Couns:	I can imagine that was quite a shock, but you did not seem to be extremely disturbed over the prospect of getting married and having another child. How did Lucille respond?
Earl:	She accused me of deception regarding the status of my vasectomy and that I did not consider her feelings at all. But I stood my grounds on rejecting an abortion. In a way, I didn't think it would be bad to have a new family and have her by my side through the bond of the baby. My daughters would profit by having female influence and monitoring in the house.
Couns:	You have very strong beliefs that seem to guide your actions as you have shown in the past. Did Lucille agree to the marriage?
Earl:	No, she has refused to see me. She wrote me a note, saying that she could not imagine herself living with someone who was so judgmental and would not consider anybody else's opinion. She also asked me not to contact her again. I tried to call her at work but was told she had taken a leave of absence for family reasons. They did not tell me where she is. I am afraid she went somewhere all by herself to have an abortion.
Couns:	How do you feel about her actions?
Earl:	I still feel abortion is wrong and I am angry at her for doing it. But I also feel sad about her going off all by herself to do this. I feel guilty as if I had deserted her,

	even though she is the one who left me. What she said in her note made me think. I always thought I knew what's right and what's wrong, and I have tried to live accordingly. How come things have worked out so badly for me? I lost my wife, one of my daughters was abused, and now I have lost another chance for happiness.
Couns:	As you said, you follow your principles on what is right or wrong and that gives you certain strength. How do you handle interactions with others when their ideas are different from yours?
Earl:	That's their business. I don't interfere with their beliefs and they better stay out of mine!
Couns:	Sometimes family members do not hold all the same beliefs. When you got married, did you discuss your beliefs and values with your bride?
Earl:	Some of them I did, but not everything in detail. I figured we had the same outlook on life. We seemed to agree on most important issues.
Couns:	Often, when we are convinced that we are right, we don't consider other viewpoints—it does not seem necessary. Yet we do not live in a vacuum, and those around us and important to us may feel differently at times. During our rather brief relationship, you have voiced several strong beliefs that I can remember. Infidelity is the end of a marriage; children belong with their mother, no matter what; abortion is a crime. It seems those three beliefs had some connection to the events that went wrong in your life, as you mentioned earlier today.
Earl:	Are you saying I should not have divorced my wife when she had an affair with another man? Perhaps I should have had an affair with another woman. Then we would have been even.
Couns:	I am not really talking about affairs. I did not even know about the overall status of your marriage and what led your wife to have an affair. You didn't talk much about your marriage. It seems to me your mind was made up the first time we met.
Earl:	That is true, and that's why I did not come back. Everything was decided and I did not see any need to talk more about the situation, although I wished I could have done something to prevent what happened to my children.
Couns:	You could not foresee what would happen. Perhaps it

would have been beneficial then to think more about your wife's involvement with the other man, such as what was the relationship between them, how they treated each other, and what was she looking for in him. At the time all that was very painful for you, and it is understandable that you did not want to involve yourself deeper in it. Apparently, the other man was not a good influence on your wife, and although she was a very good mother in your opinion, she was not able to completely protect the children. Human relationships are very complex and, at times, the best we can do is to learn from past experiences. In retrospect, is there anything you would like to have done differently in the most recent situation with your lady-friend?

Earl: I would have married her, as I told her, but she would not even listen to me.

Couns: As you said, she felt you had not been completely honest with her. Perhaps she was not sure whether you wanted to marry her for herself as a person, or because she was pregnant with your child.

Earl: I thought her being pregnant would make her want to marry me and everything would work out for the best.

Couns: What do you think her beliefs and values regarding marriage and family life may be?

Earl: I don't really know. She never talked much about it. She should have believed me when I told her we would be happy with a baby. Children are a blessing, I know that from raising my daughters. She should have trusted me and my knowledge about children. I guess, she did not love me enough to trust me.

Couns: It seems you did not really have sufficient time to know each other well enough for such a commitment as marriage, and the pregnancy forced you to make a decision prematurely. Where do you want to go from here?

Earl: I thought you could help me convince her that I am a good person. She won't talk to me, but if you wrote her a letter on my behalf, she might be more inclined to listen to me. Although I don't know where she is, I am sure mail will be forwarded to her from her old address. Seeing my name on the envelope, may lead her to throw it away without reading, but with your name on it she would at least open it.

Couns: I don't think I have the right to approach the young woman. Except for people who are ordered by the court system to engage in counseling, the therapeutic relationship is strictly based on voluntary participation. If at some time Lucille would be willing to come in with you or by herself, I would be glad to help you both sort out your feelings and make decisions that are beneficial to both of you. Besides, have you come to a conclusion on how to deal with the issue of an abortion, if she had one already, as you seem to think?

Earl: You are right, I would have to consider that before getting back together with her again. Also, there is still the trust issue. I don't know if I can forgive her for that. Perhaps I need a lot more time to think.

Couns: Significant decisions, such as the ones that have come your way recently, deserve in-depth considerations. As you said, there is a lot to think about and if I can be of help in the process, please don't hesitate to contact me.

Summary of Client-Counselor Interaction: Conflicting Values. The case study above is not representative of the usual process of reevaluating gains or losses experienced during a therapeutic relationship. The client had never engaged in counseling or therapy on a regular basis. His sporadic visits were prompted by situational factors, mostly when his beliefs collided with those of others in his environment, causing him temporary discomfort. In the past, the counselor had unsuccessfully attempted to encourage exploration of how the client's beliefs may have impeded his decision-making skills. The most recent efforts were equally futile. Although the counselor repeatedly invited the client to participate in such explorations, the client's focus remained directed toward what had happened to him instead of what he could have done differently. The counselor realized that the client was not ready to make the shift from seeing himself as a victim of circumstances and of the actions of others to being a participant in the events that occurred in his life.

Need for Therapeutic Alliance. Perhaps a more confrontational counseling approach would have been successful in this case. In this counselor's opinion, the therapeutic alliance necessary to entertain thoughts for even the mildest confrontation had not yet been formed, due to the sporadic nature of the client's attendance. Also, the counselor soon recognized that the client had come to the session with his own agenda. Normally, having an agenda can be seen as a good attempt by the client to take the initiative for what occurs in the session. In Earl's case, the agenda contained a manipulative aspect. For ethical reasons, the counselor could not participate in the client's agenda.

In the end, not much change could be recorded as result of counseling. Earl's belief system was still as intact as it had been at his first visit, but the counselor kept the door open. If the counselor had been more confronting, would Earl have been amenable to becoming more flexible in his beliefs? Perhaps he would have, and then, again, he might not have been ready for any change, and also would not have come back to counseling at a later time. He had returned to the same counselor twice after his initial visit; therefore, the possibility for future contacts seems reasonably good.

SUMMARY

Structuring a point of reevaluation into the counseling process serves many purposes. For the counseling profession, it is a reminder for accountability of our services. Have standards of care, as much as they are available, been followed? What is the client's level of satisfaction? Has change occurred in the client's coping or overall functioning?

Inviting the client to take stock of gains or losses encountered through the counseling process helps to define and emphasize the rewards of the client's work. Any gains can be used as encouragement to continue with the growth process, either in the same problem area or through application to other aspects in the client's life. Minimal gains or losses, in turn, can be used to explore the existence of hidden stumbling blocks. After resolution or removal of the stumbling blocks, work can resume with increased understanding of the significance of uncovering such hurdles.

Returning clients who were seen in counseling previously, but who discontinued for one reason or another, constitute a point of reevaluation that we normally do not think of in those terms. At least, as far as client satisfaction is concerned, the client's return to counseling can be interpreted as a positive action. Perhaps the client was pleased with the results achieved through previous work or, if the results were not as desired, the client felt comfortable enough within the therapeutic relationship to address other issues.

Although reevaluation is treated here as a discrete phase within the counseling process, as with all other phases in the hands of the skilled therapist, reevaluation will work as a smooth transition to the next phase: that of generalizing learning on to other life situations.

EXERCISES

Remember a program of goal-directed activities. After achieving or not achieving the goal, did you reevaluate your actions up to that point? In retrospect, what would you have done differently? Did you learn from the experience and continue toward the goal or did you give up the pursuit? What emotions were you aware of at the point of your reevaluation? In case you have difficulties remembering such a process, you can use last semester's course work as an example. What were your goals for that semester in terms of grades and/or learning? Did you achieve them? Was your studying approach effective? What would you change if anything? What were your feelings when you received your grades?

SUGGESTED READING

Granello, P. F., & Witmer, J. M. (1998). Standards of care: Potential implications for the counseling profession. *Journal of Counseling & Development, 76,* 371–380.
   Standards of care are discussed within the context of ethical principles, credentialing, managed care, and cost-effectiveness, issues that currently have a significant impact on the counseling profession.
Kopec, A. M., Beal, D., & DiGuiseppe, R. (1994). Training in RET: Disputational strategies. *Journal of Rational-Emotive & Cognitive-Behavior Therapy, 12,* 47–59.
   The authors describe a training exercise for skill development in cognitive disputation.

9

Generalizing Learning Onto Other Situations

OBJECTIVES

1. To reinforce previous learning.
2. To transform strategies and coping skills into stable entities in the client's repertoire.
3. To reinforce initiative and enhance the client's independence.
4. To provide the client with a general concept of learned resourcefulness.
5. To facilitate pervasive growth of skills to the enhancement of the client's overall style of life.
6. To facilitate transition to the next phase.

GENERALIZING LEARNING

As clients have emerged successfully from the reevaluation phase, they may feel encouraged to apply their new skills to different aspects of their lives. Through repeated applications of learning, the content of the lessons, as well as the behavioral expressions, becomes firmly rooted in the person's cognitive, emotive, and behavioral systems. Moreover, with additional practice, desired responses become better defined and readily available to the person.

Albert Ellis (1996), in promoting Rational Emotive Behavior Therapy (REBT) as one of the main humanistic psychotherapies, emphasized that individuals are viewed as holistic and goal-directed, having the ability to create and direct their own destinies. Cognitive-behavior therapies are not only accepting of humans as they are, but beyond that are also enhancing opportunities for significant changes in peoples' personalities if they so desire. Personalities are viewed as ongoing and changing processes, rather than stable and static entities. Therapy is a vehicle to help people live happier, more self-actualizing, and creative lives.

Behavior vs. Conduct

Bakan (1995) has emphasized the distinction between behavior and conduct. For those outside the behavioral sciences, the term "behavioral" is generally understood in terms of conduct, rather than as the narrow type of behaviors elicited in Pavlov's well-known conditioning experiments with dogs. Human conduct is mainly derived from decisions and plans people make and the goals they set. Certainly, when we as clinicians involve ourselves with personality aspects, the term "conduct" is more meaningful than "behavior." Understanding our clients' conduct requires knowledge of the clients' wishes and goals, as well as of their individual decision-making processes. To know the individual, it is necessary to know how the individual perceives the meaning and purpose of life as applied to that particular individual. In exploring the individual's perception of the meaning of life, we will learn to know the person's thinking, feeling, and acting—the person's lifestyle (Adler, 1933). Adlerian counselors believe that the key components in the therapeutic process are understanding clients' lifestyles and assisting clients to become aware of their own lifestyles (Ashby, Kottman, & Rice, 1998).

Generalizing Learning and Its Effects on Personality

The phase of generalizing learning provides excellent opportunities for the client to explore various personality aspects and make choices about emphasizing some and reducing or modifying others in the pursuit of a creative and fulfilled life. From resolution of isolated problem areas, the move is toward additional problem-solving activities and integration into the client's personality or style of life. Achieving desired changes may not be that difficult for a while, but maintaining the change requires intensive work over and over again (Ellis, 1988). Generalization consisting of repeated participation in the different counseling phases, and awareness of the lessons learned in each phase is the means for achieving pervasive and lasting changes in the individual's way of living.

Case Study

Bill: Too Many Problems

Bill, in his most recent session, had attempted to resolve his feelings of guilt regarding his ex-wife's suicide attempts and to decide whether or not to gain full custody of his sons. His homework assignment had been to consider the consequences, if he acted on his belief that prevention of his ex-wife's suicide attempts was his responsibility.

Couns:	How did you do with your homework assignment? Did it help you to resolve your feelings?
Bill:	I tried to do it, but I did not get very far. Too many things have been happening. I feel just like I did the first time that I came to see you. Where to begin? What problem to work on first?
Couns:	You sound frantic. Can you tell me what happened in addition to your attorney's recommendation that you file for full custody of your sons?
Bill:	That is not even a question anymore. I think I have to go ahead with the custody. Linda had a serious relapse. She probably had been drinking all along, but trying to keep it under some control. Last weekend was not my visitation time. On Saturday night my older son spent the night at a friend's house. Linda and my younger son were alone in the house. He woke up from a bad dream and tried to have his mother comfort him. When he went into her bedroom, he found her lying on the floor out cold. Naturally, he got scared and called 911 and after that he called me. Of course, I drove right over, but the ambulance arrived long before I did. You can imagine the rest. They took Linda to the hospital and later to another

treatment center. I stayed in the house until the next morning when my older son returned from his friend's house. After breakfast the boys and I went to my house to pack some clothes and other things I needed to live with the boys in Linda's apartment. I can't take them back to my house, even though that would be more comfortable for me, but they have to go to school. I have to drive the long way back and forth to work again, plus I had to find someone that the boys could stay with until I come back.

My sister has been really helpful to me. Several days she just packed up her own children and drove to Linda's place to stay with the boys after school. After I got there from work, she had to face the long drive back to town with her own children. Eventually she found one of Linda's neighbors who was willing to have my sons at her house after school, but only for a couple of weeks. I don't know what I would have done without my sister.

Couns: I can see that you would be distraught at this turn of events. You seem to be in control of the situation relatively well, and can take credit for that. Of course, your good relationship with your sister helped a lot. You did well in getting closer to her and helping her in the past when you were able to. But, as you said, it is a temporary solution. If you are awarded full custody, are you planning to move back to the town you lived in before, with your family?

Bill: I don't really want to do that. My attorney filed an emergency petition for immediate custody. So I am responsible for the boys on a full-time basis. I need my job and I can't see how I can spend so much time driving every day and still do all the maintenance work for the three of us. During the weekend visitations, I got some idea what it takes to be a full-time parent. But then my sister's family was close by and it was only on weekends, except for the whole month in the summer when I had the boys living with me. I took quite a bit of vacation time then. I don't know any other man who has full custody for his children.

Couns: You apparently already decided about the custody issue. Actually, you are a member of a rapidly growing group. The number of father-only families has tripled since 1974. Do you expect Linda to give you difficulties with that?

Bill: Not really. We talked about her going away for a longer treatment period. I took the boys to visit her. That was

	hard for her, but I think it is important that they see their mother, and I know she misses them terribly. She was talking about giving up her apartment and putting her things in storage for a while. She is ashamed to return to town. By now, everybody knows about her drinking problem. We discussed that it would probably be better for the boys if they moved in with me and went to school in my area. Changing schools in the middle of the school year will not be easy for them, but hearing the other kids talk about their mother's drinking problem will be very painful, too. Linda thought she might want to move a bit closer to where I live after release from treatment.
Couns:	What are your feelings about Linda now?
Bill:	I feel sorry for her. Looking back on our lives, it is so sad how everything ended up. Some of it is my fault, but I don't think I can go back to her; too much has happened.
Couns:	You have taken control in very responsible ways, and you have come to a resolution about your feelings for Linda. What other problems were you referring to?
Bill:	My mother has been concerned about my living by myself. My parents are of the old-fashioned type. My father was always the breadwinner and my mother was at home, raising us and taking care of all the chores. My mother thinks I need a wife. She introduced me to a daughter of a friend of hers. I liked her right away, but she is a widow with four children. You would never guess that she has four children, she is so tiny and as cute as a button. I have dated her for a while, usually on the weekends when I did not have my sons. I like being with her.
Couns:	You sound like you are having some conflicts in regard to the young woman. You like her and you like being with her, but something is holding you back. Does it have to do with her children?
Bill:	Yes, at first I thought it was because it did not feel right being with her and her children when I could not be with mine.
Couns:	In a way, the presence of her children could have made you miss your own sons even more. That could have amplified your feelings of loss. But you seem to have some other thoughts about the children.
Bill:	Cindy, that's her name, is younger than I am and her children are quite a bit younger than my boys are. I don't

	know that I want to start raising another family again at my age. Also, four children cost a lot of money, and even though her husband had made some provisions before his death and Cindy is working part-time, it still worries me. Her youngest one is a boy and he seems somewhat slow. I think there were some difficulties at his birth. My thoughts don't make me feel proud. If I really love her, it should not matter.
Couns:	Your concerns are certainly realistic. It takes a lot of energy and money to raise six children, counting your own two. Considering your reservations before making a commitment seems more responsible than rushing into a relationship, believing love will conquer all, only to regret it later when it becomes more difficult to correct your actions. You mentioned earlier that you met Cindy through your mother. How is your mother's opinion affecting your thoughts?
Bill:	That's another tough part of the situation. My mother thinks Cindy would be a perfect wife for me. Having four children of her own that she is raising very well would also make her a good mother for my sons. As much as I like her, I should not have dated Cindy. I was lonely and I did not know how to date again. I guess I was afraid; it's been such a long time since I was out on the dating scene.
Couns:	Many people who have been widowed or divorced after some years of marriage share your concerns about dating again. They are afraid they won't know what to say or do. Times and customs may have changed a bit. Perhaps a good way to approach dating is the way you feel comfortable in the situation, rather than to worry about what others expect of you. Is there anything to be lost by being open about it? We can talk more about dating later on. It seems to me that you are more immediately concerned about Cindy and your mother. There is nothing much you can do about what you said you shouldn't have done. The fact that your mother and her friend are involved in some way makes the situation more difficult for you. As you said, you felt lonely, and probably did not consider the consequences of what would happen if the relationship did not work out. Now is the time to resolve the conflict. Have you thought about how to handle the two situations?

Bill: I thought I should resolve my feelings about Cindy first before I even approach my mother. But I wanted to check with you, because I remember I was on the wrong track when I first came to see you. As a matter of fact, I thought about those rating scales you gave me to fill out about my marriage. At the time, they helped me to realize that the marriage was not as good as I had wanted to believe. Seeing my own marks on those scales helped me confront my unrealistic wishes. When I moved from my parents' house into my own place I lost those scales. Can you give me another set to work on?

Couns: You seem to be on the right track. Your situation may have been easier if you had not been involved with Cindy, but your idea about making a decision regarding Cindy before even talking to your mother makes sense. Your priorities are in the right order. You learned from the past how important that is. In addition to the rating scales about your relationship with Cindy, I think, we may develop one for the different aspects you are going to face as a single father. You already had some experience living alone with your sons, so you have a basis for assessing the difficulties associated with your new lifestyle. There may be an interface between the two parts you are working on right now. As you pointed out, after you have decided on your relationship with Cindy, how to communicate that decision to your mother will be the next step. The situation you are facing is far from easy, but you have made good use of your past learning. I am confident you will handle the new developments in a way that is congruent with your values.

Summary of Client-Counselor Interaction: Too Many Problems. The client had recently returned to counseling in order to work on making a decision about custody for his sons. Although that issue was resolved by circumstances beyond his control, other problems emerged affecting his life as a single parent. Initially, the client stated that he did not know where to begin, but he used his previous experience about prioritizing efforts. The counselor acknowledged the client's past learning and his good attempts at establishing the order in which the new issues needed to be addressed.

The client expressed some regret over having started to date the daughter of his mother's friend. The counselor, while agreeing with the client, also reassured him that his concerns and worries had been realistic under the circumstances, and were shared by others in similar situations. Instead of spending time in discussing whether or not the client should have done what he obviously already did, the counselor directed the focus on taking immediate steps to resolve the conflict. While outlining some of the future steps with the client, the counselor expressed confidence in the client's abilities to handle the current circumstances in an efficient manner.

Case Study Follow-Up: Additional Decisions to Make

For his next session, Bill had completed the Intrapersonal Growth Scales (IGS) reflecting his current single situation (see Figure 9.1).

Couns: I see; you have done your homework. Let's look at the scales representing your living arrangement with your sons first. You seem to see significant difficulties there. You also marked Parents, Work, and Vacations relatively high. That is surprising, because you have had opportunities to spend time with your sons on at least one vacation since the divorce, as well as your weekends. I assume that the areas with the blank scales do not represent problem areas for you. You rated the Meal area about two-thirds toward the problematic range. Your ratings on Hobbies and Money are also relatively high. The scale pertaining to Sex and Marriage is even more problematic now than before. Let's explore some of the reasons for these ratings as we go along.

Bill: The school is still an unknown factor. I imagine there will be some hassles getting my sons enrolled in a different school in the middle of the school year, and they may have some problems in adjusting to that. Their cousins are attending the same school, and that will be of some help. Coping with all the chores will be tough at first, mainly because of time. I may be able to get help from a cleaning service once a week or every other week for the big cleanings. The rest of the time all of us have to learn to pick up after ourselves. Grocery shopping may be prob-

Generalizing Learning

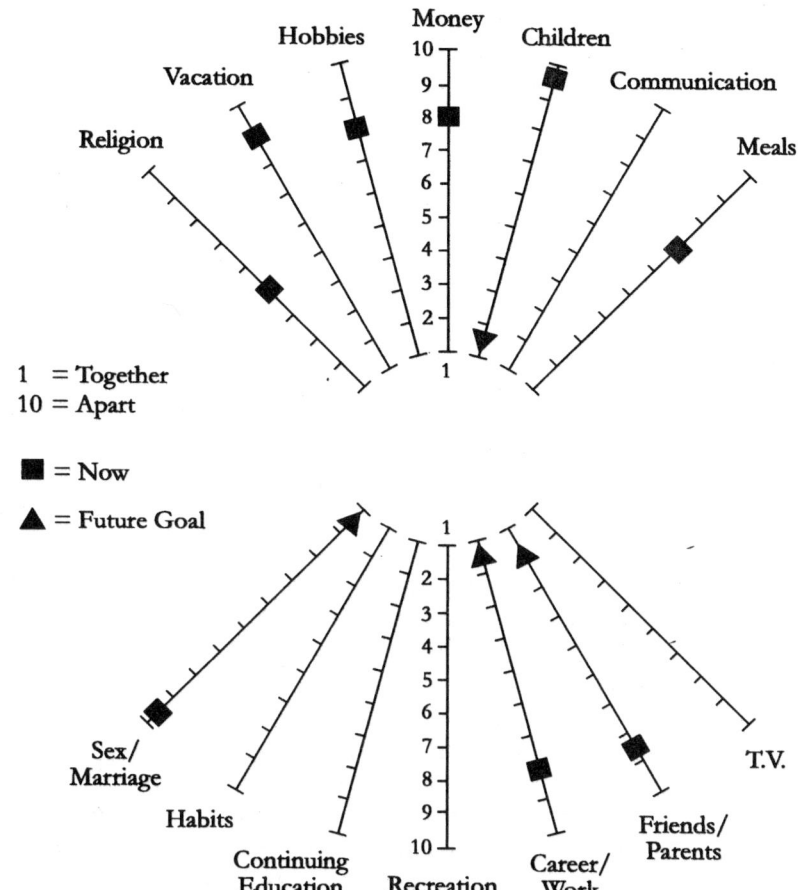

FIGURE 9.1 Ratings from Bill's Intrapersonal Growth Scale (IGS).

lematic. I don't want to take the boys away from doing their homework in the evenings by taking them shopping with me. I thought we could do that as a family on Saturdays and if need be, I could find some time during my lunch hour to do some shopping.

Couns: What a great job you did, thinking about the daily necessities and coming up with very reasonable solutions. What are your concerns with meals?

Bill: I know how to fix some simple foods and I got some recipes from my sister. I had been concerned about providing well-balanced nutritious meals. You hear more and more about the importance of balanced meals, and I have no idea about that whole area. Before I got full custody for my sons, I had enrolled in a cooking class one evening a week. The pressure was not as great, and I thought I could learn some important facts, get some tips on how to look for the best groceries, and have some time to experiment with the cooking itself. The class is much more fun than I thought. I expected to be the only man in the class, but to my surprise, there are three other men and about five or six women. In addition to learning new things, I get a lot of enjoyment being in the class and trying out new recipes. Being with a group like that is a whole new experience for me. As an adult I never had much time to make friends, because of my work and spending my time driving and being with my family. The last couple of weeks I had to miss the class because I had to go back to Linda's apartment after work. I hope I can return to the class once we are all settled in. Right now is a busy time at work, and with all the other unexpected responsibilities I am a little bit concerned about the effects on my work.

Couns: That explains your high rating on the Work area and the rating on the Meal area. Your attempts at gaining knowledge on a topic that will be so important to you as a single parent sound great. You recognized your responsibility as a parent and decided to learn more on the subject of nutrition. The social element of participating is also very important. As you already stated, you enjoyed the company of your classmates. The way you described your experience sounds like you are participating in an adventure, and get to use a sense of creativity that you did not know you had. I sincerely hope you will be able to continue with the class.

Bill: What you just said is so true. So far, I haven't told anybody how I feel about my cooking class, because I thought it sounded foolish. There is something creative about it when a dish turns out the way it is supposed to or when I know that the ingredients are healthy. There is also certain camaraderie in the class when one of us reports

Generalizing Learning

a near-disaster. The rest of us understand because it happens to all of us sooner or later.

Couns: I can't think of a more rewarding experience than what you just described. You are enriching your life as you reach out for new adventures. Let's look now at your ratings on the scale reflecting your concerns about your romantic relationship. Is there any connection to your ratings on the areas of Vacation, Hobbies, and Money? Are they all inter-related?

Bill: Yes, they are in my mind, at least. Actually, I should have added another area, that of Housing, to the scales. With six children, there will be less time and money to spend on recreation activities. Vacations may be fun, but I can't even imagine how we can handle that. Perhaps I am too cautious on that subject. The Hobby area is my own selfish pursuit of new activities, like the cooking class. With taking care of six children, will there be time for such pursuits? Also, Cindy is a good cook, and she may see it as criticism or invasion of her domain if I involve myself more in it.

Couns: You are making a good point; considering Cindy's feelings on that topic is important. With your sensitivity to her feelings, you may be able to work through that point if needed. What are your concerns about the housing situation?

Bill: By far, the biggest difficulty will be in an area I had not even been aware of prior to completing the scales. In the back of my mind I remember Cindy mentioning that no matter what, she would not move out of her house. It is a big, comfortable house with enough space for her children and another bedroom for visiting relatives. The basement could be converted into a family room, making space for another bedroom out of the current family room. She has a nice yard and likes the neighborhood. There are special services available for her youngest son. Also, it is close to her part-time job. At the time, it sounded logical and reasonable for her circumstances. When I thought about it now, it occurred to me that if we got married, she would probably expect me and my sons to move in with her. You may think this is selfish, but I like where I live now. I like being closer to my sister and her family. My sons took the news about being transferred to another school a lot better than I had expected. They seem to like

	being closer to family and I think they like our little house; it's familiar to them by now. After all they went through, I don't want to have to tell them about yet another school, another neighborhood, and another family.
Couns:	Of course, it is your right to decide where you want to live. You have been the stable influence in your sons' life and you are doing well, considering the effect your relationship with Cindy may have on their lives. So far they seem to have adapted well and you are probably right, having extended family nearby is another stabilizing factor. You are placing a high priority on your sons' well-being. How are your personal feelings for Cindy affected?
Bill:	I haven't talked to her about any commitments yet. Perhaps there will be another opportunity to find out about the seriousness of her decision not to move, but I don't want her to think that I am testing her—although, in a way, I guess, I am.
Couns:	You sound ambivalent and that is natural. There are many aspects that you like about this young woman. If you had to make a decision right now—what would it be?
Bill:	Right now, I would say "no." Something is going on in me. I don't know what to call it. Maybe you can help me figure it out.
Couns:	In connection with what you told me earlier—how you feel about your cooking class and the people in it—I would almost guess that you are seeing a new path for your life, different from the past. Perhaps other worlds are opening up, and you want to see what may be there for you.
Bill:	Yeah! Even with the increased responsibilities I have now as a single parent, I feel younger, more curious about things. The other day we went to the library to get library cards, so the boys can get books they want to read. I saw some cookbooks that looked interesting. They have storytelling programs for children on Saturdays. I did not dare ask if adults could attend too. How many years has it been since I was in a library? I can't remember. The librarian was very nice, telling us about all the services they provide for the community. She mentioned an amateur photography club that meets there once a month and I remembered that one of the men in my cooking class belongs

Couns: to a photography club. I wonder if it's the same; I have to ask him. I am rambling and I may not make sense, but the way you talked about worlds opening up, that's how I feel, like there is a door and I could open it. If I make a commitment to Cindy, I am afraid that the door will not be there for me.

Couns: You are describing a different outlook on life. Yours and Cindy's children still could be stimuli to open the doors, but as you know from your own past experiences, when so much time and energy is spent on matters of just plain survival, not much is left for developing other interests. You have worked hard today to face difficult decisions and to learn and understand more about yourself as a person. I would say that in itself is an exciting adventure.

Summary of Client-Counselor Interaction: Additional Decisions to Make. As the client had completed his homework assignment, the counselor made the decision to discuss the client's living arrangement with his sons first. The other major issue, the relationship with the young woman, could be expected to require more time, because of the client's emotional ambivalence connected with the issue. As the counselor mentioned, the client had become a member of rapidly growing father-only families (Meyer & Garasky, 1993) and had been very realistic in the appraisal of his future life as primary parent to his sons. The counselor expressed appropriate reinforcement for the client's acceptance of responsibility.

When the discussion shifted to the client's romantic relationship, the smooth transition made it easy for the client to mention his most pressing concern. Although the client expressed embarrassment about some of his feelings, he nevertheless felt comfortable enough to talk about them. The client's ability to express himself openly is a direct reflection of the counselor's skills in providing a safe, non-judgmental atmosphere. As the counselor clarified and validated the client's feelings, the client felt accepted, understood, and encouraged to explore parts of his personality that he had not been aware of until then. An important aspect to note is that the counselor did not make a predictive statement regarding the future of the client's romantic relationship, but instead referred to the client's own past experiences when mentioning the toll that survival efforts can exert on the development of creative interests.

As clients attempt to increase the range of application of their newly learned problem-solving skills, the focus may be on various areas of the overall counseling process. Bill, the client discussed above, remembered that in the past he had difficulties addressing the most significant problem area. Now he wanted to avoid repeating his earlier error. He found himself rewarded for his prior learning when the counselor confirmed that the client's order of priority of problems to be addressed was logical and efficient.

Other clients may return to the same therapeutic relationship when their problem-solving attempts yielded the desired results. They may want to apply similar strategies to other parts of their lifestyles in long-range planning for the future.

Case Study

Betty: Long-Range Planning

Betty, the suddenly widowed mother of three who was encountered in Chapters 5 and 6, returned to counseling. She wanted to increase her decision-making skills and apply them to long-range plans for the future.

Betty: Due to the choices I made when I first came here, our immediate situation is relatively stable. As you know, there were financial setbacks, but by holding firmly on to the decisions I had made, I was able to protect the rest of my property. Finally, even Tracy had to accept and live by my rules. Although I did not like having to make those decisions by myself, I learned that I had to be firm over time and stick to my decisions to make them work. Now that our life is going a bit more smoothly, I wondered about other options I may still have for myself. Eventually, I would like to get married again, but there is nobody waiting for me and I am not ready for anybody yet. I need to forge my own life first.

Couns: The results of your decision-making seem to have encouraged you to look for other options. I remember your struggle with some of those harsh-appearing decisions. Through the struggle you have become stronger and more

	courageous. What options are you considering now?
Betty:	I have lived here all my married life. It was a good life. I have many friends, a nice house, a steady job, but I feel like I am a remnant of my past. Perhaps it is because I am living in the suburbs, but it's also the climate. I want something different for the future.
Couns:	You sound restless and eager to close a chapter of your life. What options have you considered so far?
Betty:	My son Jeff is about to graduate from high school. He is excited about having been accepted by the second college of his choice. So, coming fall, he will move to a Southwestern state to start college. I have always liked that part of the country. One of my favorite cousins lives in the state with his family. On my visits there I became attracted to their lifestyle. As you had taught me in therapy, we do have options, but there are also consequences. Although I would not necessarily want to move to the location of Jeff's college, as long as I establish residence in the state, I would not have to pay the out-of-state tuition for Jeff after a year of moving there. Of course, the move would cost quite a bit of money, but I think the savings on the tuition would offset the moving expenses. One of the main factors would be what kind of a job would I be able to find? My cousin seems to think that there are good possibilities for me. Tracy is old enough, she could either move with me, or stay here. My main consideration is Lisa. She is going to start in high school next fall. She would have to get used to a new school environment anyway. Even though many of her classmates would also make the transition to high school, it is a much larger school, and their connections will be looser.
Couns:	Besides your cousin, nobody knows about your plans yet?
Betty:	That's right, even my cousin thinks I am just toying with the idea. I think he wants to encourage me to move, because he is sending me newspaper advertising and real estate brochures. I wanted to discuss my options and wishes with someone who knows me but who is objective. You have helped me so much in the past, so I came back to sort out things again with your help.
Couns:	I am glad our past work was helpful to you in your struggles to cope with the responsibilities resulting from your sudden widowhood. You certainly put your learning to good

use. The way I remember you talked about your daughter Lisa was that she was a shy little girl and did not complain much when the two older children were more resistant and challenged your authority. In fact, you seemed to think Lisa was internalizing her fears or unhappiness. I remember there was a time she did not eat much and complained of stomach pains. If you ask her about the move, she may tell you what she thinks you would like to hear.

Betty: How can you remember all those details? It makes me feel that you have been part of our lives all along. You are right, Lisa would not tell me her true feelings if I asked her directly. Thinking about that and learning from the past, I have contemplated two different plans. I increased my options. During spring break we will all visit my cousin and his family. Jeff will go to the town where his college is located and look at places to stay; possibly he will get into the dormitories. I encouraged Tracy to go with him to help him with house-hunting. Partly, I am hoping she might become interested again in going back to college, and partly, I want to be alone with Lisa during this visit. I want to observe her reactions to the area and the lifestyle. Lisa seemed to get along well with my cousin's daughter who is roughly the same age. Perhaps while we are there I can ask a few questions without letting her know what I am up to. Do you think that would be dishonest?

Couns: You are acting in her best interest. I think it shows a lot of caring on your part to make sure you know what Lisa would like. Sending Tracy with Jeff to the college town sounds like a marvelous idea. You will have more time to observe Lisa and, as you said, Tracy may benefit in other ways. You have done a fantastic job with your planning. I can hardly wait to hear about the options you have developed for yourself.

Betty: If I get the impression that Lisa would want to move before starting high school, I would have to act fast to establish a residence for us. Once we make up our minds, my cousin will be a great help. In addition to finding a home there, I would also have to get our house here ready to put on the market. I have already quietly started that by sorting out items to be sold and by painting some of the rooms. Even if I don't sell it by the end of the summer, if it is in good shape, the real estate agent would probably be able to continue to show it while we are gone.

I am also planning on selling part of the other property I still own. That would provide funds for moving and for another home in case the house does not sell as fast as I would like.

If Lisa's well-being would be unfavorably influenced by a significant geographical move before entering high school, we will simply stay here until she graduates. I would still intend to move, but would take more time to prepare for it.

I am not worried about which way it will work out. If my first plan does not seem feasible, I just switch to my alternate plan. My alternative is going to be my "safety net." Either way, I will prepare for what I want; I just don't know yet what the speed of action will be. If Plan One does not work out, I will not be disappointed. My daughter's happiness is too important to me. The time to her graduation will not be wasted, because I will use the time to prepare myself as best as I can. I even thought of taking a computer course or two here to increase my marketable skills.

Couns: I am very much impressed by the comprehensiveness and details of your planning. The development of events sounds logical and realistic. Having an alternate plan in place is especially helpful, because you can put that into action if you have to without having to waste time and energy on feeling sorry for not getting what you want immediately. You have been a great student and it may just be time to take your computer classes wherever you are going to be. You seem to be determined to grow and spread your wings.

Summary of Client-Counselor Interaction: Long-Range Planning.

The session demonstrated how clients at times return to counseling when a particular aspect of the counseling process appeals to them, because of what it may have meant to them in the overall process of problem-solving. Clients are inclined to use ideas or strategies that worked well for them in the past. Betty was intrigued by the concept of options. When she wanted to make a change in her life, she remembered to explore different possibilities for herself. After she worked out her plans as much as she could, she wanted an unbiased opinion, but from someone she knew would keep her best interests in mind. By remembering details from their past work together, the counselor reinforced the client's opinion that, indeed, the counselor was still very much interested in her well-being. Clients are usually pleasantly surprised to find out how much their therapist remembers about them from previous sessions, in spite of working just as intensely with many other clients.

Disclosure Builds Trust. In a therapeutic relationship clients disclose much about their innermost feelings and thoughts. The level of disclosure has a direct positive correlation to the degree of trust the client feels during the counseling process. Therefore, when clients return to the same therapeutic relationship, the counselor's memories aid in quickly reestablishing the previous level of trust. If at all possible, the skilled counselor will make every effort to become familiar again with the case of a returning client. In this session, the counselor was quite familiar with the details of previous sessions, and was easily able to connect with the client's concerns. As always, the counselor made use of opportunities to praise the client for her good work and to encourage her to continue with her own growth process.

Case Study

Kahla: Temporary Single Parenthood

One type of single parenthood that we normally don't think of occurs when one of the parents is hospitalized for a long period of time; when one is deployed on a military mission; or when one parent is incarcerated. Although officially still married, the parent remaining with the children struggles with many of the difficulties that other single parents face, in addition to the upset the children and spouse feel. Kahla, the young mother of a little girl, found herself in just such a situation. Kahla had met her husband in a residential treatment facility for chemical dependency where she worked as a nurse's aide. Leroy was there to overcome his cocaine addiction. Several months after Leroy's discharge from the treatment program, they were married. Kahla was eager to help her husband adjust to an alcohol and drug-free life. She knew that he had been married before and had a couple of children from that marriage, but he seemed to have no connection to them now.

Kahla's income was not sufficient for the two to live on, so they temporarily moved in with Leroy's mother. Leroy did not spend much time at home. He told Kahla that he was job-hunting and hoped to land a good job "real soon." Kahla was surprised that he did not seem concerned or worried about not having a job, but he laughingly told her she did enough of that for the two of them. Several months later, Leroy was arrested for armed robbery and possession of cocaine. Leroy was in jail when Kahla discovered that she was pregnant. Searching for options, she discussed her pregnancy with her mother-in-law. She thought it would be best to have an abortion or give the baby up for adoption. Leroy's mother told her how devastated Leroy had been after the loss of his children through the divorce. It hurt his manhood and drove him to cocaine use. Worse things would happen if he had to go through that again. Leroy's mother definitely opposed an abortion. Kahla sought counseling from another therapist at that point. From what she remembered, she wanted the counselor to tell her what to do, but the counselor put the responsibility for the decision back on her. Kahla did not continue with counseling.

After the birth of her daughter, Kahla returned to her job. For financial reasons she continued to live with her mother-in-law. One day Kahla answered the telephone while her mother-in-law was out of the house. A woman on the other end identified herself as Leroy's former wife. The woman sounded angry, demanding the money Leroy owed her in back child support. When Kahla told her that she was Leroy's present wife and that Leroy was in prison, the woman did not seem surprised but told Kahla that as the current wife, Kahla would be responsible for her husband's debts. She added that she had hired a lawyer. At her next visit to the prison, Kahla told her husband about the woman's telephone call. He admitted that he had been behind in child-support payments for years and upon his release from prison he would probably have to go to jail if he did not come up with the money. Leroy was not worried because, as he said, that was still 7 to 8 years away. Kahla was shocked at her husband's response. Before returning for other visits she sought counseling again.

Couns: On the intake form you listed quite a number of problem areas. Can you tell me what area you would want to start with?

Kahla: I think the divorce is the most important one, but I may need to look at other issues first or almost at the same time.

Couns: You stated that your husband is in prison. Is that your reason for wanting the divorce?

Kahla: Yes and no. I loved my husband and when we met at the treatment center where I work, I thought I could help him. Even before I knew that I was pregnant he relapsed without telling me. He is now in prison for 7 to 8 years. I am lucky I did not lose my job. We are not allowed to date patients. Financially, I am not able to move out of my mother-in-law's home. She is on disability, but needs to charge me for room and board for us. There is not much money left over for me to save and I was already resigned to live that way for a long time.

Couns: What you describe sounds like a very sad situation. I am wondering, would your mother-in-law still let you live with her if you divorced her son?

Kahla: No, I don't think we could live there anymore. I feel very bad about secretly thinking of divorcing my husband. It is dishonest, and yet I cannot tell her about it. I have to keep my thoughts to myself. I don't think I would divorce Leroy because he is in prison, but what shocked me was his lack of feelings for his children. When we first met, he did not tell me that he did not pay the child support as ordered by the court. I don't blame his former wife for being angry. As I drove home from the prison visit that day, I realized that Leroy would probably treat our child the same way. I also realized that my mother-in-law had not been honest with me when she told me how devastated Leroy had been over losing his children.

Couns: You mentioned on the intake form that you had been in counseling before. How did that work out for you?

Kahla: I wanted somebody to tell me what to do when I was pregnant. The counselor wouldn't do it, so I did not go back. Instead my mother-in-law told me what to do, and I did it. I am not sure it was the right thing.

Couns: In counseling or therapy our job is to help you with your decisions, such as help you explore your options and

	consider the consequences or results of different paths of action. You are the only one to make significant decisions about your life.
Kahla:	I understand that now; that's why I am back. If I had listened to the counselor, rather than insisting that somebody make my decisions, I would not have been in this predicament. I have tried to look at my situation realistically. I feel so bad about my daughter and what I have done to her. What kind of life is in store for her?
Couns:	When you first tried counseling, you probably believed that you could not make such an important decision over your life. As we often do when we believe something strongly, we do not consider the possibility that our beliefs may not have a solid basis in reality. We do not dispute our beliefs. Therefore, we do not consider the consequences that may follow when we act on some of our beliefs. You were convinced that you could not make the decision on your own and when you did not find in counseling what you were looking for, you turned to your mother-in-law, who was willing to tell you what she thought was best for you. Only later did you realize that the decision might not have been in your own best interest. Although later than you perhaps wanted to, you have learned from your first counseling experience. Now you are here to apply that learning to your current life circumstances. In thinking through your earlier experiences, you have developed a lot of insight that will be an asset to you now. Looking at your concerns for your daughter, are you troubled about her not having a father around for much of her childhood, or because her father is in prison, or because you think he will forget about your daughter as he did with his other children?
Kahla:	All three reasons are on my mind. I feel she has already three strikes against herself—and it's all my fault.
Couns:	If we want to work together, let's see what we can learn from the past, rather than continue to blame ourselves. When you married your husband, you loved him and wanted to help him. Because you loved him, you probably wanted to trust him, and did not check out whether or not he told you the truth about his previous marriage. Most young people in love do not run a check on the

other's past. That's why we say "love is blind." Again, you seemed to have acted on a belief that when you love somebody you trust him implicitly. In the future you can act differently, if you apply what you learned now. From today on, we can focus on what is best for you and your daughter. You mentioned divorce; with what you know now, what do you think would be the consequences if you stayed in the marriage? Here is a piece of paper for you to write down what we come up with.

Kahla: If I stay in the marriage, my daughter and I will have a place to live with my mother-in-law until Leroy is released.

Couns: That could be a positive consequence, at least, for now. You might want to put a plus sign next to it. What other consequences come to mind?

Kahla: My daughter will not only grow up without knowing a father, but by the time she enters school, she will know that her father is in prison. If I divorced him, perhaps I could keep it a secret by moving away?

Couns: Perhaps, but we don't know that yet. There may be a time in the future to make a decision on that. You mentioned earlier that you are concerned that even if you stay married to him, he may not concern himself more with your daughter than with his other children.

Kahla: Yes, that is true. I could not expect him to be different. Another big minus would be my feelings for him. I feel betrayed that he went back to using cocaine and then even became involved in armed robbery instead of finding a job. He could not have considered what that would do to me. My feelings have changed a lot. I don't know that I could even live with him after he is released.

Couns: Your feelings certainly are important to consider here, along with the other reasons you mentioned. What would be the likely consequences if you divorced your husband now?

Kahla: I don't know how and where we would live. I have looked at some apartments, and for the next couple of years we could probably manage something like a studio apartment, but I could not afford childcare. Another possibility might be to find an elderly person who needs some nursing care in exchange for room and board for us. That would be the last resort, because I would be almost as

	dependent as I am now. I think I need to work toward independence.
Couns:	You got a little bit ahead of our agenda here, but it is great that you already explored some possibilities. You are absolutely correct in wanting to work toward independence. Your initiative will serve you well as you go along. Do you foresee any difficulties your husband may give you in the divorce?
Kahla:	I am sorry; I got sidetracked. To answer your question about my husband giving me difficulties if I divorce him: I don't think he will, as long as I don't ask him for money. For a while, I worried about explaining the divorce to my daughter, but I have a lot of explaining to do to her anyway about what kind of a father I chose for her. In a few years, I hope, I will be ready with explanations. Now it is not part of my decision.
Couns:	Good for you! You have already learned to distinguish between what is of immediate importance to your decision and what is not. You are a good student. Today's main lessons are to always look at options, as you already did. When you are about to act on beliefs, take the time to challenge or dispute the beliefs regarding their basis in reality and the consequences resulting from acting on them. We usually take our beliefs and their role as guiding lights for granted. Also, be alert—beliefs come in different disguises. We don't always say to ourselves, "I believe such and such." Sometimes we say, "I feel" that my daughter has already three strikes against her, as you did earlier today. Most likely you expressed a belief. Can you also believe that it is possible to remove one or more of the strikes? I think you do, because you were considering some ways of approaching that, such as moving away. In that instance, you expressed a belief but you seem to have challenged it a bit, at least, to the point where you were able to consider alternatives. You could remember this example as a learning paradigm.
Kahla:	I think I tentatively understand what you mean. How can I manage to be aware of all those hidden beliefs and what they are doing to me? I need help in uncovering them; it's like a big black monster! Counseling would be helpful, but I can't afford it.

Couns: Yes, the task seems overwhelming. Not all our beliefs are hurting us: Many of them are good solid guidelines for our lives. The job is to uncover the ones that are the monster, as you said. For a moment, let's think about where our beliefs and values come from. We were not born with them. Most of them came from parents, teachers, church, friends, and other persons we looked to for guidance. Did we accept *all* the beliefs our parents, teachers, and others tried to instill in us? Probably not; we selected some that made sense to us and discarded others. The fact that we made those choices means we created our own belief and value system or we created the monster. If we created the system, then we can un-create it. I would like you to think about that for our next session. For the duration of your current decision-making process, I will work with you free of charge.

Summary of Client-Counselor Interaction: Temporary Single Parenthood. The first session with the young woman was devoted to collecting information about her current life circumstances, as well as exploring her way of thinking. The client was very open about her earlier expectations from counseling, and ready to generalize her initial willingness to other areas. On her own she had gained insight that her faulty expectations and her decision not to continue with therapy had caused her much trouble. She appeared eager to learn what did not work in the first place and how to make it work in her present circumstances.

The counselor praised her insight and initiative and acknowledged the difficulty of her situation. Rather than remain for long on the topic of the client's past self-defeating behaviors, the counselor explained the significance of beliefs and values in people's lives. Not all beliefs are in our best interests. The counselor stated as the main point that some beliefs need to be explored, challenged, and possibly replaced with more self-enhancing beliefs before we act. In addition, the counselor emphasized that people in general create their own belief system and, are capable of modifying the system. With those explanations the counselor diverted the focus from blaming—something in which the client was already an expert—to formulating actions that would guide the client in future decision making.

Pro Bono Therapy. Realizing the truly difficult life circumstances the client was in and the financial struggles she was facing in addition to her emotional struggles, the therapist offered *pro bono* services to the client. Individuals in the helping professions give a certain amount of service free of charge as part of their professional obligations and ethics.

SUMMARY

Generalizing learning onto other areas occurs in various ways when clients return to counseling for different reasons. Broadening the scope of applications of learning invariably renders the strategies and skills more stable and more readily accessible in the client's behavior repertoire through the general effect of repetition. Whether the client returns to counseling because of additional problems, as in the case of Bill, or because the client appreciates the idea of having options and wants to explore future alternatives in her long-range planning, as in the case of Betty, the result is that the client's initiative is reinforced. A learned resourcefulness develops that ultimately pervades the client's style of life.

Kahla's return to counseling after a brief prior exposure reflected her recognition that her past unrealistic and unhealthy expectations had prevented her from making desired gains at that time. On her own, she realized how she had programmed herself for failure. Her awareness and desire to generalize her initial willingness to seek counseling paved the way for the real beginning of the process. Thus, in the absence of learned coping skills to generalize, her initiative was reinforced and generalized onto problems in her current life circumstances.

EXERCISES

An appropriate exercise for generalizing learning onto new areas would be the application of studying skills from one subject area to another. Can you think of an example where a particular studying strategy brought you the desired grade? Could those skills that were so helpful in mathematics (or another subject) be equally useful in studying for a psychology (or other subject) test? Many people are more likely to generalize their procrastination skills from one area onto another by telling themselves, "I work or study best under pressure." With repeated application, this sentence grows into a belief, guiding (or misguiding) the individual into acting on the sincerely held belief, only to receive grades that are substantially lower than the desired ones. How would you challenge the belief? Possibly, the challenge would work if you design an experiment that would lead you to start studying early on in the semester, designating certain study periods over the course of your days, and strictly adhering to the schedule. Oh yes—refuse to yield to tempting distractions. Choose one subject area for the whole semester and follow the schedule. If your grades in that subject area are better than they were in the past or better than expected, would that refute the validity of the belief? Would you consider generalizing your success to other subject areas?

SUGGESTED READING

Bakan, D. (1995). The crisis in psychology. *The General Psychologist, 31,* 77–80.
   The author discusses losses regarding subject matter, method, and mission in the field of psychology and emphasizes the distinction between behavior (in the Pavlovian sense) and the larger domain of human conduct.
Ellis, A. (1996). The humanism of Rational Emotive Behavior Therapy and other cognitive behavior therapies. *The Journal of Humanistic Education and Development, 35,* 69–88.
   The article constitutes a comprehensive outline of humanistic principles inherent in the philosophy and application of cognitive-emotional-behavior therapies.

10

Reconceptualizing the Self

OBJECTIVES

1. To provide opportunities for explorations of clients' self-concepts.
2. To assist clients to refrain from rating themselves as persons along a good-bad continuum.
3. To facilitate clients' acceptance of themselves as human beings who make mistakes.
4. To encourage clients to view small steps as evidence that change is possible.
5. To facilitate adoption and integration of new perceptions and values into a consistent self-concept.
6. To aid clients' understanding and perceiving of the self as a process rather than a static entity.

THE SELF

How does the idea of the self come into existence for people? According to McCrone (1993), special aspects of the human mind, such as memory, imagination, self-awareness, and others are actually skills we learn. They are not innate traits or capacities that unfold during the developmental process of maturation. It is through the power of speech that we develop patterns and habits of thinking. Our thoughts take on the role of an inner voice with which we talk silently in our heads. We use words to construct pictures of ourselves, the world around us and the other people in it. Information about how others perceive us adds another dimension and can be obtained by simple verbal means or by interpreting others' behavior toward us. The impact on the individual can be positive and beneficial or negative and detrimental.

Katz and Beach (1997) studied the connection of self-verification to depression. They hypothesized that self-verifying feedback will result in more stable self-views, and that in individuals with high self-esteem, self-verifying feedback will lead to decreased depression. Conversely, for persons with low self-esteem, self-verifying feedback will result in increased depression. As part of a larger study, 138 married women responded to mailed questionnaires. Another part of the study involved 258 undergraduate females who were involved in dating relationships. Instruments used included the Beck Depression Inventory (BDI), a 21-item self-report measure of depressive symptomatology; the Partner-Specific Support Scale (PSSS), a measure of social support adapted for marital partners; the Quality of Marriage Index (QMI), a six-item scale assessing a unidimensional evaluative aspect of marital satisfaction; and, the Rosenberg Self-Esteem Scale (RSE), assessing global self-esteem. In both married and dating women, self-esteem and depressive symptoms were more strongly related among women who experienced self-verification from their partners than among women who did not experience self-verification. The authors interpreted their findings to mean that self-verifying feedback may intensify the degree of self-esteem on depression. For women with high self-esteem, the self-verifying feedback reinforces their positive self-views, whereas for women with low self-esteem, higher levels of depressive symptoms result from receiving self-verifying feedback.

According to Self-Verification Theory (Swann, 1983), people are strongly inclined to have others view the self in a manner that is consistent with their own preexisting self-conceptions, apparently looking for both positive and negative aspects of a person's self-view to be confirmed or verified by others. The desire for consistency of one's own self-concept with the view of others seems to function in a way similar to confirmation bias, where a tendency is noted to give preferential treatment of evidence supporting existing beliefs or opinions (Nickerson, 1998). Considering the detrimental impact confirmation bias or desire for consistency between self-concept and self-verification may have on an individual whose self-concept is already poor, intense work in counseling to overcome the maladaptive behavior would seem to be of extreme importance.

Threatened Egotism

Other hypotheses regarding patterns of self-defeating or self-destructive behavior have focused on threatened egotism or self-regulation failure as possible explanations (Baumeister, 1997). The author uses the term "egotism" in a generic sense, meaning all the favorable views of self, whether or not they are justified. Synonyms for favorable self-views include such desirable terms as self-confidence and high self-esteem, but also less desirable entities, such as arrogance, narcissism, or being conceited. The notion of threat refers to any event implying some reduction in one's self-appraisal. Receiving an unfavorable appraisal in an area previously invested by a very favorable self-evaluation would be a typical example.

Instead of defending the threatened self-view by engaging in self-promoting behaviors, the individual may experience emotional distress in the form of anxiety or depression, preventing the calm and rational consideration necessary to respond in an enlightened self-interest manner. People with high but unstable self-esteem are most likely to engage in self-defeating behavior in the event of ego threats. Ego threats have little impact in people who have stable, high self-esteem.

Failure of Self-Regulation. Self-regulation is the mechanism that keeps the individual in a position to employ behaviors that result in positive outcomes. Self-defeating behaviors that result in negative outcomes may either be brought on by an incident of underregulation, where the individual fails to make the effort necessary to achieve the desired outcome, or by misregulation, where concerted efforts at changing the self are used, but some contingencies in the situation have not been properly understood by the person.

Self-Efficacy. In his attempts to explain and predict psychological changes as functions of different modes of treatment, Albert Bandura

(1977b, 1997) stated that psychological procedures change the level and strength of individuals' self-efficacy. In his opinion, cognitive processes mediate the acquisition and regulation of human behaviors, but the most powerful procedures for effecting psychological changes are performance-based.

A common cognitive mechanism is thought to bring about changes achieved by different methods. People's beliefs and expectations about their ability to achieve desired goals and their ability to deal effectively with obstacles that may stand in the way of those goals determine the degree and duration of efforts expended toward the goals. Thus, an outcome expectancy is the person's estimate of how effectively a certain behavior will lead to a given outcome, but an efficacy expectation is the degree of the person's conviction that the person can successfully perform the behaviors necessary to yield the outcome. Both expectancies are seen as working together in influencing people's decisions about what behaviors to initiate. In most cases, the expectancies are defined in terms of likelihood, rather than in "either-or" terms. What are the chances that a particular behavior will lead to a desired outcome and that the person will be able to perform that behavior? Bandura sees efficacy expectations as coming from four sources: performance accomplishments (our own actions), vicarious experiences (actions of others we observe), verbal persuasion (what others tell us), and emotional arousal (what we feel).

Self-Concept and Self-Esteem. Both self-efficacy expectancies and outcome expectancies are specific cognitions or thoughts that can only be defined in relation to specific behaviors in specific situations. They are not personality traits, but self-efficacy expectancies are related to people's self-evaluations, such as self-concept and self-esteem (Maddux, 1991). People's self-concepts consists of all their attitudes and beliefs about themselves, including all their likes and dislikes, their capabilities, talents, and inabilities. People's self-esteem is their evaluation of what they are worth as persons and how much or how little they like the person they think they are. Self-esteem evaluations are usually independent of self-concept assessments. Similarly, Blascovich and Tomaka (1991) see self-esteem as an affective assessment of one's own worth, also referred to as self-regard or self-acceptance, whereas self-concept has a broader meaning, including cognitive and behavioral self-perceptions and beliefs. Bandura's (1977b) concept of self-efficacy expectations would be a component of the self-concept.

Self-esteem in client-centered therapy (Rogers, 1961) is the goal of counseling, and is also referred to as self-acceptance or unconditional self-regard, the congruence of one's ideal and real selves. Counseling interventions are centered on the client's psychological distress arising from a discrepancy between the real and ideal selves. In the course of counseling, the therapist is thought to provide unconditional positive regard to the client as a means to assist the client in the move toward unconditional self-regard.

In a series of studies, Betz, Wohlgemuth, Serling, Harshbarger, and Klein (1995) developed a measure of unconditional self-regard based on Rogerian theory. The Unconditional Self-Regard Scale (USRS) is a 20-item scale with the following salient features: The client perceives self as a person of worth and places standards of evaluation within self; self-acceptance does not depend on one's own performances in various behavioral domains, although the individual may strive for improved performance in those areas. After completion of validity studies using various other instruments, the USRS was used in combination with a version of the Barrett-Lennard Relationship Inventory (BLRI). The BLRI (Barrett-Lennard, 1962) was developed by Rogers' colleagues to assess client perceptions of the provision of the Rogerian core conditions (empathy, genuineness, and regard). In the current study, only the scales evaluating level and unconditionality of regard were used.

Subjects were 164 undergraduate students (83 female, 81 male) from an introductory psychology course. Before completing the instruments, the students were instructed to select the three most important older persons in their lives as they were growing up for use as target persons on the inventory. By far the most frequently mentioned important persons were parents, followed by other relatives, a teacher, and, among the male students, a coach. Among the female students, their unconditional self-regard was significantly related to both the level and unconditionality of regard perceived from significant others in general and from mothers in particular. No statistically significant correlations were obtained among the male students, although those between the student's self-regard and that of brothers and coaches were high in absolute magnitude. The authors explained the lack of statistically significant findings for the male students with the fact that small sample sizes resulted from the breakdown by both gender and category of significant others, thereby limiting findings of statistical significance. On the other hand, it could be argued that, in general, men are more independent of significant others in forming their unconditional self-regard than women.

Reviewing empirical research in the literature related to the psychological well-being of individuals in connection with gender role orientations, Burnett, Anderson, and Heppner (1995) found that masculinity seemed to be a strong correlate of self-esteem, while femininity was relatively unrelated to self-esteem. The authors considered the possibility of a cultural bias toward masculinity in the American culture, where individuals who are masculine receive more positive reinforcement and therefore develop higher self-esteem. Attempting to measure the effects of environmental or situational influences on masculinity and femininity traits and self-esteem, the authors designed a study to test their hypotheses that individual masculinity would be more strongly related to self-esteem than individual femininity; that environmental press for masculinity would be rated higher than the press for femininity; and that there would be a person-by-environment interaction, resulting in the lowest self-esteem in individuals low in personal masculinity but living in an environment with high demand for masculinity.

Participants in the study were 236 undergraduate students (90 male and 146 female) at a large Midwestern university. The instrument used to assess participants' individual sex-role orientation was the Personal Attributes Questionnaire (PAQ), developed by Spence, Helmreich, and Stapp in 1974 (Burnett et al., 1995). The Personal Attributes Questionnaire-Environmental form (PAQ-env) was employed to assess environmental presses for masculinity and femininity. The Coopersmith Self-Esteem Inventory (SEI), a 25-item self-report measure of self-esteem, was used to obtain individuals' evaluations of themselves as persons. Participants were able to complete all three instruments in about 30 minutes. Statistical evaluation of the results revealed that individual masculinity was significantly correlated with self-esteem for all subjects as well as within each sex. Significant correlation for individual femininity scores and self-esteem across all subjects or in either sex group was not obtained.

Individual-by-environment interaction was found to be significant for women but not for men. Thus, the lowest self-esteem ratings were found in women with low individual masculinity living in environments that rewarded high amounts of masculinity. While it is not surprising that women with low masculinity traits in an environment with high demands for those masculinity traits will suffer some loss in psychological well-being, it is noteworthy that men are apparently able to distance themselves sufficiently from the environmental presses to avoid experiencing significant reduction in their psychological well-being. Obviously, women's greater vulnerability to environmental and social pressures is an important factor to be aware of when counseling female clients (see also Highlen & Hill, 1984).

Self-Consistency. Prescott Lecky (1969) has argued that there is coherence in the behavior of individuals that indicates an organized dynamic system pointing toward self-determination, but that the organization cannot be revealed in experiments focusing on attitudes toward any single situation. Instead, the organization of the system becomes apparent when looking at the consistency of attitudes toward a variety of situations. Bakan (1995) echoed Lecky's concerns when he pointed to psychology's uncritical expectancy that applying statistical methods to aggregated measures of behavior, rather than to studying behaviors in dynamic relationship to each other, will reveal meaningful psychological information.

Similarly, proponents of Contextualism caution that empirical data resulting from psychological investigations are applicable, in principle, only within the limits of the conditions when the observations were made. Applications of data to situations beyond the limits of the original experimental set represent a faith not grounded in ordinary science (Deese, 1996). Lecky pointed toward the total organization of the individual, as one would think of when using the terms "lifestyle," "character," or "personality." People's behaviors are consistent, or "in character," because all the different acts of those people are performed with the goal of maintaining the same structure of values.

Individuals' personalities are systems of organized conceptions of the world within the unique framework of values peculiar to each particular individual. In order to preserve its essential integration and unity, the personality system resists change. Standards for acceptance and rejection of new experiences are automatically created, congruent with the requirements of preserving the system. The degree of success in rationalizing some values, and making them seem consistent with the system while rejecting others, may lead to resistances that are not in the best interest of the individual. Knowing an individual's self-concept can provide information about the nature and level of resistance that can be expected when introducing new values or ideas.

In the field of counseling and education, concerns about changing individuals' self-concepts have focused on participation in intervention programs as a means to enhance self-concept or self-esteem (Hattie, 1992). Particular attention was given to implementing self-enhancement programs in schools. In order to measure and record behaviors indicative of self-esteem, Burnett (1998) developed and validated an instrument, the Behavioral Indicators of Self-Esteem Scale (BIOS), to be used by teachers. The teachers' perceptions of the frequency of self-esteem related behaviors in their students were found to deviate widely across teachers, indicating the need for further research.

In a response to Martin Seligman's "The American way of blame" in the July, 1998, President's column of the *APA Monitor*, discussing the relationship between self-esteem and aggression, Ervin Staub (1999) raised the issue that knowing the level of self-esteem in children and youth is not as meaningful as knowing what self-esteem is based on. Roy Baumeister (1999), in discussing the same issue, seems to support Seligman's disagreement that low self-esteem causes aggression. He also is congruent with both Seligman and Staub in his opinion that programs promoting indiscriminate self-esteem boosting may be helpful in some instances, but may also lead to a sense of entitlement for just existing as a human being rather than promoting the value of actual achievements. Instead, Baumeister proposed a system of self-control that enables individuals to regulate their own impulses, emotions, and goal-directed activities, as mentioned earlier in this chapter.

Categories for Psychological Study. Meaningful categories for psychological study have been proposed by Gregory Kimble (1995). His three broad-scale categories encompass the fundamental faculties of knowing, feeling, and doing, commonly attributed to Aristotle's triarchic view. Kimble seems concerned that contemporary psychology regards a person's self-concept as consisting of partly cognition or self-knowledge, partly affect or self-esteem, and partly reaction tendency or self-efficacy—only to lump them altogether in the literature, often making analysis too difficult to attempt.

Interestingly, Kimble considers the different therapies available for helping persons in strengthening their self-concepts as having different consequences. For instance, reinforcement of competent behavior is seen as instrumental in improving self-efficacy in behavior therapy. Engaging in existential or humanistic approaches may result in enhancement of self-esteem. Cognitive therapy is regarded as helpful in modifying people's knowledge of themselves. Kimble is looking for a complete therapy that would do all of the above and would focus on organizing the components as important aspects of an individual's self-concept. No matter how accurate Kimble's perception of currently available therapy approaches may be, the steps outlined in the phases of the present therapy process do just that, focusing on the person's thoughts and beliefs, feelings, and actions regarding their own personal concepts of themselves as well as in relation to the worlds at large.

Case Study

Kahla: Self as Single

In the previous chapter, Kahla turned to a new counselor after an earlier unsuccessful attempt, when she was faced with additional complications in her already difficult life situation. Following her first session with the new counselor, Kahla almost decided that a divorce from her incarcerated husband would be the best solution for her and her little daughter's future.

Kahla had refrained from visiting her husband in prison when she received a phone call from him, complaining about her absence. Kahla told him she could not afford the money for gasoline for the long trip. Leroy did not accept her explanation and accused her of not caring about him. He felt neglected at a time when he needed her support more than ever. One of the inmates that Leroy had become friendly with was about to be released. Leroy had told this man in detail about his own arrest, trial, and conviction. The other man thought Leroy had a good chance for filing an appeal, but he would need a smart lawyer. His own lawyer had been quite helpful in getting him a reduced sentence and would be Leroy's best bet. Money for a retainer was needed. Leroy instructed Kahla to be there at the next allowed visitor's day, bringing the money along. Leroy wanted Kahla to meet the other inmate, so they could work on Leroy's behalf after the prisoner's release. Kahla felt a big wave of anxiety come over her after she hung up the phone.

The next day at work, she saw a man in the hallway of the treatment center who had been a patient there at the same time Leroy was treated. The man had apparently relapsed and returned to treatment. He asked her about some of the former patients, including Leroy. Kahla stared at him; she could not answer; panic, even stronger than the day before, engulfed her. After a while, she started to shake and tremble, gasping for air. Finally, without a word, she turned around and went into the ladies' room. She tried to calm herself down by letting cold water run over her head. Then she left without telling anybody, got into her car and drove off. The counselor was called from the emergency room of a local hospital. Kahla's car had hit a tree. She was not seriously hurt beyond a broken shoulder, but she appeared to be in a state of shock and did not recall any details of the accident. She responded only with her own and her counselor's name to most questions.

After her shoulder had been attended to, Kahla was transferred to the psychiatric ward. Her mother-in-law was called and agreed to take care of Kahla's daughter. Kahla was terminated from her job. She could have appealed, but did not. Kahla's counselor held privileges as allied health professional at the hospital, and was able to see her from time to time without interfering with the hospital program.

Couns: After you told me what happened to you, I can understand your desperation. Can you remember any of the thoughts you had after your husband had called you and the next day at work? It must have been extremely upsetting for you.

Kahla: After I saw you, I had some hope that I could get out of my situation by divorcing my husband. As you know, I did not want to go back to the prison to visit him and was trying to buy time. When he called I felt like a big black

	cloud was swallowing me up. I remember thinking "I can't get away!" The cloud was suffocating me, I couldn't breathe. After it passed, I felt some guilt for wanting to abandon him, but also some threat.
Couns:	Where do you think the threat came from—anything your husband said to you?
Kahla:	Yes, it wasn't just the money he wanted, but that he wanted me to meet this other prisoner. That made me feel as if I was sinking deeper and deeper into the hole and the cloud kept pushing me down. I just kept thinking, "I can't get out, I can't get out."
Couns:	Somehow you were able to function again to take care of your daughter and to go to work the next day.
Kahla:	That is true; I tried to tell myself to look around and there was no hole. I tried to hold on to reality, thinking if I could discuss it with you at our next appointment, there would be a solution I could see with your help.
Couns:	You still felt some hope that you would be able to resolve your situation, but the next day that hope was apparently destroyed.
Kahla:	When the client at work asked me about Leroy, I could not handle that. I know he did not mean to frighten me. He did not even know that I am married to Leroy. The black cloud seemed to swallow me up again and I heard in my head my voice saying, "You'll never get away. You are too dumb to be alive. You messed up your life and your daughter's life. You are too stupid to live." That voice drowned out everything else in my head. It seemed like everybody else could hear it. I had to run away, but I did not know where to run to.
Couns:	That was a terrifying experience for you. When you were driving, did you still hear your voice in your head as you just described it?
Kahla:	No, it was different after I had the water run over my head. Actually, I felt numb, but I knew that it was hopeless; I was incompetent to live. I also knew that I did not want to drive up to the prison to see my husband anymore, not ever!
Couns:	All this went on in your head when you had the accident?
Kahla:	Yes; oh, no! Do you think I ran into the tree on purpose?
Couns:	All I know is that you were extremely upset. Anybody in that condition could have an accident. Driving a car in a

	state of such emotional upheaval can be very dangerous. I am glad you are here and I am glad you remember some of your thoughts. They will be helpful when we continue our work. We also want to see if you ever felt anything like this panic before in your life and when. For now, I want you to promise me something: Whenever you feel that upset, call me before you do anything that dangerous, no matter when your next appointment is.
Kahla:	I did not want to bother you between appointments, because you are already so kind to see me for free when I don't really deserve it.
Couns:	Let's not worry about whether or not you deserve it; we will find out more about that later. For now I want your promise.

Summary of Client-Counselor Interaction: Self as Single. The counselor was very careful in offering support and understanding of the client's emotions. At the same time, it was important to obtain the client's thoughts at the time they occurred. The counselor needed to know what had triggered her panic and her actions, so the thoughts could be recorded for work in the future, as there was a possibility for an underlying panic disorder. The other reason for the exploration was to see how deep the client's state of shock had really been. The counselor was certainly aware of the possibility that the client's accident may have been a suicide attempt. Considering Kahla's fragile emotional state, the counselor decided not to confront her overtly with the question of a suicide attempt, but raised her awareness to that effect in a gentle manner. Explaining that people in such state of emotional turmoil can easily become involved in accidents, the counselor used that moment to obtain a promise from the client that in the future she would contact the counselor before taking any action whenever she felt that emotionally stressed. Kahla's concept of herself was so negative that an open confrontation about a suicide attempt would not have helped improve her self-esteem, as she could have interpreted that as just one more failure on her part.

Case Study Follow-Up: Taking Control

The recent events as described above had not improved Kahla's situation. She had lost her job and, except for her mother-in-law's home, she had no place to live. For a while, she and her baby daughter had to stay in a homeless shelter, because she did not want to continue living with her mother-in-law. In counseling, she worked on her anxiety and panic attacks as well as on her decision whether or not to divorce her husband.

Kahla contacted vocational rehabilitation services and was able to obtain financial assistance for studies at a vocational college, and for continuing therapy. She completed a 2-year program in secretarial and bookkeeping training combined with data entry skills. After graduation, she secured an entry-level position with a progressive local pharmaceutical company that provided child care services for their employees. Another decision point arose when her ex-husband asked her to relieve him of all child support payments in exchange for staying out of her and her daughter's life forever. Apparently, he was eligible for parole in about a year and he wanted to be free of financial obligations from this marriage.

Couns: You have done extremely well so far, and now you want to work on another decision. As most decisions in your life, this is a significant but difficult one. Tell me a little bit about your reasoning and expectations for the various outcomes as you see them now.

Kahla: As I have learned in counseling, I have looked at the different sides to consider in this decision. The way I see it, is if I relieve Leroy from any responsibility for child support, I may relinquish my child's rights for additional money and deprive her of some needed resources in the future. With my training, I hope to be able to provide for the two of us in a very modest way, but something could happen to me where I cannot work. On the other hand, even if he were released from prison, there is no guarantee that Leroy would ever pay any child support, just as he did not do for his other children. I would have to take him to court every time.

Couns: You have made a good analysis of the situation so far, using lessons of past experiences as part of your reasoning. I agree with you, your child has some rights of financial protection, whether or not she actually gets this from her father. It also makes sense to consider that you may not always be able to provide that financial protection. You may consider asking for some legal advice about what

	might happen to you and your daughter in such a case. What are the benefits you see in relieving Leroy from his responsibilities?
Kahla:	Thank you for reminding me that I could seek legal advice for some of the questions. The most important benefit in my opinion is to have him completely removed from our lives. My experiences during those prison visits were so traumatic; I don't ever want to be involved in something like that again. With your help, I have overcome my panic attacks and I have started to build up a new life. I do not want to jeopardize what I have gained.
Couns:	You have worked hard in overcoming your anxiety, and you have worked very hard in starting your future after going through those traumatic experiences. Your wish to cut all this out of your life is certainly understandable. Have you thought how to handle questions from your daughter regarding her father?
Kahla:	I have thought about that a lot. She will start asking about her father when she will still be too young to understand. I could lie and say he died, but I don't want to risk losing her trust. Perhaps I can say he went away and I don't know where he is, hoping that will be the truth at the time. As soon as she is old enough to understand, I will tell her the truth and let her decide if she wants to see him. If she wants to meet him, I will make every effort to find him and take her for a visit. Of course, he could try to find us before my daughter is ready for it. Again, going by past experiences with his other children, the possibility is slim. If it should happen, I will deal with it then.
Couns:	It sounds like you are very close to making your decision. Your plan not to lie to your daughter shows a lot of courage and I am sure you will exercise good judgment as to when the time has come for her to know the whole truth. Going so far as to help her find her father, if that's what she desires, shows great strength on your part. It says a lot about your sense of dignity.
Kahla:	Dignity is something I have learned here. I remember you used the word some time ago and I looked it up in the dictionary to get the correct meaning. Yes, I want to have the sense of being worthy and conduct myself accordingly. That is how I want to see myself and I want to teach my daughter.

Couns:	How do you feel about your life with your daughter now?
Kahla:	I have wondered if you would ever ask me that question and I am grateful that you waited until now. I love my daughter dearly and I would not want to give her up for adoption now that she is here. That does not mean I would have made the same decision in the past with what I know now. I still think it would have been better for me not to have a child at that time and, for that matter, not to have a husband like Leroy. From those mistakes in the past, I have learned that it is my responsibility to make the best decisions for myself; nobody else can do that. I have also learned that it takes time and a lot of thinking to make good decisions, at least for me.
Couns:	I can see you have considered the events in your life with a sincere attitude of wanting to learn from the past. Your thoughts about your daughter sound honest and realistic. You are acknowledging the difficulties caused in your life by having a child at that time and under those circumstances. You are honest enough to admit that you would have been better off without those difficulties, but you are now ready and willing to accept your responsibility for whatever decisions you made at the time and making the best of it now. You have grown so much. I will always think of you as a person with dignity.
Kahla:	Thank you, those words coming from you mean a lot to me. You were there when I was ready to give up on myself. I'll never forget that. You invested in me and I want to make your investment grow.
Couns:	I like your analogy of an investment. It is yours to grow into whatever you want. You have made good use of it so far in creating opportunities for yourself.
Kahla:	You mentioned opportunities: I had not planned to talk about this today, but the word "opportunity" reminded me of what has been on my mind lately. While I was getting my training through vocational rehabilitation, I learned about myself that I like to work with numbers. The bookkeeping classes were so interesting, and, at the same time, reassuring. I knew everything had to come out even at the end, unless I made a mistake. I wonder if I could work toward a degree in accounting?
Couns:	When you started to talk about your interest in bookkeeping, I liked the way you said "I learned about myself."

That is so true—you learn about yourself, one of the best subjects to study. Awareness about yourself, knowing your likes and dislikes, your talents, your abilities, and even your weaknesses, is an important basis for making decisions. As for the accounting, there is no reason why you could not try it. Perhaps your employers would even assist you financially if you could use those skills in their employment. Considering going back to college to get an accounting degree shows how much your self-confidence has grown, and it has grown realistically because it is based on what you have already accomplished. You have a healthy outlook toward the future and your opportunities.

Summary of Client-Counselor Interaction: Taking Control. The interaction in the session reflected the degree of self-confidence the client had gained through her achievements. As the counselor pointed out at the end of the session, the client's self-confidence had a sound basis in reality. Significant progress was demonstrated in the client's willingness to make her own decisions and accept the responsibility for the consequences. When she introduced the concerns she wanted to work on in the session, apparently she had already done most of the groundwork for her decisions. She had considered alternatives and their possible consequences. The counselor used every opportunity to praise her for her initiative and encouraged her to continue, occasionally pointing out additional resources of which the client could avail herself.

A significant emotional moment came when the counselor inquired into the nature of the client's current feelings about her daughter. The most interesting point was that the client had expected the question for some time, and that expectation apparently had served as a catalyst for her own explorations regarding the issue. Her response reflected the depth of the therapeutic relationship and the trust and protection she felt within that relationship. The counselor's response confirmed the client's concept of herself and facilitated the discussion of the client's future goals.

WELFARE MOTHERS, THEIR SELF-CONCEPTS, AND CONCEPTS REFLECTED BY OTHERS

In the context of self-concept and self-esteem, a part of the population most at risk is probably the group of welfare recipients. One study demonstrated that intervention designed to develop coping skills reduced depression and increased self-esteem, except in women who had been on welfare the longest (McKeehan, 1992). Dependent children and their unmarried mothers constitute the majority of welfare recipients who, until recently, received financial assistance through the Aid to Families with Dependent Children (AFDC) program. The program has been replaced with the new Temporary Assistance to Needy Families (TANF) program that sets lifetime limits of about 5 years maximum on welfare payments.

Although several changes have been incorporated into the new program, the social stigma attached to the large group of single mothers and their children will probably not change rapidly. Society at large holds on to the many stereotypes of able-bodied but lazy persons receiving welfare benefits. The majority of those are obviously single mothers. Seccombe, James, and Battle Walters (1998) conducted a study examining how women on welfare interpret their own and others' welfare use. From in-depth interviews with 47 women who received cash assistance in 1995, the authors learned that the respondents were aware of their stigmatized status and tended to blame the social structure, the welfare system itself, or fate for their own economic circumstances and their reliance on welfare benefits. When discussing the reasons for other women's dependence on financial assistance, the respondents seemed to concur with the opinions inherent in society at large. Many women believed the popular descriptions of welfare mothers as being lazy and unmotivated, but saw their own circumstances as distinctly different. In their attempts to obtain explanations for the finding that their respondents' opinions were congruent with the popular opinion where others were concerned, but incongruent in their own cases, the authors turned to various social theories. Their conclusion was that the hegemony of the individual perspective represents a strong barrier to dealing constructively with poverty and welfare use, and that the individual perspective may be deeply rooted in the psyches of the poor within our society.

Whatever the reasons may be for the respondents' congruence with the popular stigmatizing opinions of other welfare mothers, on an individual level it can be expected and understood that they would disagree in order to defend or protect their images of their selves, their self-concepts and self-esteem, especially when interviewed by strangers from the other side of society (or the railroad tracks). In the privacy and protection of an individual counseling session, people would be more inclined to search deeper within themselves for reasons determining their own actions.

As was seen in the case of Ruth—encountered in previous chapters—she was keenly aware of her own decisions and actions that rendered her in need of public assistance for herself and her children. She felt harshly judged by her mother and felt ashamed and inferior to her sister-in-law and most of the people in town. Although angry and depressed about her circumstances, Ruth did not blame society or the welfare system for her predicament. Had she insisted that the responsibility lay outside herself, she might not have been able to conceive of anything she could do to help herself. Indeed, she and her friend Becky saw their situations as hopeless many times in the past, but there was enough sense of responsibility in both of them to bring them in to counseling to explore options.

Letter From Ruth

Years had passed since Ruth and Becky had been in counseling. Their therapist had moved away. Ruth had been accepted with a scholarship at the college of her choice. Ruth had been able to obtain the therapist's new address and the therapist received the following letter:

> Dear Doctor:
> A lot has happened since Becky and I last saw you. As you may remember, I was accepted at college and received the scholarship that made it possible for me to pursue my studies. It has been hard but very exciting and gratifying work. In addition to my studies and part-time participation in the child-care program, I have been very active in writing for the student newspaper and being Becky's representative for her creations at our bookstore and a local boutique. Business is good and her work is very much in demand. My children are doing very well here. My daughter is really blossoming. It was a good move!
> My writing for the student newspaper has been helpful in securing an internship in a local government agency last summer and I hope I will be able to repeat the experience this summer, possibly leading to a part-time position. People in the agency have been very supportive of me.
> It is almost graduation time; I think I will be graduating with honors (straight A's all the way). Who would have thought about this years ago (except probably you?) I am still the same person, but I feel so strong and powerful, powerful enough to shape my own destiny and possibly make an impact on

the community that we live in. Because studying has been so exciting for me, I decided to go on for a graduate degree. It may take me longer because I will need to earn money for us to live on, but I have some support in the community, as I mentioned.

It would be such an honor if you could come to my graduation. You and Becky are the people whom I would like to have with me on this important occasion. Becky has promised to come. She will be getting married again soon. She will probably want to tell you about it herself. However, I know you are very busy and it is quite a distance to travel, and I understand if you cannot attend. Just in case, I am enclosing an invitation with the graduation announcement; there is always room for hope. Incidentally, the graduation announcement is for Ruthanne. I remember years ago when I mentioned that my real name was Ruthanne, you said it had a special ring to it. You never mentioned it again, but it remained in my memory. Now, I think, I have grown enough to carry that ring. Thank you for everything, thank you for my new life—I doubt it would have been possible without your guidance,

Ruthanne

The letter does not need much interpretation. Obviously, Ruthanne's concept of herself has changed drastically: from a welfare mother, to an active and contributing member of her community and a powerful role model for her children. She sees herself as having grown in the awareness of her abilities, talents, and performances, and possibly some personality traits. As she said, she is still the same person. She has learned not to rate herself as a valuable or not-valuable person, but to accept herself as that person. The acceptance had freed her to spend energy on exploring what she could do, rather than to worry about who she should be. The incident with Ruthanne's name serves as an example of how seriously some clients take their therapists' words. Although not all clients respond in the same way, therapists are well advised to be aware of what they say and how they say it. Clients interpret and misinterpret and assign significance in their own characteristic way to statements made by their therapists.

As a solution for the problem of dealing with human worth, Albert Ellis (1973) recommended that it was better for people to avoid rating themselves at all. People are not good and they are not bad; they are merely human beings, with all their frailties. People possess many traits that are ratable. If people so desire, they can give their talents, personality traits, or their various performances report cards;

but they better abstain from giving themselves report cards as persons. When people become self-accepting instead of self-evaluating, they gain the freedom to inquire about what they really want in life and go out to find and enjoy those things. Instead of being concerned only with symptom-removal solutions to human problems, cognitive therapies—according to Ellis—deal with personality-restructuring solutions.

In accepting themselves, individuals may form a concept of self-identity much in the way what George Kelly (1963) refers to as "role constructs." Kelly does not use the term role in the way often used by sociologists and social psychologists to mean a series of behavior prescriptions outlined by the culture and filled by people who play these roles. For Kelly, the role construct is an ongoing process in which individuals define their roles. When individuals face new life events that do not fit in well with the construct of themselves, or when newly formed constructs are inconsistent with older ones, a need for change or "reconstruction" is indicated.

Constructivist vs. Rationalist Views

Restructuring one's personality or identity of one's human self is a lifelong process, intertwining experiences from one's past and present interactions and relationships with others and one's internal and external reactions to those experiences. The self and the system within which it exists continually interact and co-construct in a developmental process as shapes and substances of their boundaries change (Mahoney, 1991).

Constructivists acknowledge the self as a lifelong organizing process that embodies patterns of affect, meaning construction, action, and other experiential aspects. Ultimately, all experience is thought to come from the realm of the self, where its possibilities and limitations are determined. In comparing constructivist theory with rationalist psychotherapies, a term used by Mahoney (1991) to group cognitive, behavioral, and other approaches together, he interprets rationalist therapies as emphasizing the control of self by means of ritualized techniques. Where constructivist therapy considers intense emotions as powerful allies and expressions of peoples' past and future development, Mahoney believes that rationalist approaches regard intense

Reconceptualizing the Self

and undesired emotions as constituting the clients' problems, and that the central goal in therapy is the modification of these emotions. For that reason, Mahoney sees rationalist therapists as operating from an authority-based perspective, justifying their practices as interventional or corrective measures. Most rationalist-interventionist approaches are also teleological (goal-directed), ahistorical, and homeostatic (pursuing a return to a static equilibrium), according to Mahoney, while the evolutionary, developmental, and constructivist perspectives are teleonomic (directed, but not by a single, explicit goal), historical and socioculturally sensitive and homeorhetic (dynamically self-organizing).

The purpose of this book is not to defend one therapy approach against any others, but to explore them briefly within the context of the overall counseling process. As before, case studies serve well in the illustration of the formation of an individual's concept of self.

Case Study

Kent: Changed Outlook

Kent, the widowed father of two children last encountered in Chapter 7, made a follow-up appointment with his counselor. He was defining himself differently.

Couns: Thank you for the note you sent me, filling me in on your success at the family conference some time ago. I was pleased to know that your hard work in preparing yourself really paid off. What would you like to discuss today?

Kent: For once, I don't have a real problem. The kind of preparation I did for the family conference worked so well, as I told you, I have used similar approaches in different situations. In my job, I find it much more helpful to prepare myself when I have to discuss one of our author's works with the author. Of course, I have always known the content of the discussion, but now I take the time to think about how the author would feel about a certain statement, how he or she would likely respond to suggested changes, and how I want to act and feel in the situation. People at work have commented that I am very

	supportive of the authors and that any changes or suggestions are usually well accepted. I enjoy my work and I am about halfway through on my first draft for my book.
Couns:	That sounds exciting. I remember you were thinking about writing a book when we first met. Now you are actually on your way. Also, the way you are describing your interactions with your authors, it seems that the process of preparing and considering what others may feel and say has become almost second nature to you.
Kent:	Right. It feels almost natural now, not like an act or like manipulation. The way I see it, is that I take the time to think more in depth about the person I am going to interact with. In considering the other person's feelings, I can avoid unfriendly confrontations even if we happen to disagree. In a way, I conduct the meetings through my preparations, but I try to do it in such a way that nobody loses. I am using that approach more with my children, too, and it works well. I am much more open with my feelings now. I remember that when I first saw you, I was convinced I had to put my feelings aside when making decisions; now they are an integral part of the whole process.
Couns:	At the time, you wanted to be sure to make the best decision for your children. You took your responsibilities as a father very seriously.
Kent:	I think I was afraid then. Deep down, I did not think I was a good person. I put myself down for getting Marilyn pregnant before our wedding and for not giving her the promise she asked of me when she died. I was not emotionally open because I thought people would find out what a bad person I really was. Now I have learned that I am all right as a person; I am not a saint, but I am not an evil person either. Some of my behaviors in the past have been wrong, but I am trying to learn from them, hoping to avoid making additional mistakes. One source of great satisfaction for me is my relationship with my children. They are great kids and Marilyn had done a wonderful job of raising them as long as she could. I feel I am continuing to raise them according to our values. The three of us have a close and comfortable relationship. I am not hiding my feelings from them and encourage them to tell me how they feel.

Couns: You have learned a lot. I am glad you have accepted yourself as a person who makes mistakes at times, as we all do. We can evaluate our actions and behaviors, but if we evaluate ourselves as persons in terms of the behaviors, we would flip-flop back and forth from good person to bad person and back to good person as our behaviors fluctuate. There are so many facets of a person, so many roles as a husband, father, employee, friend, child of your own parents, and many others. If we don't do well as an employee for some reason, does that mean all the other facets of our person are not good either? It is not a workable concept to rate oneself as a good or bad person. You have done a marvelous job as a father and you can pass on to your children your ideas about self-acceptance as persons and to rate or measure only their traits and performances.

Kent: That is a very good lesson, and it was high time I learned it. I am trying to look at my children the same way, and I want them to love me as their father but to be able to realize that I am as fallible as any human being. They are growing up fast now. In less than 2 years my daughter will set out to go to college. My son is going to camp this summer. I hope my daughter will decide to go to a local college. Not only would it be cheaper on the tuition, but I would like to be able to have her around us a little longer. Those are selfish reasons and if it is in her best interest to go to college in another state, we will work on that.

Couns: It sounds like you are preparing yourself to let them go. In your situation, the bonds you have formed with your children are especially close and strong. Letting go while keeping the mental and emotional closeness does take some preparation for your relationship with your children and for you yourself, as your daily life changes without them. Your daily responsibilities will be reduced, but some feelings of loneliness may appear. It will take another adjustment for you to go through.

Kent: Indeed, it will be an adjustment. I have thought about it and I don't want to be a possessive parent who keeps the children from reaching their independence. Also, I have thought about finding a companion for myself again. I liked married life. At the family meeting, I saw Marilyn's cousin again. There is still an attraction for me. She is divorced now and I would like to get to know her again. Before taking any steps, I wanted to make sure that my children will be safe emotionally. There will be situations in which they may not want to share all their thoughts with me, and I would like for them to have an objective listener whom they can trust. I want them to meet you. They already know a lot about you and the help you have given me. Would you think it appropriate to bring them in to meet you, not for any current therapy, but to make a connection for the future in case it is needed or wanted? I thought if they get to know you and feel comfortable with you, it would be so much easier for them to call on you if they need guidance.

Couns: That is an excellent idea. You are taking your parenting responsibilities very seriously by planning ahead for possible future needs. I feel privileged that you trust me with your children's happiness. Getting to know them will be both a pleasure and a challenge, a pleasure because they are your children and a challenge because we want them to be the happiest they can be with their lives. We will set up a convenient meeting time whenever you are ready.

Summary of Client-Counselor Interaction: Changed Outlook. In this session, the client described the changes in his self-perception from the beginning of therapy to the current time. The problem-solving approaches that he had learned in his sessions he had applied to his personal and his professional life. In both areas, he had made significant strides to the point that the adopted behavioral approaches had become part of his natural way of thinking and acting. The client found that his method of preparing himself mentally and emotionally for important interactions had increased his sense of competence and effectiveness in professional encounters, as well as in his role as primary caregiver to his children.

The counselor praised the client for his progress and emphasized the importance of accepting ourselves as human beings without evaluating ourselves as good or bad, but instead focusing on actions and behaviors as ratable entities if appropriate. True to his new pattern, the client expressed his plans of preparing himself and his children for their increased independence in the future and for his own search for a new companion. Based on his own experiences, he thought it best to provide his children with an objective and understanding listener who would be able to guide them toward their own goals if they wanted to avail themselves of professional assistance.

SUMMARY

The timing of explorations of self or reconceptualizing the self is crucial to the success of the overall learning process. Confronting clients with issues of self-concept or change thereof could be extremely frightening and discouraging. First of all, the often painful challenge of looking at oneself is better accomplished when a supportive and trusting therapeutic relationship has been established. The client needs to feel safe in order to disclose and share with anyone the deepest thoughts and feelings of self. Secondly, the notion of possible changes in the structure of self is a threatening one, considering the emotional investment that people have in their own self-concepts. Again, a safe and trusting atmosphere is necessary to embark on this task. Thirdly, it is easier to help people realize that change is possible after they have already made some strides and seen small successes. Reconceptualizing the self at this point in the counseling process leads to the conceptualizing of the self in the larger framework—the worlds we share with significant others in our environment and the world at large around us—both stretching beyond the sphere of our own intrapersonal worlds.

In the view of self-consistency theory, most problems are due to defects in the major philosophy of individuals, rather than due to unhappy experiences (Lecky, 1969). The constellation of the person's system of values and attitudes, in combination with the individual's actions, may give rise to inconsistencies in the person's awareness of self and thereby lead to discomfort. A fundamental characteristic of human nature seems to be the tendency to maintain a self-consistent organization. In accepting one particular value, the person is opposed to accepting other values that are not consistent with the already accepted value. The therapist's task is to assist the client in reexamining and modifying old values that block the individual's further development, generating a new and more congruent general outlook.

The young woman Kahla could not conceive of herself as a person who could make decisions, even where the most important areas of her own life were concerned. When her first attempt at seeking help from a therapist did not bring about the desired response, namely telling her what to do, she turned to another person, her mother-in-law, for her needs. Resisting inconsistencies in her awareness of herself came at a high price, and only after several painful consequences of her actions was she willing to look at alternatives. Rather than avoiding making decisions altogether, as she had done in the past, Kahla slowly learned to consider possible outcomes of choosing one or another path before selecting the one that held the best promise for a desirable outcome. Owning the responsibility for the outcomes gradually not only increased her sense of self-confidence, but also became congruent with her self-concept of a single and independent woman and mother of her young child.

A similar process can be traced in Ruth's case. As a "welfare mother," her assessment of herself as a person caused her much shame and embarrassment. Her initial self-concept had been that of a victim of her mother's treatment of her. She saw herself as absolutely helpless in the pursuit of her own goals. Regarding the few decisions she had made as wrong decisions only confirmed her low estimation of herself. Although she acknowledged that her own actions, such as to marry her husband to get away from her mother, were instrumental in her ultimately being dependent on welfare assistance, she still considered herself as helpless. Through her work in counseling, she learned to explore opportunities and take well-calculated risks, behaviors that had been inconsistent with her old self-image. Gradually, she reconstructed herself in the image of an independent, goal-oriented woman and mother and active participant in her community. She symbolized the process of her growth by assuming her full given name instead of using a shortened version she had responded to for most of her life.

Finally, Kent, the young widowed father who believed that emotions were inappropriate considerations when making important life decisions, learned the value of including his own feelings and those of others into the process of choosing and planning. By doing so, he was able to prepare himself for selecting his best options and to explain his choices to others when appropriate to gain needed support.

EXERCISE

Construct your own self-concept. At what age did you become aware of a concept of self? Has it remained the same since then? If not, what changes have you become aware of over the years? What factors initiated the changes—internal? External or situational? How does your self-concept compare with the perceptions others may have of you? Is it congruent with your own view of yourself? Is it different? If so, what might be different in the way others perceive you? Is there anything you would like to change about your concept of yourself? If so, what would you like to change? Do you think, changes are possible? If so, how would you start?

List the characteristics that in your opinion are or would be significantly related to your self-esteem. On your list, mark the ones that you think you possess with a "p," the ones you desire but may not have yet with a "d." Do the "p's" outnumber the "d's"? If not, devise a plan of action on how to accomplish that.

SUGGESTED READING

Bandura, A. (1977b). Self-efficacy: Toward a unifying theory of behavioral change. *Psychological Review, 84,* 191–215.
   The author presents a theoretical framework to explain and predict psychological changes achieved by different treatment modalities. Psychological procedures are thought of altering the level and strength of self-efficacy. Hypotheses on how expectations of personal efficacy influence initiation, maintenance, and persistence of coping behaviors are presented.
Ellis, A. (1973). *Humanistic psychotherapy: The rational-emotive approach.* New York: Julian.
   The author discusses the advantages for people in refraining from rating themselves at all as persons and instead accurately assessing their traits and deeds.
Mahoney, M. J. (1991). *Human change processes.* New York: Basic Books.
   The author examines basic assumptions about human change processes, identifying common themes and experience patterns associated with change. The roles of emotionality and cognitive processes are emphasized. Chapter 9, "The Self in Process," is of particular interest here.

Rogers, C. R. (1961). *On becoming a person.* Boston, MA: Houghton Mifflin.
Chapters provide an account of client-centered theory and the role of therapist's unconditional positive regard in facilitating the client's unconditional regard of self. The author discusses emotional distress as resulting from incongruence between a client's ideal self and real self.

11

Coordinating and Balancing the Worlds We Live In

OBJECTIVES

1. To facilitate clients' general comprehension of functioning in the different spheres of their lives.
2. To aid clients in their recognition of the significance of a healthy balance among the different spheres.
3. To promote clients' understanding that maintaining the balance is an ongoing process.
4. To introduce the idea that different sets of values are appropriate for functioning in the three spheres.
5. To integrate the stages of the counseling process into its culmination: a holistic and balanced view of the client's overall life.
6. To signal the termination of the counseling process for the present.

THE WORLDS WE LIVE IN

As clients have moved through the counseling process, having identified and selected problem areas to work on; have become aware of why some of their approaches in the past have not brought the desired results and have gained knowledge from those past experiences; have learned various coping skills, have tried them, and fine-tuned them with continued practice; have evaluated their new skills and frequently applied them to other problem areas; and, finally, have reorganized in their minds their perceptions of themselves and their capabilities, the time has come to integrate all those individual experiences with the world at large. Most people do not live in vacuums, and whatever new behaviors and skills clients have incorporated into their own repertoires, undoubtedly, there will be effects felt in the clients' environments. The counseling process cannot be regarded as finished or complete without giving attention to clients' continuing interactions with others around them.

THE EFFECTS OF ROLE BALANCE ON VARIOUS INDICATORS OF WELL-BEING

When discussing individuals and their adaptation to their environments, the literature has focused on various aspects. Marks and MacDermid (1996) consider the ways that people create and organize their roles and identities as an empirical question. In their opinion, people have an implicit knowledge of how their different roles fit together. Their choices of what to do next, what role to attend to, is seen as following episodic rather than continual patterns. In conjunction with their work toward a middle-range theory of role balance, the authors conducted two studies on role balance, using planned comparisons to test their hypotheses that people with more balanced role systems will report less role strain, more role ease, greater well-being, and more positive role-specific experience than people with less balanced role systems. They expected no significant association between role balance and restriction of one's overall activities.

Role Balance and Role Ease Defined

The authors' conceptual innovations of role balance and role ease were explained as follows: Role balance is seen as a general orientation across roles rather than a role-specific one; role balance consists of a behavioral pattern of acting across roles in certain ways and a cognitive-affective pattern of organizing multiple selves in one's conception; role ease is the ease felt by the individuals in carrying out their role performances. The authors proposed as a theory linking these variables together, in that role ease is generated by role balance and the lack of role balance results in role strain.

Study 1. For the initial test of their theory, the authors had a sample of 65 employed wives and mothers, each having at least one child under age 18 years living at home. The average age of the participants was in the mid-thirties, and they had been married on the average for 15 years. Their work experience in their current positions had been 34.4 months on the average.

The instruments employed were a single-item measure related to enjoyment across the role system to be rated on a five-point scale for the role balance variable and four pairs of different role combinations for the role ease variable. In addition, role overload was assessed with an eight-item role-strain scale. Other indicators of well-being, tapping depression, mastery, and innovativeness were used. On the basis of their ratings on the single role-balance item, the participants were placed in three groups. The findings supported the predictions that the women in the more role-balanced group would score significantly higher on most measures for role ease and positive functioning than would the women in the less role-balanced group. In addition, the more balanced group showed significantly less tendency to restrict their avocational activities than did the nonbalanced group.

Study 2. A second study, involving 179 male and 123 female full-time college students, most of whom were employed and were either married or in a serious romantic relationship in addition to leading an active social life. Participants were presented with an eight-item role balance scale (expanded from the previous single-item measure), an eight-item scale for role overload (the same as in the previous study), and a five-item role-ease scale to assess the independent variable (role balance) and the key dependent variables (role overload and role ease). Other measures covered self-esteem, depression, and, for positive role functioning, academic grade point average and number of friends with whom the participant has weekly good times. A tension scale, consisting of eight items and to be rated on a four-point scale, was also included.

Forming groups based on the single-item measure as in the previous study, it was found that the role-balanced students had significantly higher role ease and self-esteem, but less role overload and depression, than the students scoring lower on role balance. Using a median split on the eight-item Role Balance Scale produced two groups for planned comparisons across all the dependent variables. Analysis of variance revealed that all hypothesized mean differences were significant. The role-balanced students reported significantly lower role overload and depression, as well as significantly higher self-esteem and role ease, than was found for the students with lower scores on role balance. The role-balanced students also had significantly higher grade point averages than the less role-balanced students. No significant differences were found between male and female students.

On purpose, the authors avoided considering a hierarchical role organization, where people are assumed to experience more enjoyment when they are engaging in some roles than when participating in others. Their decision was based on the notion that the more balanced individuals felt about all their roles, the higher their self-esteem would be. The authors cautioned that their findings do not predict causality concerning their key variables. While greater role balance is positively correlated with role ease and negatively correlated with role strain, it cannot be said that greater role balance causes individuals to experience less strain and more role ease. The possibility exists that higher role balance is a consequence of less role strain and increased role ease.

In an analysis of single mothers in Canada (Morrison et al., 1986), the authors said that single women represent a large constituency with specific characteristics and needs. They recommend training in job-search skills and peer counseling that would be directed toward role strain, family benefits, and employment.

Another aspect to consider is the fact that the configuration of roles changes over the individual's life, not only as a function of maturation, but also due to declining abilities or reduced need for some of the roles as people go through the aging process. Rather than a static entity, role balance then must be conceptualized as a process that may require periodic adjustments. When people who have previously been parenting partners emerge as single parents through divorce, widowhood, or other life circumstances, their role balances become labile and unbalanced for a while until a new equilibrium or balance is achieved.

Role Reduction and the Effect on Personal Identity

For many people, work furnishes them with a role or personal identity and also creates a sense of community and belonging. The working person is part of a group and has a role in the community of coworkers. Even better, when one is engaged in productive work activities that provide focus and purpose, the benefits extend well beyond the rewards of a paycheck. Thus, working people may adjust somewhat easier to being single again than non-working individuals, even with the added responsibilities that come with single parenthood.

On the other hand, unemployed individuals who return to a single life may experience a feeling of emptiness, even while busy with activities of daily living, caring for their own and their children's needs. Their time may be occupied, but their skills and talents may remain insufficiently challenged. They may feel bored amidst anxiety about making time for all the necessary but not intrinsically rewarding daily activities. According to Csikszentmihalyi (1990), between boredom and anxiety, an optimal state of "flow" exists where both our time and skills are engaged in a meaningful challenge. The concept of flow came out of Csikszentmilhalyi's studies of artists who engaged for many hours with great concentration in their activities of painting or sculpting. As they immersed themselves in their projects, nothing else seemed to matter. The author concluded that joyful absorption in meaningful activities is a major source of happiness and well-being that lies within the individual.

Case Study

Lynn: Perceived Lack of Personal Competence

Lynn was first encountered in an earlier chapter when she worked on resolving fears and anxiety relating to her church attendance.

During her marriage, Lynn had not been employed outside the home. She had devoted all her time to the well-being of her husband and their two sons. After the family was settled in their new environment, having been relocated through her husband's employer, Lynn started to do some volunteer work at the local art museum. She had a Bachelor's degree in fine arts, but never perceived herself as sufficiently talented to be successful as an artist. Her perceptions were shared and encouraged by her husband. After the divorce, she worked in a part-time position as sales associate in an up-scale department store to supplement the child-support payments from her husband. She continued with her monthly volunteer work at the museum because it was something she enjoyed just for herself. Lynn could not afford regular counseling sessions and after she had overcome her disabling anxiety attacks, she kept in contact with her therapist on an as-needed basis.

Couns: You sounded upset when you scheduled this appointment yesterday. What happened to cause your discomfort?

Lynn: Thank you for making time for me on such short notice. I had a discussion with my former husband and I just lost it. I cried all the way home when I picked up the boys from his place. My sons were very concerned about me and called their father while I was in the bathroom washing my face. That made me think it was time to come and see you.

Couns: What led up to this? Can you tell me, or do you need a few minutes to calm yourself down?

Lynn: It's a long story, but those deep breathing exercises you taught me helped me to get myself calmed down enough to go to work and come here. Perhaps you remember that I still volunteer at the art museum. One of the women has been doing a newsletter for the group of volunteers to keep us informed about various events and activities. She had an accident and will be unable to continue with the newsletter for quite some time. She asked for help from the rest of us. I offered to do what I could to keep the newsletter going.

Couns: Yes, I remember your activities at the museum and the enjoyment you derived from that. Offering to help with the newsletter was very kind of you, and I hope it will be

	a source of additional enjoyment for you along with the stress of the added responsibility.
Lynn:	Yes, it is more work, but I feel good about it. I feel like I am creating something. I know, "creating" is a big word for a little thing like a newsletter. While my sons are doing their homework, they let me use their computer. Of course, they know much more about computers than I do, but they try to help me. In fact, I had quite a few compliments for my attempts. One of the people in the commercial arts department, where museum brochures are produced, suggested that I take some classes in graphic design and computer artwork, because she thought I showed talent in that area. When I was in college, we did not have much exposure to computer artwork; it was too new.
Couns:	That sounds great. I am sure the lady recognized your talents and did not say that only to make you feel good. She is a professional in the field and she would know. Are you planning on acting on her suggestions?
Lynn:	I did. I found out about two classes that are given back to back at the art school. One is on graphic design in general and the other is computer applications in graphic design. The instructor recommended that I take both classes at the same time, because one builds on the other and it would enhance the practice of studies. I was ready to enroll when I realized that the classes were both given on Thursday evenings. With paying for the tuition I could not really afford a weekly babysitter.
Couns:	You seem quite excited about taking the classes. It sounds like a good opportunity for you to try out how far your talents will lead you. Is there anyone who might be able to help you out with supervising your sons?
Lynn:	My ex-husband has the boys on Wednesday night and I thought he might be willing to trade nights with me. When I told him about my plans of taking the classes, he said spending the money on taking art classes was a complete waste. I would never amount to anything. All I could think about is spending money and if I had time left over to volunteer and to go to classes, I would be better off working full-time as a sales clerk to meet my financial responsibilities.
Couns:	Your attempt to exchange visitation nights seems like a

	reasonable approach on your part. It is sad that he would not be agreeable to that.
Lynn:	That's not all. He told me that he could not continue indefinitely to pay as much child support as he does now. In fact, he is planning to get married again. His current girlfriend is pregnant and wants a family. After all, she is entitled to have children of her own. He may have to go back to court to have the child-support payments lowered. I am just selfish and not a good mother if I think of my own interests before taking care of my children. I should consider myself lucky to be able to work as a sales clerk. That's the best I could ever expect to do with my shortcomings.
Couns:	That was a terrible experience for you, no wonder you were so upset. How do you feel now?
Lynn:	I still feel awful, but he is probably right; I had my hopes up too high. He knows me and is more objective than I am about my abilities, and as a good mother I should put my children's well-being first.
Couns:	Are you saying you believe him? If you do not consider your children first at all times, that makes you a bad mother? Where do you draw the line in considering your own needs? Does it make him a bad father if your ex-husband does not agree to take care of your children when needed? Regarding your talents, what about the lady who praised your work? She would seem to be just as objective, possibly more so than your ex-husband.
Lynn:	Perhaps she was just being nice to me. She has not known me as long as my husband has.
Couns:	I can't tell you who is more neutral, your husband or the woman at the museum, when it comes to evaluating your talents. You seem to ascribe some predictive qualities to your ex-husband's pronouncements, though. I wonder how warranted that is. Can you think of any predictions he made and that have come true, as far as you know?
Lynn:	Well, he did say that I would probably ruin the car by forgetting to bring it in for oil changes and other services. That was his reason for giving me our old Toyota van and keeping the Mercedes for himself. He also thought the boys would lose all sense of discipline living with me and that he would have a hard time straightening them out again on his weekends with them. Oh, I remember an-

other occasion. We had just moved into our house and neighbors of ours had bought several young magnolia trees for their yard. They ended up having one more than they had space for, and she asked me one morning if I wanted it. She did not charge me anything for it. I was so happy about her kindness that I planted it the very same day. When I told my husband, he said it was planted in the wrong spot, there wasn't enough sunshine and it would probably die soon anyway. I pleaded with him to help me replant it in a better spot because I would feel guilty if I did not take good care of the tree the neighbor had given me. He was too busy to do it, preparing for a business trip he was going to take in a couple of days.

Couns: Did you ruin your car?

Lynn: No, it's running fine. I always mark it on my calendar when to take it in for service.

Couns: I haven't heard you complain about your sons' being out of control. You never mentioned having any problems with them, is that correct? And how is your magnolia tree doing?

Lynn: Oh, I see what you are doing. No, my sons are not out of control. Sometimes they get a bit excited with an activity and don't want to stop when I tell them to, but all in all, they are pretty good kids. And my magnolia tree is doing just fine; it had beautiful blossoms last spring. Next spring I'll take a picture and show you.

Couns: Please do that, I think that would be an excellent thing to do. You can use it as evidence that your ex-husband is not always right. Perhaps it is possible that the predictive quality of his statements is mixed with some wishful thinking. You would probably know that better than I.

Lynn: Are you saying that he puts me down because he does not want me to succeed and not because I am not able to do anything right?

Couns: As I said, I don't know him, but it appears to me that you are as capable as anybody. For some reason you don't seem to have as much confidence in yourself as would be desirable. We could explore the underlying reasons for that. I think the picture of your magnolia tree would be a good start for collecting evidence of what you can do. Actually, you may wish to take a picture of the tree right now and then take another one in the spring? Now is the time to start looking at your abilities in a realistic way. Have you thought about your sister as a resource person to look after your sons on Thursday evenings? From what you said, the classes seem to be something of great personal interest to you and they may lead to other rewarding activities.

Lynn: I will ask my sister. I just thought it would be easier to trade days with my ex-husband. After his remark I felt so crushed that I did not have the courage to even think further about it. As you said, it is something important to me personally. When my ex-husband called me selfish, I felt guilty for wanting this training for myself instead of just being there for my children. I need to learn what is appropriate for me to want for myself without harming my children.

Couns: Under the circumstances, it is natural that you felt guilty, because you have been in the habit of not only seeing yourself as less competent than you are but also as selfish if you wanted something for yourself. You are right, now is the time to take the next step in your divorce. In order to assess your competencies and talents realistically and independently from your former husband, you need to reinforce the mental and emotional separation from him. It is your responsibility and opportunity to create your own worlds, the one that is your very personal sphere and the ones you are sharing with others around you.

Summary of Client-Counselor Interaction: Perceived Lack of Personal Competence. As the above session demonstrated, the client perceived herself as lacking competence when confronted by her former husband. She also did not have a well-defined concept about herself as being in a position to fulfill some personal interests. The counselor expressed understanding for the pain she experienced in the confrontation with her ex-husband, but used every opportunity to examine the validity of and evidence for her beliefs that her ex-husband's knowledge of her competence, or lack thereof, was correct. When suggesting that she not wait until Spring, but take a picture of her magnolia tree now, the counselor emphasized the client's need for assuming control and fortifying her actions with evidence immediately.

Because the client was still vulnerable to her ex-husband's criticism, the therapist indicated that as a completion of the divorce process, her responsibility was to achieve mental and emotional independence. As another future-oriented goal-directed activity, the counselor introduced the opportunity of creating her own worlds for herself and for the significant others around her.

Subjective Well-Being and the Balance of Interests. New research on psychological well-being has focused on various components contributing to a theory of happiness. Values and goals constitute one such component. As people identify goals for themselves and are able to progress toward them without significant interference from other goals, they are predictors of people's subjective well-being (Emmons, 1986). Involvement in valued activities and progress toward identified goals is more likely to result in happiness than existing more or less passively in a desirable situation or environment (Diener & Larsen, 1993). In proposing a balance theory of wisdom, Robert Sternberg (1998) defined wisdom as the application of practical intelligence to the process of establishing a balance of various self-interests of individuals with the interests of others and of other aspects of the environment.

In other words, wisdom is seen as a balance of intrapersonal, interpersonal, and extrapersonal interests or goals. Wisdom, as a special case of practical intelligence, requires the equalizing of multiple and often competing goals or interests. Individuals using practical intelligence may pursue outcomes that are of benefit to the individual and significant others, but not necessarily to the world at large. Through a balance of adapting, shaping, and selecting environments, intrapersonal, interpersonal, and extrapersonal interests are equalized toward the achievement of a common good.

Self in World

The notion of intrapersonal, interpersonal, and extrapersonal interests seems reminiscent of Ludwig Binswanger's (1962) little-known—or little-used—concept of the human existence occurring in three worlds, the *Eigenwelt*\\'ī-gen-velt\ or personal world, the *Mitwelt*

\'mit-velt\ or interpersonal world, and the *Umwelt*\ 'úm-velt\, the environment or larger world around us (see Chapter 3). Looking back into the literature, there seem to have been some incomplete understandings or misinterpretations of Binswanger's concept. For instance, Rychlak (1973) mentioned that Binswanger's *Eigenwelt* refers to the person's bodily sphere of experience. Basically this statement is not incorrect, but it fails to include other significant aspects of intrapersonal experiences.

In reading Binswanger's (1962) original version, the understanding emerges that all aspects of a person—the body, the mental life, the emotions, and all the experiences—constitute the individual's *Eigenwelt*. Similar incomplete interpretations (Needleman, 1963; Rychlak, 1973) are reflected in defining the *Umwelt* as being the environment, including both animate and inanimate features of existence. The *Mitwelt* is referred to as the social world, including all those things we mean when we speak of "society." Following those interpretations, there would hardly be a distinction between the worlds, because the *Mitwelt* would then be a part of the *Umwelt* (which at times it is) including the animate features of the social world.

Three Worlds. To fully understand the distinctions and meanings Binswanger assigned to the three worlds, one would have to remember that Binswanger tried to comprehend and explain human nature in terms of care and love. The *Umwelt* is the sphere of care, as people care what happens around them; but in the *Mitwelt* the emphasis is not on social relations, but rather on being together with individuals in a loving way. In Binswanger's opinion, the world of love is completely different from the world of care. Both worlds have different aspects of space. The space of care is bounded all around; it is an exhaustible and finite space. In contrast, the space of love is boundless, inexhaustible, and endless. Understanding of this contrast has to occur on a logical level, but also on a phenomenal level. While the *Dasein* (existence) as care is caring about something in a certain situation, therefore, always being a limited kind of totality, the *Dasein* in the sense of love exists in a limitless, unrestricted, unconditional being-with-each-other.

Existence. Binswanger conceptualized that all phenomena occur within a meaning-matrix. Within this matrix they take on relevance for the *Dasein*, but when there are only a few dominating themes, the *Dasein* is constricted to one or two world-designs. World-designs are the modes of the individual's perceptions and reactions to the total environment. As the world-designs become fewer, existential anxiety grows until the individual's *Dasein* may exclude all but one world-design, the *Eigenwelt*. For instance, if *Mitwelt* and *Eigenwelt* are not compatible, the mounting anxiety will cause the individual to withdraw completely into the *Eigenwelt*, as is the case in psychosis. Also, the individual—due to a constricted *Dasein*—may be unable to explore future possibilities. Inability to transcend the circumstances in which the individual is positioned (or "thrown") prevents the individual from gaining any sense of achievement. As a result, drifting back—or regression—instead of expanding and growing occurs. In agreement with existentialism, Binswanger maintained that the individual is free to choose whether to transcend the difficult experiences of life, or whether to surrender to the "thrownness."

Binswanger viewed the client-therapist relationship as extremely important. In the turmoil of the client's present situation, the therapist is the steady element, aiding and protecting the client in the process of rescue. In helping the client in reconstructing the *Dasein*, *Daseinsanalyse* (existential analysis) involves more than empathy. The therapist "lives along with the client," experiencing the client's struggles with the client. Binswanger tried to find the client's particular world-design and the client's being-in-the-world. The focus in therapy is on the self-understanding of the client's current existence. The goal is the individual's freeing from the unfreedom of finite human existence, so that the individual can transcend the present situation. In obtaining a future orientation, the client becomes able to regain independence and authenticity.

Existentialists, in general, have been accused of employing a vocabulary that is regarded by many psychologists as being poetic and esoteric. Binswanger is no exception; his writings assume extremely patient readers, and are not readily interpretable. Binswanger's particular use of language probably accounts for the scarcity of translations of his works in this country. Therefore, for our purposes in counseling, we may think of human existence as occurring in three worlds or three spheres. In consideration of the overall goal of counseling or therapy, this is a useful concept. These three worlds can be more or less independent, but they frequently overlap and intersect. The client's existence as a healthy balance in the three worlds is the goal of therapy and the culmination of the successful counseling process.

While balanced existence is the goal, it is not a static goal, because the aspects of the three worlds change periodically or even continually (Maass, 1996). The goal is a process of adapting to the fluctuating elements within the individual's life spheres. As therapists, aiding clients in gaining self-understanding and ability to transcend their current troubling situations, we need to remember that dissonance and harmony among the worlds occur as functions of the various values operating in the clients' different worlds.

ILLUSTRATIONS OF THE INTERCONNECTEDNESS AND RECIPROCAL INFLUENCES OF THE THREE WORLDS

Because this phase of the counseling process is the logical conclusion of the work accomplished in previous sessions, descriptions of the progress made by clients encountered in earlier chapters will serve well to illustrate the progression to the natural culmination of the overall process. The clients presented different problem situations, aspired to different goals, and proceeded along different paths in order to reach their goals. A function of this chapter is to illustrate the concluding steps on the journeys to their goals.

Focusing on the case of Lynn, we observe that prior to her divorce, the biggest sphere of her existence was the *Mitwelt*. Here she interacted with her husband, her children, and her sister. In her *Umwelt*, activities such as talking to neighbors, interacting with sales clerks while shopping for the family's needs, and attending church and school functions for her children, occupied this sphere. Her *Eigenwelt* appeared to be rather small; in fact, it seemed to be defined and limited by forces in her *Mitwelt*. Only the time and money resources not exhausted in her *Mitwelt* were available for use in her *Eigenwelt*. Her volunteer activities at the museum seemed to be the most notable involvement in her *Eigenwelt*.

After her divorce, remarkable shifts for her occurred in the *Mitwelt* and *Umwelt*. Her husband physically moved from the *Mitwelt* into the *Umwelt*, the sphere that also had an addition from her part-time employment. Her *Eigenwelt* remained small. Perhaps that accounts in part for her anxiety attacks, because she also felt pain and insecurity from having to change her perceptions of herself as wife and mother to only mother. Her anxieties in the past indicate that she allowed the reduction in her roles to affect her concept of herself in her *Eigenwelt*. By not having a sound foundation in her *Eigenwelt*, she became increasingly more vulnerable to influences and perceptions from the other worlds. She did not have a well-defined concept of herself and her abilities and desires.

At the time of her most recent counseling session, the effects upon her *Eigenwelt* from the dominating influence of her ex-husband's opinion of her were apparent. As she tried to increase the sphere of her personal world by taking some additional art training, he not only dismissed that as selfish, but also attempted to further reduce her personal world by threatening to reduce his financial obligations. If he were successful in realizing his threats, Lynn would have to take a full-time job, leaving little time and energy for herself. Lynn's effort to involve her ex-husband in the solution for her difficulties by exchanging scheduled visitations with his children seems logical and appropriate on the surface. Her mental and emotional reactions to his response and criticism of her were understandable but not appropriate. As her ex-husband had removed himself from her *Mitwelt*—the sphere Lynn shared in loving relationships—into her *Umwelt*—the world of caring, but not loving, relationships—she allowed him entirely too much influence over her personal world.

The focus of the counseling session centered on shifting the balance of Lynn's worlds. The significance of her *Eigenwelt* was increased by adding activities that were of personal enjoyment to her, by increasing her decision-making skills, and by reducing undesirable influences from the other worlds around her. In the comparison of Lynn's ex-husband's opinion with that of the professional graphic designer at the art museum, the ex-husband was placed in the same sphere of influence with the designer (*Umwelt*), where Lynn was able to explore competencies and qualifications of both in her decision regarding the degree of impact she would allow them on her personal sphere. As the counselor pointed out, mentally and emotionally Lynn had not yet divorced herself completely from her ex-husband's influence. Placing him more firmly in the world around her, instead of keeping him in the loving sphere of the *Mitwelt*, enabled Lynn to objectively collect evidence for or against his opinions.

In comparison, the change or reduction in roles had a very different effect on Bill, the divorced father of two sons, last encountered in Chapter 9. He experienced two transitions in his worlds. Immediately after the divorce, his roles as husband and father underwent dramatic changes. He was no longer a husband, and the father role changed to a part-time role. Some of the losses in his *Mitwelt* were compensated for in becoming closer to his sister and her family and to his parents. His *Umwelt* remained generally the same for a while, until he made changes that enriched both his *Eigenwelt* and his *Umwelt* by participating in cooking classes.

The second transition occurred when Bill assumed total custody for his sons. His sons occupied a larger part of his *Mitwelt* again, but involvement with his sister's family remained as before or even increased. Functioning as a full-time single parent, mutually beneficial interactions with his sister's family increased in frequency as well as in level of intimacy. Even though time pressures and the possible consequences of an ill-advised relationship threatened part of Bill's *Eigenwelt*, he was not ready to relinquish his newly found interests. In fact, he was considering increasing his interests from cooking and nutrition to include photography. As he enlarged the boundaries of his *Eigenwelt*, his *Umwelt* grew to accommodate the people in the cooking class, the library, and possibly a photography class into the world previously occupied mainly by job-related relationships and activities. As a single parent, he also had more interactions with his sons' schools, his new neighbors, and clerks in stores where he did the family's shopping. Linda, his former wife, was still part of his and his sons' life, but she now occupied a space in his *Umwelt*, rather than as before in his *Mitwelt*. A graphic presentation (see Figure 11.1) shows the status of Bill's worlds at the end of counseling (Maass, 1996). His *Eigenwelt* includes not only such hobbies as cooking, nutrition, reading, and fishing, but also some aspects of work. In many cases, people derive a sense of personal pride or achievement that is connected to job activities, but goes beyond the interest of the paycheck because it is inherently rewarding to the person. In counseling, it is helpful to have blank poster-size diagrams of the three worlds available for clients to fill in the contents of their worlds as they proceed through the stages.

For Kent, the young widowed father of two children, the most significant changes occurred in his *Mitwelt* when his wife suddenly

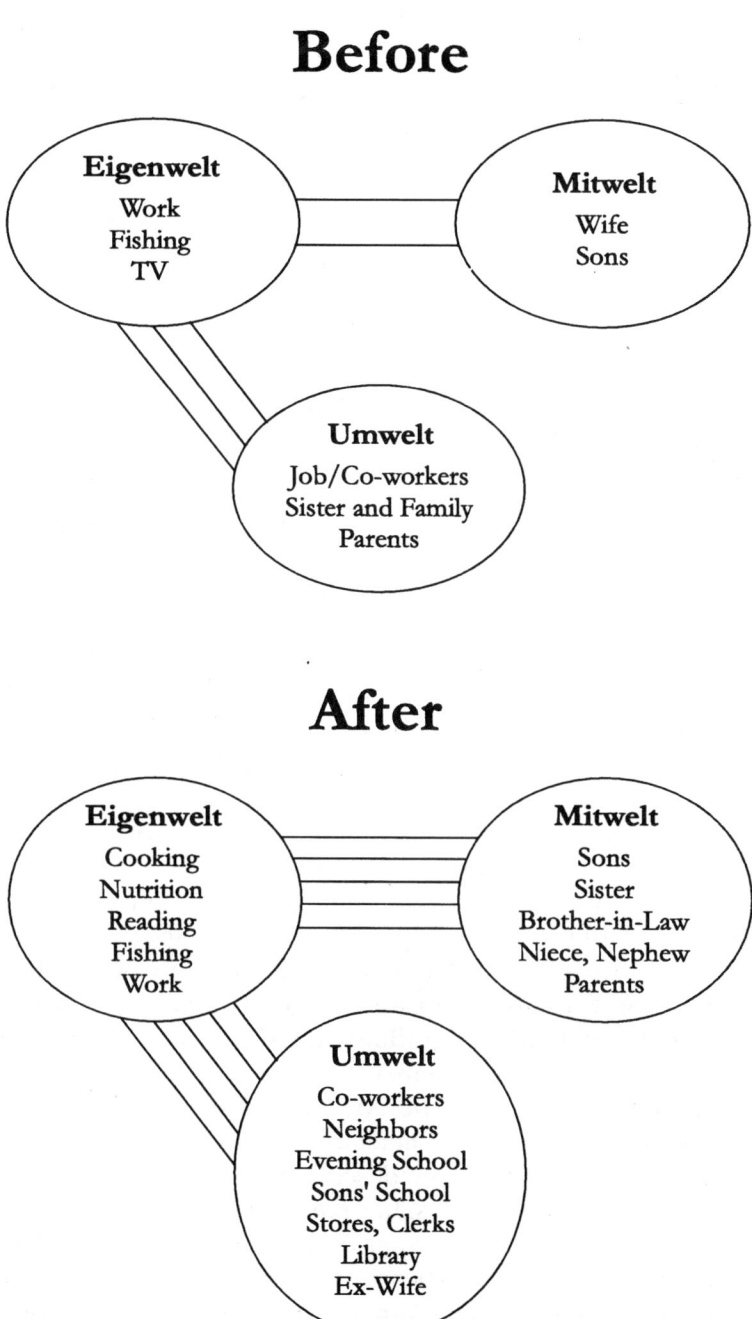

FIGURE 11.1 Bill's three worlds—before and after therapy—reveal changes in his lifestyle.

died and left him with the sole responsibility for his children. Some of the aspects of his wife's death certainly influenced his personal sphere as he struggled to resolve his guilt feelings that were connected to his wife's request for a promise and also her premarital pregnancy. In spite of increased demands on his time as the sole care provider for his children, he managed to achieve a balance between his *Mitwelt*, the sphere of his parenthood, and his *Umwelt*, the work-related world, that actually increased his opportunity for goals in his *Eigenwelt*, his writing. In addition, the attention and preparation he devoted to tasks enabled him to function quite successfully in his three spheres of living. At his most recent visit to the counselor, he was in the process of balancing his roles even more when he took steps to prepare his children for more independence while at the same time attempting to enrich his *Mitwelt* by bringing another significant person into it. He understood the fluctuating nature of his worlds and the advantage of planning and preparing as effective tools in adapting to changes.

Although changes accompanying transition to single parenthood have significant impact on both men and women, for women they often constitute opportunities for sweeping changes in their concepts of self and their roles. In other words, their *Eigenwelts* may be more profoundly affected than is the case for most men. Women, usually more so than men, perceive their personhood as connected to and reflected by the significant others in their lives, such as husbands, parents, and children. Even after divorce or widowhood, this perception lingers on, as was demonstrated in Lynn's story above and other case histories. Rather than bemoan this phenomenon as a shortcoming, the skillful therapist will help interpret and welcome the situation as an opportunity for improvement in the person's overall life.

For instance, Ruthanne, last heard from in Chapter 10 when she invited her therapist to her graduation from college, had not been able to free herself from the label of incompetent "welfare mother" bestowed upon her by her mother. In counseling, she was encouraged to explore other options for herself and finally break free of her mother's opinion. As Ruthanne described in her letter, her *Eigenwelt* had grown through her studies, her part-time work in child-care, her writing for the student newspaper, and similar activities. Although some were work-related activities, in themselves they were very exciting and stimulating as they connected to her innermost interests.

Coordinating and Balancing 319

Her *Mitwelt* still mainly consisted of her children and her close friend Becky, but her *Umwelt* had grown tremendously, as it now included interactions with people at college, at work, and the community at large that she wanted to shape in some ways. In her letter she expressed the strength and power she had gained that would enable her to shape her own destiny and perhaps make an impact on the community. Taking possession again of her full name was her way to symbolize and celebrate her identity in her worlds.

Case Study

Kahla: Final Steps to Graduation

Similarly significant changes in self-perception occurred with Kahla, whose single parenthood started out on a temporary basis at her husband's incarceration. Since then she had to make many decisions, a task she initially thought she could not handle. Her increased sense of competence brought her to yet another decision, namely to extend her single parenthood for an indefinite period of time.

Couns: The last time we met you were considering divorcing your husband, and you had explored reasons for and against the divorce. I was impressed with the thoroughness of your weighing your options and the possible consequences of choosing one over another. Have you come closer to a decision?

Kahla: Yes, I have decided to go ahead with the divorce. I thought you would be proud of me. To be absolutely sure, I decided to visit Leroy in prison one more time to discuss the terms of the divorce, but also to make sure that I was not completely acting out of my bad memories from my last visit there.

Couns: That trip must have been difficult for you, considering your previous experience. You are a courageous person, and I agree with you, looking at your husband again gives you more information about your own feelings for him.

Kahla: Information, that is what I learned in counseling about making decisions, to collect as much information as possible. You are right; the trip was very difficult. Several times along the drive I became anxious when I thought about seeing my husband again. A couple of times I had to pull over to the side of the road to calm myself down. The deep-breathing exercises came in handy. I was taking the time to challenge my thoughts and to remind myself of my goals. The drive to the prison took considerably longer than the trip back.

Couns: I am glad you were able to use the techniques you learned to your advantage. You had worked hard on your lessons. Apparently, you reaped the benefits of your work in this difficult endeavor.

Kahla: In our conversation, I was calm, but not unfriendly. I did not want to antagonize Leroy. He did not seem upset that I had not visited him. Actually, he started out by saying that he thought we had rushed into marriage too fast. Although he liked me, he realized that he was not ready to take on the responsibility of another family. He admitted that he did not want to be tied down.

Couns: Not wanting to antagonize was a wise decision on your part. The purpose of your visit was a difficult task and you did well to make it as calm as you could.

Kahla: Being calm helped, because I felt a small twinge of anger when I realized that the fact that I am not making much money in my job seemed to have cooled down his feelings for me. I was able to remind myself that the purpose of my visit was to collect information. Leroy was willing to go along with the divorce if I agreed not to ask for child support. My attorney's opinion had been that if at some time in the future I could not support my daughter, there would be a way to try for financial help from him because paternity had been established. Of course, there are no guarantees, but I thought that was about the best I could expect. My intention is to work hard enough to take care of our needs and getting any money out of Leroy seems unlikely anyway.

Couns: I am glad you considered the advice of an attorney before you acted on your plans. What were your feelings about Leroy during your visit? Did you find out what you had gone there for?

Kahla: That part was a bit surprising. My expectations, or perhaps my hopes, were that I would dislike him intensely. In spite of the brief anger, there were moments when I had some warm feelings for him. More than anything, his voice had

	always made me feel that I wanted to be near him. I was shocked to realize that. What saved me from becoming weak was when I told myself to listen to his words rather than to be carried away by the sound of his voice. I didn't like the words; it was like hearing a song with a beautiful melody but empty lyrics.
Couns:	What a beautiful and fitting analogy! Your thinking has served you well. You took a big step and you came out with big gains. It sounds as if you are ready to put that part of your life aside.
Kahla:	Yes, the agreements are signed and my attorney filed the papers for the divorce. Everything is moving smoothly. My reasons for wanting the divorce to be in effect soon are that I think I need to go on with my own life, but also that I was getting worried that Leroy would want to live off of my little income after his release from prison. I admit, it was not a nice thought.
Couns:	Considering the sad experiences of your short marriage, thoughts like the one you mentioned are understandable and actually quite rational. From what you told me in the past, he never supported you financially, except for the room and board you received from his mother. How is your relationship with your mother-in-law now? Does she know about the divorce?
Kahla:	I told her as soon as the papers were filed. For the help she has given me and my daughter, I thought she deserved to know the truth. Her reaction was another surprise. She thought that I was abandoning her son in his time of need, but she seemed to have expected that after we had moved out of her home. She added that she would always be there for Leroy, even if everybody else deserted him. What was strange is that she did not ask at all about my daughter. She acted as if she had forgotten her granddaughter. Although I don't quite understand it, I think it will make it easier to end that relationship.
Couns:	With all the pain inherent in your decisions and living through them, you seem to have put another part of your past aside. What are your plans for the future? I remember you mentioned the wish to obtain more training in the field of accounting.
Kahla:	You remember everything your clients tell you, like you are living with us between sessions, even if we don't see

you. Considering all the detours I had placed in my life, I decided not to waste any more time. I picked up some information about studies in accounting. If I get accepted, I could start with one or two classes. They would count some of my secretarial and bookkeeping classes toward the degree. After I got that information, I talked to my boss. He was very encouraging and told me to write up a proposal about my plans. He was willing to support it and pass it on to the next higher level in the company. According to him, my plans seemed sound, and most likely the company will assist me because they could use my future skills somewhere within the company.

Couns: Great work! You are making great strides within your life. You are busy planning and changing several parts of your life at the same time.

Kahla: That's exactly how I feel. My life has become different. There seems to be so much more of it than before. I don't quite know how to say it.

Couns: Perhaps I can help you to conceptualize it. Most peoples' lives occupy different spheres—almost like different worlds. One part we share with those we love, usually our spouses, children, parents, siblings, and perhaps very close friends. In another part, we interact with others in less intimate but still caring ways, such as friends, teachers, more distant relatives, colleagues, neighbors, and so on. The third part is for ourselves our own feelings, interests, desires, hopes, goals, and accomplishments. To live and function in all three worlds is necessary for a healthy and meaningful existence. Our own personal world is where we get a lot of strength and where healing takes place. That does not mean that we are isolated there. Strength and healing also occur through interactions in the intimate world we share with significant others and, to a degree, in the larger world around us.

Kahla: That makes sense to me. The kind of intimate world, as you described it, was supposed to be shared with my husband, my daughter, and maybe my mother-in-law. With the divorce it will be a very small world, just my daughter and myself and my close friend from my previous job—is that correct? The larger world would be the people where I work and my classmates if I go to school. Some of my neighbors, the people where I shop, and the librarian

	where I get my books and videos, would be in there too. My goal to become an accountant—would that be in my very personal world, even though the school, teachers, and classmates would be in the larger world?
Couns:	Yes, that is correct. You really seem to understand the concept well. In addition to our functioning in those three worlds, we need to be aware that different values are operating in the different worlds. Usually, the values operating in our own personal sphere are of a competitive nature, involving things we want for ourselves, such as your degree in accounting or books you might read for your own benefit and enjoyment. In the world we share with our significant others, just acting out of a competitive value system would not lead to a harmonious life with those important to us. Here we employ a more cooperative value system, because we want our interactions to be mutually beneficial and enjoyable. If we were to only consider our own desires and not pay attention to the wishes of those important to us, we would end up taking advantage of them and possibly losing them in the end. In the larger world around us both types of values come into play, depending on the situations.

Let's take the situation of your going to school as an example. There will be a certain amount of competition for grades, but cooperation with your classmates will also be needed, as you may have to work as teams on some projects. You may also need their help in getting notes for classes that you may have to miss for some reason. Especially in your situation, being the single parent of a small child, there may be times you have to stay at home when your child is ill. At those times, the help of a classmate will be very important to you and, in return, you may want to be there for others if they want your assistance. |
| Kahla: | You are saying that in my own personal world I am thinking mostly of my wishes, but in the other two worlds there are give-and-take situations. That sounds logical to me. If I were to think only of myself in those worlds, people would shy away from me and not be there for me when I need them. |
| Couns: | You have a good understanding of the concept. Another aspect to remember about the worlds we live in, is that although we strive for a healthy balance of all three of our |

worlds, the balance is not a static situation that remains the same once we have achieved it. In fact, as situations and circumstances change in our lives, different people enter and exit the world we share with significant others and the world we share with those around us in the larger context. To successfully accommodate for those shifts, our beliefs and values that operate within our worlds may need adjustments from time to time. Therefore, the balance is really a process of continually selecting for and adapting to experiences that occur in the worlds we live in.

Kahla: What you just explained really helps me understand my situation. I have always been pretty much alone, but lately I have thought that I would want to be with other people. Not only to have someone to ask for help when I need it, but also to exchange some ideas about what is going on in the world. Although I won't have much time, I want to make some friends and I know I will have to give and do my share. If I had not been so isolated in the past, I might have recognized the risky situations I was getting myself into, believing I had found the great love of my life.

Couns: You have grown so much as a person. The price you paid was high, but you have learned a lot about yourself. The whole growth process, starting with identifying problem areas, finding out about attempts that did not bring the desired results but could serve as learning experiences, to practicing your skills and techniques and applying them to other situations, to finally reevaluating your perception of yourself and your competencies has brought you to the knowledge of yourself and how you function in relation to the worlds around you. The last step is a point of graduation for all the learning that occurred up to this point. Graduation to this point will be a solid foundation from where to build your future life.

Summary of Client-Counselor Interaction: Final Steps to Graduation. With the decision to divorce her husband, the client started to prepare herself for an indefinite period of single parenthood. The client's initiative in gaining information about her options and about her feelings was reinforced by the counselor's statements. The skills and techniques she had learned in counseling were put to good use in the client's preparations for the big step of divorcing the father of her child. The counselor acknowledged the difficulties she had just overcome and then directed the focus to the future by asking about her plans to avail herself of additional training.

Values Balanced Among Worlds. With the shift in focus, the therapist was able to help the client conceptualize the idea of how people live and interact in different spheres of their lives, according to the values appropriate for each of the spheres. The counselor also explained that these worlds are in flux, and that keeping a healthy balance among them is really a process rather than a one-time achievement. The fluctuating nature of the balancing process requires some flexibility in the individual's value system because of episodic shifts throughout the three worlds. The client was able to comprehend that the different worlds of her existence had not been balanced as well as would have been desirable for her own well-being. She realized that she had the responsibility for enlarging and balancing her worlds. In emphasizing the personal growth the client had experienced and the solid foundation she had laid in the way she had restructured her thinking, the counselor encouraged the client to continue on the path to her goals.

Worth of Human Beings

For individuals to understand the worlds they live in, they first have to have a good knowledge of themselves and what determines their behaviors in all areas of their lives. As discussed in the previous chapter, people attempting to comprehend their own actions often entrap themselves in evaluating themselves rather than the nature of their behaviors. Albert Ellis since 1973 has cautioned about the pitfalls of rating oneself as a person. Explaining how Rational-Emotive-Behavior theory has built on some of Alfred Adler's work and carried it through to a logical but perhaps better defined conclusion, he stated that in Adler's opinion, the individual's character is not a basis for moral judgment, but an indication of the individual's attitude toward the environment and the individual's relationship to society. Adler warned about judging the moral worth of a human being.

Despite these early warnings, people seem to hold on the notion of rating themselves and others along the good-bad continuum. As was discussed in Chapter 10, professionals in the field of psychology and counseling are concerned with different techniques to raise people's self-esteem without necessarily agreeing what the self-esteem is or should be based on. Existential philosophers have attempted to resolve this issue by accepting a person's goodness in terms of the person's existence as a human being. While this notion sidesteps the problems of rating oneself as good or bad, it raises other problems, such as regarding people as good or worthwhile no matter how many not-so-good actions they may have performed. In general, people have difficulties accepting that premise, and usually return to the ways they have rated themselves and others in the past. The notion that individuals can believe in goodness as persons merely based on the fact that they exist is considered by Ellis (1973, 1996) to constitute an inelegant solution. Instead, he offers the more elegant approach of helping clients accept the fact of their existence as people who will make mistakes. That is, they can enjoy their lives and measure or value their traits and performances without bothering to value or rate their selves.

The purpose of repeating here parts of what had been discussed in the previous chapter is not only to remind us to abstain from rating our own personhoods, but also to apply the same reasoning regarding the other people we encounter in the worlds we live in. It is not uncommon for people to say, "What a rotten person my ex-spouse is. How could I have been so stupid to fall for this person? I am a complete idiot!" Thus, in the most efficient way, people accomplish putting down ex-spouses and themselves as well. Most people don't get married because they know their spouse to be a bad person; they see some desirable qualities in the other person. They may in the beginning overlook some not-so-desirable traits, but, in general, we can assume that people are not looking for a bad or rotten person to get married to. In staying away from evaluating personhood, therapists can help their clients to free up time and emotional energy to focus on beliefs, attitudes, and behaviors in themselves and others that may lead to overall improvement.

SUMMARY

Requirements for successful balancing of the three worlds can be envisioned as described below, using Lynn's case study. Her attempts at increasing her personal world by developing some of her talents were attacked by influences from her *Umwelt*, her ex-husband who accused her of being selfish, incompetent, and not a good mother. Moreover, he threatened that he would withdraw some financial assistance that, in turn, would make it even more difficult to pursue her own interests. In her *Eigenwelt*, she operated out of a set of competitive values to achieve cooperation in her *Mitwelt* about having her sons taken care of while indulging in *Eigenwelt*-related activities. Her approach to accomplish this was to enlist assistance from the *Umwelt*, her ex-husband. On the surface, her choice appeared logical, but expecting her ex-husband to respond in a cooperative manner to her competitive wishes was not realistic. In their past relationship, Lynn could think of few occasions where her former husband had operated out of a cooperative value system with her. Instead of cooperation, she faced an attack on her personhood. She was ready to accept her ex-husband's evaluation of herself and to give up on her plans to the point where she did not even consider other possibilities, such as obtaining assistance from her sister in her *Mitwelt*, where interaction based on cooperative values can be expected to occur more readily.

Lynn's willingness to accept her ex-husband's rating of her personhood shows that she had not yet learned to distinguish herself from her behaviors, but it also demonstrated that the boundaries of her *Eigenwelt* were largely undefined. Definition of the boundaries of the different worlds belongs to the individual. How to balance them is the individual's responsibility. That responsibility requires significant groundwork in self-knowledge and in understanding the value systems in which self and others operate in the different worlds.

EXERCISE

Consider the following scenario: You are a non-traditional student, divorced with two children. Both you and your ex-spouse have jobs. Last fall you returned to graduate school to go for your master's degree. Now, during the summer, you have decided to take one elective course that is not closely related to your major area of studies, but that has always been of great interest to you. You are excited about this class, and you are glad you decided to take it in the summer where there is no interference from studying for other classes. Your ex-spouse complains about your involvement in the summer class, saying that now in the summer with the children being out of school, more time should be spent in visitation with the children and similar family responsibilities.

1. Design a map of your three worlds: What people, interactions, and activities occupy your *Eigenwelt,* your *Mitwelt,* and your *Umwelt?*
2. How would you balance the three worlds? How much time and energy to devote to each world?
3. Design a schedule for a typical weekday accommodating activities in all three worlds. Do the same for a typical weekend. Are there differences between weekdays and weekends in your allocations of time and energy?
4. What value systems (cooperative vs. competitive) may have determined your allocations? Describe your reasoning for your choices.

SUGGESTED READING

Ellis, A. (1996). The humanism of Rational Emotive Behavior Therapy and other cognitive behavior therapies. *Journal of Humanistic Education and Development, 35,* 69–88.
   The article is a discussion of REBT as one of the main humanistic psychotherapies. The author explains how as a theory of personality and therapy REBT emphasizes emotional health and self-actualization for individuals and the social group they are part of by their own choice.
Rychlak, J. F. (1973). *Introduction to personality and psychotherapy.* Boston: Houghton Mifflin.
   The author gives a basic description and overview of Binswanger's work.
Sternberg, R. J. (1998). A balance theory of wisdom. *Review of General Psychology, 2,* 347–365.
   The author presents a theory of balance mediated by values toward the achievement of a common good through a balance among intrapersonal, interpersonal, and extrapersonal interests.

12

Where We Have Been— Where Are We Going?

OBJECTIVES

1. To provide a brief history of the development of psychotherapy.
2. To integrate selected theoretical viewpoints into a current cognitive framework.
3. To trace themes used by the counselor throughout the phases.
4. To reiterate the involvement of the client in the process.
5. To highlight certain ethical constraints encountered by the therapist.
6. To describe the importance of the counselor seizing teachable moments.
7. To emphasize the importance of the therapeutic alliance throughout counseling.
8. To introduce the therapist as a person.

OUR ANTECEDENTS

This book focuses on single parents, a special population. However, the content is applicable to the client population at large. Useful ideas and techniques from other approaches have been philosophically translated and integrated to fit into a cognitive therapy framework. The authors considered the cognitive approach to be most beneficial in working with a special population. This chapter also focuses on the population of therapists, clinicians, and students who have decided to make the field of therapy and counseling their life work. Issues connected with theory, research, and clinical experience, are integrated to provide closure to the practical application developed throughout the book.

Freud: A Century Ago

Most therapists would agree on the point of departure in psychotherapy. The beginnings of psychotherapy are found in psychoanalysis and Sigmund Freud's work. Freud's theory is constructed on a mind-body dualism. Struggling with the impossible task of describing man in purely physical terms, he turned to the writings of anthropologists, archeologists, and sociologists for stimulation. Although he considered some social and psychological explanations and relied less on physico-medical models, he continued to stress the importance of biological factors in trying to understand human behavior. Freud's psychotherapy is based on the ideas of psychopathology, and his theory of cure centers on providing the client with insight rather than on removal of symptoms. Freud informed patients from the onset that therapy would take a long time—a year or more, at the least, with three to five or six sessions per week, each lasting 50 minutes. Freud treated clients' financial responsibility equally openly. Clients were informed at the outset that they were expected to pay for each scheduled session, including any sessions they missed (Rychlak, 1973).

Adler's Theory

The medical-physical models of human behavior had several proponents at the time. Reacting to and struggling with the issue of physical vs. psychological explanations, Alfred Adler formulated his individual (in the sense of highly unique) psychology that evolved into a psychology of use, or applied psychology, when he became instrumental in creating Individual Psychology Clinics. These clinics were child guidance clinics, associated with the state schools in Vienna, and included entire families in counseling. Adler's nonauthoritarianism and sympathy with the underdog made him a psychologist for the common man. He believed that therapists should contribute some time without pay. Many of his clients came from the lower classes, as contrasted with Freud, whose patients were predominantly from the upper social classes.

In Adler's view, man is a holistic organism. Mind-body interactions can only be understood within the totality of the holistic process. Mind and body are connected and united through the law of movement, and mentality is understood in terms of directed movement. Direction of the movement comes from man's ideas and the meanings they reflect. Although people's actions originate from their ideas and are part of the overall style of life, Adler warns against evaluating people on the basis of what they think and say of themselves but rather measure their actions. Among Adler's motivational constructs, the best known is perhaps the notion of overcompensation for a particular deficiency or inferiority. It is also often called "striving for superiority." Adler later modified the construct from overcoming deficiency to fulfilling innate potentiality. The shift in emphasis from overcoming to fulfilling defines the person in a more powerful or active way. The person, or the self, moves the mental life and determines the direction of the move (Rychlak, 1973).

In 1934, Adler closed the child guidance clinics in Vienna and moved to New York, where he lived until his death in May of 1937. Adler's work has stimulated other theorists. Albert Ellis (1973) readily admits that Adler, with his hypothesis that individuals' emotional reactions are closely correlated with their basic ideas, beliefs, and attitudes, was one of the main mentors in the formulation of RET. In his discussion about the influence of Adler's individual psychology, Ellis (1973) mentions that Adler, more than any other modern therapist, stressed the significance of education as a general method for changing individuals' self-defeating emotional reactions. He maintained that psychotherapy is education and that education would better be psychotherapeutic. The client is the scholar.

The Concept of Community Psychiatry

Adler's Individual Psychology Clinics in Vienna seem like forerunners of the child guidance clinics and community mental health centers in the United States. The concept of community psychiatry as a health service delivery system was authorized by the federal Mental Retardation Facilities and Community Mental Health Centers Construction Act of 1963, also known as the Kennedy Bill, providing a coordinated program of continuing mental health care to a specific population, usually all the residents of a designated geographical area, called the "catchment area." The programs of the centers were supposed to accept responsibility for all the mental health needs of the community and were thus dictated by the needs of the population. Mental health services were to be made available to everybody in the community. The right to treatment became an entitlement, rather than a privilege.

The bill providing federal funding for the construction of community mental health centers and for the salaries of the staff covered a period of 4 years. After that, it was expected that local funding would replace federal funding. Many centers had difficulty with the transition of their financial responsibilities, especially if they were located in poor communities. Today many of them compete with private practitioners for clients with private pay and insurance coverage. The notion of "catchment area" has become obsolete.

Classification of Disorders: Medical Model vs. Developmental Model

Quality of care is a multidimensional concept, defined on collections of standardized data regarding the various aspects of service delivery. In order to arrive at treatment protocols and other performance indicators that serve as guidelines for a given level of quality of service, agreement needs to be obtained about the problem areas that the service is targeted for. The fourth edition of the Diagnostic and Statistical Manual of Mental Disorders (APA, 1994), known as *DSM-IV*, is a classification system that is widely accepted as the standard source for diagnosis of mental disorders and for referral and treatment decisions. Therapists in mental health agencies, schools, hospitals, or private practice are required to use it (Hohenshil, 1994). Insurance companies require the appropriate code number of the diagnosed disorder when considering eligibility for reimbursement (Tavris, 1995).

Proliferation of Treatment Categories. From 1952, when the first edition was published as an 86-page pamphlet, the current DSM has expanded to 886 pages. The DSM describes symptoms of various mental illnesses in great detail and with distinguishing criteria. The number of categories of mental disorders keeps expanding as the field of psychiatry and clinical psychology grows with increasing numbers of mental health professionals. Since the original nine general categories were published in 1952, each revision of the DSM has included more and more categories of mental disorders, some of them coming from the domain of everyday problems in living rather than being manifestations of true psychopathology (Tavris, 1995).

Mental health counselors see their function as delivering preventive services, rather than the treatment of disorders or abnormalities. They focus on health care instead of being preoccupied with illness care, and believe that people do not have to be sick to get better (Smith & Robinson, 1995). According to Ivey and Ivey (1998), professional mental health counselors experience some cognitive dissonance in using the DSM, because in their opinions it appears to be a description of pathology within individuals without stressing etiology and treatment. They contend that the psychoeducational integrity of the American Counseling Association's emphasis on developmental issues is better served by a developmental counseling and therapy approach that considers the individual's distress as a consequence of biological and developmental factors. As an alternative to the pathology-oriented model of the DSM, counseling professionals proposed the Developmental Counseling and Therapy (DCT) approach that considers individual biological and psychological history in a developmental context.

Proliferation of Treatment Specialties. Concurrent with proliferation of treatment categories is the proliferation of specialties among service providers. Various specialty groups have developed within the American Counseling Association (ACA). The development of specializations seems to have led to separate ethical standards for some of these groups (Herlihy & Remley, 1995).

Moreover, an ever-growing variety of disciplines seems to provide future psychotherapists. The fields of nursing, social work, marriage and family therapy, counseling and guidance, spiritual counseling, drug and alcohol counseling, sex therapy, art and music therapy, and biofeedback, as well as dance and movement therapy, provide training for individuals to become psychotherapists (Hayes & Heiby, 1996).

Decisions Facing Therapists. A long time has passed since Freud and Adler provided clients with their own brands of psychotherapy. Therapists of tomorrow still have to make choices about how they view their own therapeutic approaches. Are they seeing themselves as curing diseases, following the medical model, or are they prescribing to a model of educating people to live fuller and more meaningful lives? What type of clientele are they going to serve, the upper classes or underprivileged people? What are the consequences of either viewpoint? When subscribing to a medical or curative approach, how much and what responsibilities do clients have in the process of improving their condition? When embracing an educational approach, what are efficient teaching and learning modalities to stimulate clients' interest in achieving independence and control over their lives? Therapists' own values will significantly determine their choice of approach, and therapists need to be cognizant of the impact of their own values on their choices as well as on their behaviors. Whatever the approach of their choice, they need to have visions of what is possible and stretch that vision to help clients grow in the direction they want to grow.

Therapists' and Clients' Attitudes: Are They Compatible? As therapists create and maintain their helping relationships with clients, what are therapist attitudes that are particularly beneficial in this endeavor? Therapists' understanding of themselves is essential to avoid interference from their own personal problems with the therapeutic relationship. In addition to therapists' self-awareness, respect for and understanding of clients' backgrounds and current situations are basic elements in the formula for establishing helping relationships.

Therapists, however hard they may try, cannot create therapeutic relationships in a vacuum; clients have to have the capacity to benefit from what the therapist has to offer (Orlinsky & Howard, 1986). Clients have to see some value for themselves in participating in counseling. Often, at least initially, therapists are not aware of the real reasons why clients come to their offices. Some may have been following demands of significant others and—given a choice—would rather not be there. Reluctant clients rarely accept any responsibility for their participation, including payment. One case comes to mind where a couple with a history of marital problems finally resorted to marital counseling, initiated by the husband and reluctantly accompanied by the wife. Divorce was inevitable. Months later the therapist was contacted by the formerly reluctant wife. She found herself in a crisis situation with her new, physically violent companion. After several sessions, when presented with a bill, she exclaimed, "People keep urging you to seek help, but when you finally do so, you are expected to pay for it!" Obviously, she regarded her request for help as a favor to the therapist.

The attitudes of clients are important elements in building a therapeutic relationship, but they are not always what therapists expect. Thus, therapists need to know for themselves what type of clients they can work with effectively and what type of clients would be inappropriate for their therapy approaches. Therapists' conviction of their ability to help includes the ability to recognize when there is a need for referring clients to more appropriate treating sources.

Therapists' and Clients' Characteristics: Are They Compatible?

What therapist characteristics will convince clients of the credibility of their therapists? Therapists need to be in control of their own life situations in order to be convincing teachers about problem-solving methods. When the opportunity arises, therapists should be able to model problem-solving behaviors. This is not to say that therapists should burden clients with their own stories, although at times that may be helpful and appropriate, if used sparingly. During sessions, therapists' undivided attention needs to be focused on clients and their situations without lingering interfering thoughts regarding other clients.

If the therapist is involved in an ongoing crisis situation concerning another client and the therapist has reason to expect an interruption during the session, it would be advisable to inform the current client at the beginning of the session about the possibility of having to take a call. Most clients will be quite agreeable and will respond with, "I know you would do the same for me if I were in need." Rather than feel neglected, most clients will feel comfortable about their therapist's concern and caring for clients even outside their scheduled sessions. Therapists' honesty about circumstances without compromising confidentiality demonstrates respect for clients' dignity. In addition, the therapist's disclosure of the situation may actually make the client feel stronger; the in-session client had been able to handle matters between sessions without need for a crisis call.

Above all, therapists' behavior should be congruent with their theoretical approach. Clients are able to detect inconsistencies, usually better in other people's behaviors than in their own. Therapists who are not consistent within their own background will have a difficult time convincing clients to be consistent in their problem-solving approaches.

Given clients' desire to modify behavior and willingness to work at changing, counselors out of their own sound theoretical framework make an assessment of the clients' major themes of emotional disturbance and their personal tendency to cling to self-defeating behaviors and then select the most useful techniques for cognitive restructuring. As pointed out by Albert Ellis (1979), the effectiveness of therapists depends partly on theoretical outlook; the correctness of therapeutical guess and implementation of effective techniques; an artistry in teaching and persuasion when relating to clients; and persistence at assessment of clients and application of selectively chosen ways of helping them with their emotional problems. Ellis refers to Alfred Adler's notion that people's self-defeating emotional reactions can be changed through education.

Because therapists will not be successful with every type of client, it would be beneficial to devise a screening device for clients to complete at the onset of treatment. The instrument could tap the values, attitudes, and characteristics held by the client when considering counseling. When clients' attitudes and characteristics are too incongruent with those of the therapist, early referral to a more compatible treatment source would be beneficial for both therapists and clients.

Applying Theory. Theorists who regard behavior change as a function of conceptual-rational processes emphasize that individuals are not captives of their past, but can help determine their own fate (Ellis, 1984). Clients' faulty ideas or conceptions that are relevant to psychological problems can be changed in the direction of greater congruence with reality, thereby eliminating or reducing maladjustments, according to Victor Raimy (1975, 1976). Therapists help individuals recognize and change misconceptions in the process of cognitive review. For people to change a concept of any kind, they must be given opportunities to repeatedly examine all available evidence that is relevant to the concept. Considerations of the cognitive aspects of affective responses are necessary in the cognitive review, as emotions are seen as products of faulty conceptions. In Raimy's opinion, most therapists utilize the principle of repeated cognitive review, regardless of their theoretical approaches. Some therapists may have a repertoire of formal techniques for facilitating repeated cognitive reviews of clients' misconceptions, while others proceed in less formalized ways. Also, there is much borrowing of techniques back and forth among various therapies.

When clients automatically question themselves regarding the evidence for their beliefs and encourage themselves to look for alternate ways of conceiving a given situation, one can say that they have learned the cognitive review process, or that they have incorporated the teacher in their minds. As one client reported, "I often say to myself and others, 'You can also look at the situation in another way,' but in my mind the words are spoken in your (the therapist's) voice."

THEMES FLOW THROUGHOUT

The counseling process follows a general path, but proceeds at different speeds. The needs of the individual client and the particular problem under discussion determine the time spent in different phases. Variations occur from phase to phase, from theme to theme, and from client to client.

The composite cases in earlier chapters describe some of the variations to the process. Bill wanted advice on how to get his wife back. His wishes may have initially slowed the pace of work. The therapist, by refraining from being pulled into goals of unexamined value, redirected the flow of the process along a realistic path. Kent, in contrast, had an urgent need for a solution, disregarding important issues, such as the role played by emotions. The therapist avoided confrontation by initially focusing on the client's request and returned to work on emotionally charged beliefs later, when the client had achieved some relief. Gina and Earl wanted the therapist to advocate with someone else, and did not appear ready or interested in becoming involved in the therapeutic alliance.

INVOLVEMENT

Although presenting problems are different and sometimes vaguely defined, the logical flow of the phases provides a natural rhythm for the learning process. When clients introduce new problems or return after some time with another difficulty, both the process of decision-making and the examination of actions, emotions, and consequences are already part of their repertoire of skills. Clients develop the ability to generalize learning onto new situations. Their capacity to tolerate change prepares them to expect future changes to occur. Stanley Strong (1968), in his seminal article on social influences in counseling, used one word to describe a client's role in therapy: "involvement." Involvement is the client's role as taught by the therapist. This role means the client takes on responsibility, completes homework, and engages in exploration.

Single-parent clients are guided through the phases of counseling by the therapist's skill and experience. The therapist's role, in addition to monitoring client progress through the phases, involves professional decisions, ethical constraints, teachable moments, and maintenance of the therapeutic alliance.

CLIENT'S ROLE

The client's role is different from most other interpersonal interactions. In counseling sessions, the client is the focus. Through discussion and homework, clients learn to identify antecedents to the current problem. With the counselor's guidance, clients explore beliefs and emotions; they recognize consequences, and gain new skills for analyzing problems. Clients who are nondefensive and willing to explore the dynamics of their presenting problems, including doing homework, achieve the greatest success (Orlinsky & Howard, 1986).

Responsibility

Clients assume responsibility from the beginning when they agree to certain contractual conditions and limitations. They must become involved in the safe therapeutic environment, or therapy will not proceed apace.

Responsibility for action always remains with the client. Clients' identification of unsuccessful strategies can serve as lessons about what does not work. Exploration of feasible alternatives that are congruent with clients' value systems constitutes the next step. Clients describe barriers and consequences of acting on beliefs or on well-meaning advice. Environmental cues are identified regarding the feasibility of various approaches. A chosen strategy is checked against reality and with an estimation of its effect on others.

Once a new behavior has been attempted, clients can recognize successes and how they have exerted control in the situation. They have opportunities to challenge self-defeating beliefs and replace them with more effective and self-enhancing beliefs. Analysis of successes and failures promotes revised perceptions and behavior. Clients assume responsibility for replicating the revisions in other segments of their lives, thereby reinforcing the new approaches. Indeed, clients can engage in long-range planning and further analysis of their personalities. Repeated generalization of learning to other life areas may bring about changes in the client's self-image. Clients' references of self to others change when they refrain from judging themselves and others as good or bad, but instead focus on behaviors that can be evaluated.

The reconceptualization of self has resulted in recognition of the shift in roles assumed by single parents. Outcomes are integrated in the worlds that the parent now inhabits. Much of this responsible work goes on outside the therapy sessions.

Homework. Completion of homework assignments is a responsibility of the client. The assignments serve to keep clients focused between sessions on the work to be done in therapy. Homework takes on many different forms. Instruments such as the Intra-Interpersonal Growth Scales can be used by clients to rate specific issues. Lists of options, with inclusion of the forces operating for and against each item, are helpful in stimulating clients' thinking about alternatives. Journals provide a way of recording antecedents, beliefs, emotions, actions, and outcomes of present strategies. On the other hand, autobiographies provide a historical account that can be used to shorten the actual time spent in sessions.

Checklists and questionnaires are additional forms of homework that stimulate clients' explorations. For the use of behavior rehearsal techniques, a client's creativity is utilized in writing scripts for anticipated interactions.

As a summary of the changes that have occurred in the single parent's life, the diagram representing the three worlds people live in can be used to record the changes. The diagram shows the linkages between self and the rest of life. Because the client has become used to change, the flexibility in shifts among the three worlds is nonthreatening. Additional shifts can be explored.

Exploration. Although not always in sequence, the links between beliefs, actions, emotions, and consequences must become clear to the client to effect change. The exploration includes observations, both from an inner perspective and from reference to others' reactions to one's own behavior (Hollon & Beck, 1994; Orlinsky & Howard, 1986). The client becomes involved in examining strategies, but applying the strategies requires initiative. Here the single parent explores another issue: Is the solution of the problem worth the time and energy to learn new behaviors? Only the supportive and reinforcing alliance with the therapist helps the client through this difficult period.

If initial efforts are unsuccessful, clients need to recognize the bits that were successful (e.g., simply having the courage to act). Earlier explorations and prioritizations of various strategies provide backup plans. Exploration of strategies becomes integrated into the single parent's repertoire of behaviors.

THERAPIST'S ROLE

Early in professional training, counselors learn the basic interviewing skills (e.g., active listening, empathy, theory-based strategies). This book, designed for advanced students and professionals already working in the field, demonstrates that therapists' ability to grasp nuances and act upon professional judgment is a function of their experience. Professional judgments shape practice decisions, ethical behavior, teachable moments, and the therapeutic alliance.

Professional Decisions

Counselors are aware of the standard of care that is appropriate for the client. Some decision points illustrated in previous chapters are when to vary pacing, dispute beliefs, or handle crises.

Pacing. Counselor and client develop a contract about timing of sessions and contractual obligations. Therapists explain that their role is that of a neutral listener and guide. The expert therapist senses when the time is right to either lead or follow clients' responses. Listening means that the client is the focus. Pacing means waiting for the client to muse and continue and to skillfully navigate around roadblocks.

When the counselor discerns that the time is right, the sessions move through explorations of client self-perceptions, emotional investment, and the threat of change. Clients are assisted in identifying historical sources of beliefs that they hold. Responsibility is transferred to the client for decisions, actions, and outcomes. Maintaining the client's independence is shown by the responsibility placed on the client for actions and consequences. Appropriate pacing allows clients the freedom to explore options and choose strategies, try out their priorities, and reexamine successes, trials, and changes in their worlds.

The final element in pacing is preparing the client for termination of therapy. Implicit in the alliance has always been the knowledge that therapy would end, but clients are often reluctant to leave the supportive atmosphere. The client should be reminded a few sessions ahead of time that termination is on the horizon, although the door will remain open. At times, it is beneficial to schedule a trial vacation from therapy for this purpose.

Occasionally, a client does not want to enter the decision-making process. The time is not right for the work they must take on. In that case, the counselor leaves the door open for the future, when the client may be ready to work. For example, single parents may have expected that the counselor would take on the role of a surrogate parent or partner and are disappointed when that expectation is not met.

Disputing Beliefs. A major concept in cognitive therapy is helping the client identify dysfunctional beliefs. The beliefs may have worked at an earlier stage of life, but as single parents take on new roles, old myths and advice no longer pertain. The exact point when examination of disabling beliefs takes place depends upon the thrust of the counseling, and is part of the overall pacing under therapeutic control. As the appropriate time arises, counselors provide feedback that demonstrates the blocks engendered by emotionally charged beliefs. When a client ventilates, emotion can be directed into constructive channels. The experienced therapist is able to acknowledge distress without reinforcing it. As unresolved affect becomes apparent, the counselor uses it as an opportunity to explore additional underlying beliefs that had remained hidden until then.

Handling Crises. The phases of counseling are set aside if a single-parent client presents a critical situation. Regular session schedules are modified to accommodate more intensive work as may be required by the crisis situation. Any shifts in regular procedures or schedules occur in response to the client's state of mind.

Professionals such as attorneys, physicians, psychiatrists, school liaisons, and agency workers may be used in managing a case with the permission of the client. Other professional expertise supplements and complements that of the therapist working with a client.

Ethical Constraints

Therapists subscribe to and operate under explicit ethical codes. In practice, the ethical decisions that arise require therapists to know and be aware of the rules described in the ethical standards of their professions. Therapists have the responsibility to operate within the scope and limits of their knowledge and competence and to inform clients when the need for referral to other professionals is indicated.

Counselors explain to clients the boundaries of the therapeutic relationship as well as the boundaries of confidentiality of records. In other words, the therapist explains the boundaries of safety and the limits of protection of privileged communication. In family or group sessions, it is wise to remind all participants that confidentiality for what is occurring in the session becomes the responsibility of each member in the session.

Therapists should initiate periodic evaluation of clients' progress and their satisfaction with the therapy process. Cognitive therapists place a strong emphasis upon their own accountability. While doing so, the therapist uses the opportunity to give credit to client's work and initiative, thereby reinforcing the efforts made by the client so far. If gains have been smaller than expected, the situation can be used for exploring additional hidden stumbling blocks or to consider alternate paths of action. If neither approach seems beneficial, referral to another treating source may be appropriate.

Ethical standards provide a framework for the standard of care that any reasonable person could expect. They are guidelines for therapists' conduct in the pursuit of their profession.

Teachable Moments

Teachable moments occur when the client is ready to comprehend new perspectives. The counselor is aware of the client's frame of reference when introducing new concepts. For example, the single parent may have wanted the therapist to predict the outcome of a romance, when instead the moment is one in which the client is reinforced for initiative and behaviors that establish control and independence. These behaviors include having a plan of action, congruent intent and values, and the awareness of affect. The focus is on feasibility, as perceived by the client, not predicting the client's desired outcome in the world outside the session.

Some teachable moments occur when clients complete their homework assignments, especially written assignments. Hidden connections, hidden strengths and talents, hidden motivating forces or unrealistic beliefs, and other uncovered issues may make surprising appearances in the client's written notes.

Single parents need recognition that they are handling responsibilities normally handled by two people. Letting clients report success in their own words is often a stronger reinforcement than when the recognition comes from only the counselor. Clients learn to recognize and express positive feelings about themselves and their abilities. Evidence collected from others in the client's environment regarding the client's new self-enhancing behaviors strengthens the confidence and the behaviors. This is especially rewarding to a single parent who is used to hearing derogatory remarks from a former spouse.

Another use of the teachable moment is to explain dynamics that are operating. Some of these are blocks and anger, myths and folklore advice, enmeshed parenting style, and the picture of self one holds. Describing the use and function of the skillful will is another example.

Teachable moments sometimes can be scheduled, but more often they are anticipated on short notice. By keeping current on research, the counselor has the background to inform the client of reasonable explanations for happenings. The impact of teachable moments is greatly enhanced by the therapist's familiarity with clients' cognitive styles of learning.

Maintenance of Therapeutic Alliance

The therapeutic alliance is the foundation for the overall therapy process. Making an appointment for counseling does not guarantee a sound working alliance. Both parties must invest themselves in the counseling. Both must affirm their mutual goal of reaching for change and satisfaction in the client's life. A good working alliance needs to be in place before using any confrontational techniques, even mild ones. Clients need to feel trust in order to perceive therapists' confrontations as something that is happening for the client's benefit rather than being punishment.

Clients' trust starts when therapists provide accurate and well-defined information. Factual information regarding fees, time schedules, canceling procedures, limits of confidentiality and the goals and functions of authorization for release of information, as well as the roles and expectations of clients and therapists, provides the framework covering technical issues. Another level of trust will be established when counselors demonstrate absence of judgment of others' actions, beliefs, and loyalties, and refusal to reinforce blaming and pain. Therapists' punctuality and reliability also foster trust. Returning clients quickly reestablish trust when counselors have familiarized themselves with past progress notes.

Patience is another therapist trait called into play when clients need to identify problems, waffle about settling them, suggest vague solutions, or forget to do homework. With patience, the counselor keeps the focus on the client's ultimate responsibility for change and satisfaction.

Clients' trust and therapists' patience are important ingredients in the development and maintenance of the therapeutic alliance and are, in turn, necessary prerequisites for reduced resistance on the part of clients (Orlinsky & Howard, 1986). Resistance also is reduced when clients can identify successes from previous attempts to deal with children or former spouses, when they can identify behavioral changes that resulted from goal-directed actions, and when they experience the inner support that results from confidence in their ability to plan. Control, self-efficacy, independence, and knowledge regarding exploration are reinforced throughout the sessions. Outcomes are summarized and integrated into connectedness amongst self, love, and care worlds. Changed definitions of family, self, and environment are reflected upon.

The therapeutic alliance succeeds when the client achieves desired change and satisfaction. The client has been validated throughout the sessions. With the therapist's guidance, the client has learned new skills and has graduated through the process of decision-making strategies. The therapy comes to a conclusion for now, but the door is always open.

THERAPIST AS PERSON

Thus far, the professional and educational background of therapists with their required knowledge and skills has been described to some degree. What are therapists like on a personal level? Do they face problems similar to those their clients experience? Perhaps of even deeper interest is the question of what persuaded them to become therapists.

Motives for Practicing Psychotherapy

Mental health practitioners or therapists face issues that will have significant impact upon their professional and personal lives. The outcomes are highly unpredictable. What are the motives for studying and practicing psychotherapy or counseling? Practitioners' self-reports regarding their motives for selecting a career in mental health cover a wide range, from financial and pragmatic issues to philosophical and humanitarian concerns (Mahoney, 1991). The images practitioners hold of the psychotherapy process include those of treatment, education and guidance, correctional or reform process, and search for spiritual development. Whatever the reasons for embarking on a career in the mental health field, they can have a significant impact on the therapist's own well-being. Early burnout can befall a therapist whose schedule is heavy but the rewards are not congruent with initial expectations.

For some therapists, clients' growth in independence and self-sufficiency is rewarding. They are able to compensate for the lack of desired growth in some clients when they find meaningful change in a few others. Therapists, who demand of themselves to be successful in reaching their goals with every one of their clients, will face disappointment early on in their careers. After all, it is the client's choice and responsibility what changes to make—if any.

The Stress of Practicing Psychotherapy

Among the most frequent sources for therapists' stress are clients' suicide (or attempts), negative affect, and resistance to change. Therapists need to be aware of the level of stress they are experiencing and of the impact of the stress upon their effectiveness with their clients. Stress-impaired therapists can be a hazard to themselves and those they are trying to help. Long before this point is reached, therapists should have an armament of self-preservation measures in place. The measures can consist of scheduled personal time off, relaxation exercises, engaging in activities not related to therapy, to applying therapy—one's own or from another provider. Therapists, as much as clients, need to keep a healthy balance within and among their three worlds.

The Challenging Privilege of Helping

What are the rewards for living with the stress of practicing counseling and therapy, of being responsible, at least in part, for our clients' mental and emotional well being? Aside from the financial aspects, there are rewards not found in many other professions. The realization of having made a difference in somebody's life is gratifying. The recognition that clients have progressed significantly in their quest for independence is invigorating because it confirms the effectiveness of our teaching skills. The communications we may receive from clients years after completion of therapy, informing us about their continued progress and happiness, are inspiring. They are needed. When the money from collected fees has long disappeared in the requirements for our own maintenance, and the memories about uncollected fees and less successful cases haunt us, we need those communications to remind us that our work does make a difference and to motivate us to continue. As therapists, our legacy to our clients consists of inspiration for change and provision of the tools necessary to accomplish it.

SUMMARY

Therapists need to be equally cognizant of their clients' values, attitudes, and characteristics as they may determine the success or failure of establishing therapeutic relationships. How therapists conceive of and structure the therapeutic process is a function of many variables. Philosophical considerations, theoretical background, personal values, attitudes, and characteristics all play significant roles. Today, as was in the past and most likely will be in the future, the work of a therapist is both a challenge and a privilege. The task of envisioning possible solutions to clients' problems, of guiding clients to explore those possibilities, and finally to adopt as their own the solutions that satisfy them is a formidable and challenging one. That task continually taxes the therapist's knowledge, resourcefulness, creativity, and patience. Helping clients along the path of gaining autonomy over their lives becomes a privilege when therapists recognize the significance of their contributions to their clients' well-being.

This chapter has described important aspects of the therapy process that are necessary for a successful outcome. The roles of clients and therapists are outlined. The need for congruence between the therapist's choices of theory and techniques and the therapist's own lifestyle is emphasized. Attitudes and characteristics of both clients and therapists significantly influence the degree of involvement and the flow of the process and, ultimately, the outcome of the counseling experience. Both come with their own sets of expectations. With patience, trust, compassion, and mutual respect they can arrive at the common goal—the client's growth in independence, competence, self-confidence, and a degree of happiness.

Finally, who are therapists? How are they different from other professionals? A brief look at therapists as persons concludes the chapter. In the eyes of clients, various roles are attributed to therapists; some of them are beneficial to the overall therapy process, others can be harmful. Roles that therapists should resist from assuming—although clients all too often attempt to assign those roles to their therapists—are the ones of parent or friend. Both, the authoritarian position of parent and the casualness and intimacy inherent in friendships, interfere with the emotional neutrality necessary for the successful implementation of the growth process.

Constructive roles of therapists include those of educators, teaching clients new reasoning and behavioral skills. Therapists also function as guides and conductors, when they monitor the ebb and flow and direction, as clients move smoothly or more hesitatingly through the phases of the therapy process. At other times, therapists are innovators when they design homework projects and create opportunities for explorations and experimentation, pointing to new adventures. Therapists are also the client's best audience, ready to applaud and cheer when clients report their successes. Those are some of the functions therapists perform. Ideally, the therapist's personality will encompass the characteristics required to expertly and convincingly carry out those functions for the benefit of the client who is striving to achieve a harmonious and balanced lifestyle.

SUGGESTED READING

Hohenshil, T. H. (1994). DSM-IV: What's new. *Journal of Counseling & Development, 73*, 105–107.
   The author describes changes found in the latest edition of the DSM classification system with focus on mental disorders frequently encountered in counseling.
Ivey, A. E., & Ivey, M. B. (1998). Reframing DSM-IV: Positive strategies from developmental counseling and therapy. *Journal of Counseling & Development, 76*, 334–350.
   The authors discuss the use of a developmental counseling and therapy classification approach as an alternative to the pathology-oriented model of the DSM-IV.

Tavris, C. (1995). Diagnosis and the DSM: The illusion of science in psychiatry. *The General Psychologist, 31*, 72–76.
The article presents a brief historical account of the classification system and focuses on positive and negative aspects of the current edition.

References

Adkins, A. W. H. (1960). *Merit and responsibility.* London: Oxford University Press.
Adler, A. (1933). *The meaning of life. (Der Sinn des Lebens).* Frankfurt am Main: Fischer Taschenbuch Verlag GmbH.
Allen, K. R. (1993). The dispassionate discourse of children's adjustment to divorce. *Journal of Marriage and the Family, 55,* 46–49.
Almeida, D. M., Wethington, E., & Chandler, A. L. (1999). Daily transmission of tensions between marital dyads and parent-child dyads. *Journal of Marriage and the Family, 61,* 49–61.
Amato, P. R. (1991). The 'child of divorce' as a person prototype: Bias in the recall of information about children in divorced families. *Journal of Marriage and the Family, 53,* 59–69.
Amato, P. R. (1993). Children's adjustment to divorce: Theories, hypotheses, and empirical support. *Journal of Marriage and the Family, 55,* 23–28.
Amato, P. R., & Booth, A. (1991). The consequences of divorce for attitudes toward divorce and gender roles. *Journal of Family Issues, 12,* 306–322.
American Psychiatric Association. (1994). *Diagnostic and statistical manual of mental disorders* (4th ed.). Washington, DC: Author.
Ashby, J. S., Kottman, T., & Rice, K. G. (1998). Adlerian personality priorities: Psychological and attitudinal differences. *Journal of Counseling & Development, 76,* 467–474.
Assagioli, R. (1973). *The act of will.* New York: Viking Penguin.
Bagarozzi, D. A., & Anderson, S. A. (1989). *Personal, marital and family myths: Theoretical formulations and clinical strategies.* New York: Norton.
Bakan, D. (1995). The crisis in psychology. *The General Psychologist, 31,* 77–80.
Bandura, A. (1976). Social learning, perspective on behavior change. In A. Burton (Ed.), *What makes behavior change possible?* (pp. 34–57). New York: Brunner/Mazel.
Bandura, A. (1977a). *Social learning theory.* Englewood Cliffs, NJ: Prentice-Hall.
Bandura, A. (1977b). Self-efficacy: Toward a unifying theory of behavioral change. *Psychological Review, 4,* 191–215.

Bandura, A. (1997). *Self-efficacy: The exercise of control.* New York: Freman.
Bank, L., Forgatch, M. S., Patterson, G. R., & Fetrow, R. A. (1993). Parenting practices of single mothers: Mediators of negative contextual factors. *Journal of Marriage and the Family, 55,* 371–384.
Barber, B. K., & Buehler, C. (1996). Family cohesion and enmeshment: Different constructs, different effects. *Journal of Marriage and the Family, 58,* 433–441.
Barrett-Lennard, G. T. (1962). Dimensions of therapist response as causal factors in therapeutic change. *Psychological Monographs, 76,* (Whole No. 562).
Barrios, B. A. (1988). On the changing nature of behavioral assessment. In A. S. Bellack & M. Hersen (Eds.), *Behavioral assessment* (pp. 3–41). New York: Pergamon Press.
Bart, M. (1999). Rising numbers of single fathers reflect changing attitudes in society. *Counseling Today, 41,* 14–16.
Baumeister, R. F. (1997). Esteem threat, self-regulating breakdown, and emotional distress as factors in self-defeating behavior. *Review of General Psychology, 1,* 145–174.
Baumeister, R. F. (1999, January). Low self-esteem does not cause aggression [Counterpoint]. *APA Monitor,* p. 7.
Beamish, P. M., Granello, P. F., Granello, D. H., McSteen, P. B., Bender, B. A., & Hermon, D. (1996). Outcome studies in the treatment of panic disorder: A review. *Journal of Counseling & Development, 74,* 460–467.
Beck, A. T. (1976). *Cognitive therapy and the emotional disorders.* New York: Meridian Books.
Beck, A. T. (1988). *Love is never enough.* New York: Harper & Row.
Beck, A. T., Emery, G., & Greenberg, R. L. (1985). *Anxiety disorders and phobias: A cognitive perspective.* New York: Basic Books.
Beck, A. T., Rush, A. J., Shaw, B. F., & Emery, G. (1979). *Cognitive therapy of depression.* New York: Guilford.
Bester, N. (1995). The consequences of urbanization and westernization on black family life in South Africa. In P. L. Lin & W. Tsai (Eds.), *Marriage and the family: A global perspective* (pp. 269–275). University of Indianapolis Press.
Betz, N. E., Wohlgemuth, E., Serling, D., Harshbarger, J., & Klein, K. (1995). Evaluation of a measure of self-esteem based on the concept of unconditional self-regard. *Journal of Counseling & Development, 74,* 76–83.
Binswanger, L. (1962). *Grundformen und Erkenntnis menschlichen Daseins* [Foundations and understandings of the human existence]. München/Basel: Ernst Reinhardt Verlag.
Blascovich, J., & Tomaka, J. (1991). Measures of self-esteem. In J. P. Robinson, P. R. Shaver, & L. S. Wrightsman (Eds.), *Measures of personality and social psychological attitudes* (pp. 115–160). San Diego, CA: Academic Press.

Bogolub, E. B. (1995). *Helping families through divorce.* New York: Springer.

Brock, T. C., Green, M. C., & Reich, D. A. (1998). New evidence of flaws in the Consumer Reports study of psychotherapy. *American Psychologist, 53,* 62–63.

Brown-Azarowicz, M. F. (1986). *Analysis of the individual.* Chicago: Nelson-Hall.

Burnett, J. W., Anderson, W. P., & Heppner, P. P. (1995). Gender roles and self-esteem: A consideration of environmental factors. *Journal of Counseling & Development, 73,* 323–326.

Burnett, P. C. (1998). Measuring behavioral indicators of self-esteem in the classroom. *Journal of Humanistic Education and Development, 37,* 107–116.

Cannon-Bowers, J. A., Salas, E., & Pruitt, J. S. (1996). Establishing the boundaries of a paradigm for decision-making. *Human Factors, 38,* 193–205.

Coleman, M., & Ganong, L. H. (1990). Remarriage and stepfamily research in the 1980s: Increased interest in an old family form. *Journal of Marriage and the Family, 52,* 925–940.

Coley, R. L., & Chase-Lansdale, P. L. (1998). Adolescent pregnancy and parenthood: Recent evidence and future directions. *American Psychologist, 53,* 152–166.

Cooksey, E. C., & Fondell, M. M. (1996). Spending time with his kids: Effects of family structure on fathers' and children's lives. *Journal of Marriage and the Family, 58,* 693–707.

Corsini, R. J., & Wedding, D. (Eds.), (1995). *Current psychotherapies (5th ed.).* Itaska, IL: Peacock.

Crosbie-Burnett, M., & Pulvino, C. J. (1990). Children in nontraditional families: A classroom guidance program. *The School Counselor, 37,* 286–293.

Csikszentmihalyi, M. (1990). *Flow: The psychology of optimal experience.* New York: Harper & Row.

Danahar, B. G., & Thoresen, C. E. (1972). Imagery assessment by self-report and behavioral measures. *Behavior Research and Therapy, 10,* 131–138.

Davies, L., Avison, W. R., & McAlpine, D. (1997). Significant life experiences and depression among single and married mothers. *Journal of Marriage and the Family, 59,* 294–308.

Davis, D., McLemore, C. W., & London, P. (1970). The role of visual imagery in desensitization. *Behavior Research and Therapy, 8,* 11–13.

Deese, J. (1996). Contextualism: Truth in advertising. *The General Psychologist, 32,* 56–61.

Demo, D. H., & Acock, A. C. (1988). The impact of divorce on children. *Journal of Marriage and the Family, 50,* 619–648.

Diener, E., & Larsen, R. J. (1993). The experience of well-being. In M. Lewis & J. M. Haviland (Eds.), *Handbook of emotions* (pp. 404–415). New York: Guilford.

Driscoll, A. K., Hearn, G. K., Evans, V. J., Moore, K. A., Sugland, B. W., & Call, V. (1999). Nonmarital childbearing among adult women. *Journal of Marriage and the Family, 61,* 178–187.

Dryden, W. (1994). Reason and emotion in psychotherapy: Thirty years on. *Journal of Rational Emotive & Cognitive-Behavior Therapy, 12*(2), 83–99.

Ellis, A. (1962). *Reason and emotion in psychotherapy.* New York: Lyle Stuart.

Ellis, A. (1973). *Humanistic psychotherapy: The rational-emotive approach.* New York: Julian Press.

Ellis, A. (1979). Rational-emotive therapy. In A. Ellis & J. M. Whitely (Eds.), *Theoretical and empirical foundations of Rational-Emotive Therapy* (pp. 1–6). Monterey, CA: Cole Publishing.

Ellis, A. (1984). Rational-emotive therapy. In R. J. Corsini (Ed.), *Current psychotherapies* (3rd ed., pp. 196–238). Itasca, IL: Peacock.

Ellis, A. (1988). *How to stubbornly refuse to make yourself miserable about anything—yes, anything!* Secaucus, NJ: Carol Publishing Group.

Ellis, A. (1994a). Post-traumatic stress disorder (PTSD): A Rational Emotive Behavioral Theory. *Journal of Rational Emotive & Cognitive Behavior Therapy, 12,* 3–26.

Ellis, A. (1994b). *Reason and emotion in psychotherapy* (2nd ed.). New York: Lyle Stuart.

Ellis, A. (1995). Rational Emotive Behavior Therapy. In R. J. Corsini & D. Wedding (Eds.), *Current psychotherapies* (5th ed., pp. 162–196). Itasca, IL: Peacock.

Ellis, A. (1996). The humanism of rational emotive behavior therapy and other cognitive behavior therapies. *The Journal of Humanistic Education and Development, 35,* 69–88.

Ellis, A., & Harper, R. A. (1975). *A new guide to rational living.* Englewood Cliffs, NJ: Prentice-Hall.

Emmons, R. A. (1986). Personal strivings: An approach to personality and subjective well-being. *Journal of Personality and Social Psychology, 51,* 1058–1068.

Epstein, N. B., Bishop, D. S., & Baldwin, L. M. (1982). McMaster model of family functioning: A view of the normal family. In F. Walsh (Ed.), *Normal family processes* (pp. 115–141). New York: Guilford.

Featherstonaugh, H. G., & Maass, V. S. (1979, April). *Values and marital conflict.* Paper presented at the Symposium on Strengthening Family Relationships, University of Arizona, Tucson.

Fischhoff, B., & Downs, J. (1997). Accentuate the relevant. *Psychological Science, 8,* 154–158.

Foster, M. E., Jones, D., & Hoffman, S. D. (1998). The economic impact of nonmarital childbearing: How are older, single mothers faring? *Journal of Marriage and the Family, 60,* 163–174.

Garfinkel, I., & McLanahan, S. S. (1986). *Single mothers and their children: A new American dilemma.* Washington, DC: The Urban Institute.

Gaylin, W. (1984). *The rage within.* New York: Simon and Schuster.

Glasser, W. (1998). *Choice theory: A new psychology of personal freedom.* New York: Harper-Collins.

Good, G. E., Dell, D. M., & Mintz, L. M. (1989). Male role and gender role conflict: Relations to help seeking in men. *Journal of Counseling Psychology, 36,* 295–300.

Goodnow, J. J., & Collins, W. A. (1990). *Development according to parents: The nature, sources, and consequences of parents' ideas.* Hillsdale, NJ: Erlbaum.

Granello, P. F., & Witmer, J. M. (1998). Standards of care: Potential implications for the counseling profession. *Journal of Counseling & Development, 76,* 371–380.

Hagan, J., Simpson, J., & Gillis, A. R. (1988). Feminist scholarship, relational and instrumental control, and a power-control theory of gender and delinquency. *The British Journal of Sociology, 34,* 301–336.

Haines, J. M., & Neely, M. A. (1989). *Parents' work is never done.* Far Hills, NJ: New Horizon.

Hall, L. D., Walker, A. J., & Acock, A. C. (1995). Gender and family work in one-parent households. *Journal of Marriage and the Family, 57,* 685–692.

Hattie, J. (1992). Enhancing self-concept. In J. Hattie (Ed.), *Self-concept* (pp. 221–240). Hillsdale, NJ: Erlbaum.

Hayes, S. C., & Heiby, E. (1996). Psychology's drug problem: Do we need a fix or should we just say no? *American Psychologist, 51,* 198–206.

Henderson, A. J. (1981). Designing school guidance programs for single-parent families. *The School Counselor, 29,* 124–132.

Henken, E. R., & Whatley, M. H. (1995). Folklore, legends, and sexuality education. *Journal of Sex Education and Therapy, 21,* 46–61.

Heppner, P. P., & Krauskopf, C. J. (1987). An information-processing approach to personal problem solving. *The Counseling Psychologist, 15,* 371–447.

Herlihy, B., & Remley, Jr., T. P. (1995). Unified ethical standards: A challenge for professionalism. *Journal of Counseling & Development, 74,* 130–133.

Hetherington, E. M., & Anderson, E. R. (1987). The effects of divorce and remarriage on early adolescents and the family. In M. D. Levine & E. R. McCarney (Eds.), *Early adolescent transitions* (pp. 49–67). Lexington, MA: D. C. Heath.

Hetherington, E. M., Bridges, M., & Insabella, G. M. (1998). What matters? What does not? Five perspectives on the association between marital transitions and children's adjustment. *The American Psychologist, 53,* 167–184.

Hetherington, E. M., Hagan, M. S., & Anderson, E. R. (1989). Marital transitions: A child's perspective. *The American Psychologist, 44,* 303–312.

Highlen, P. S., & Hill, C. E. (1984). Factors affecting client change in individual counseling: Current status and theoretical speculations. In S. D. Brown & R. W. Lent (Eds.), *Handbook of counseling psychology* (pp. 334–396). New York: Wiley.

Hines, A. M. (1997). Divorce-related transitions, adolescent development, and the role of the parent-child relationship: A review of the literature. *Journal of Marriage and the Family, 59,* 375–388.

Hinson, J. A., & Swanson, J. L. (1993). Willingness to seek help as a function of self-disclosure and problem severity. *Journal of Counseling & Development, 71,* 465–470.

Hodgkinson, H. (1985). *All one system: Demographics of education, kindergarten through graduate school.* Washington, DC: Institute for Educational Leadership.

Hogan, M. J., Buehler, C., & Robinson, B. (1983). Single parenting: Transitioning alone. In H. I. McCubbin & C. R. Figley (Eds.), *Stress and the family, Vol. 1: Coping with normative transitions* (pp. 116–132). New York: Brunner/Mazel.

Hohenshil, T. H. (1994). DSM-IV: What's new. *Journal of Counseling & Development, 73,* 105–107.

Hollon, S. D., & Beck, A. T. (1994). Cognitive and cognitive behavioral therapies. In A. E. Bergin & S. L. Garfield (Eds.), *Handbook of psychotherapy and behavior change* (4th ed., pp. 428–466). New York: Wiley.

Ivey, A. E., & Ivey, M. B. (1998). Reframing DSM-IV: Positive strategies from developmental counseling and therapy. *Journal of Counseling & Development, 76,* 334–350.

Jackson, B. J. (1995, December). *Counseling for life transitions in work and family relationships.* Paper presented at the Fifth International Conference on Counseling in the 21st Century, Hong Kong.

Katz, J., & Beach, S. R. (1997). Self-verification and depressive symptoms in marriage and courtship: A multiple pathway model. *Journal of Marriage and the Family, 59,* 903–914.

Kelly, G. A. (1963). *A theory of personality: The psychology of personal constructs.* New York: W. W. Norton & Company, Inc.

Kelly, J. B. (1988). Longer-term adjustment in children of divorce: Converging findings and implications for practice. *Journal of Family Psychology, 2,* 119–140.

Kimble, G. A. (1995). Psychology stumbling down the road to hell. *The General Psychologist, 31*, 66–71.

Kitson, G. C., & Morgan, L. A. (1990). The multiple consequences of divorce. *Journal of Marriage and the Family, 52*, 913–924.

Knaus, W. J. (1983). *How to conquer your frustration.* Englewood Cliffs, NJ: Prentice-Hall.

Kohut, H. (1984). *How does analysis cure?* Chicago: University of Chicago Press.

Kopec, A. M., Beal, D., & DiGiuseppe, R. (1994). Training in RET: Disputational Strategies. *Journal of Rational-Emotive & Cognitive-Behavior Therapy, 12*, 47–59.

Krech, D., Crutchfield, R. S., & Livson, N. (1969). *Elements of psychology.* New York: Alfred A. Knopf.

Lambert, M. J., Ogles, B. M., & Masters, K, S. (1992). Choosing outcome assessment devices: An organizational and conceptual scheme. *Journal of Counseling & Development, 70*, 527–532.

Langs, R. (1991). *Take charge of your emotional life.* New York: Henry Holt.

LaRossa, R., & Reitzes, D. C. (1993). Continuity and change in middle class fatherhood, 1925-1939: The culture-conduct connection. *Journal of Marriage and the Family, 55*, 455–468.

Larson, R. W., & Gillman S. (1999). Transmission of emotions in the daily interactions of single-mother families. *Journal of Marriage and the Family, 61*, 21–37.

Lazarus, A. A. (1984). Multimodal therapy. In R. J. Corsini (Ed.), *Current psychotherapies* (3rd ed., pp. 491–530). Itasca, IL: Peacock.

Lazarus, R. S., & Lazarus, B. N. (1994). *Passion and reason: Making sense of our emotions.* New York: Oxford University Press.

Lecky, P. (1969). *Self-consistency: A theory of personality.* Garden City, NY: Doubleday.

Li, E. B. C. (1994). Modernization: Its impacts on families in China. In P. L. Lin, K. Mei, & H. Peng (Eds.), *Marriage and the family in Chinese societies: Selected readings* (pp. 39–52). University of Indianapolis Press.

Lipson, A., & Perkins, D. N. (1990). *Block: Getting out of your own way: The new psychology of counterintentional behavior in everyday life.* New York: Carol.

Maass, V. S. (1979, November). *The use of imagery in the treatment of phobic patients.* Paper presented at the Third American Conference on the Fantasy and Imaging Process, New York, NY.

Maass, V. S. (1986, February). How do you score? Giving and getting in love relationships. *Indianapolis Woman*, p. 46.

Maass, V. S. (1991, June). *A new look at single parent families: The weaknesses and strengths.* Paper presented at the Third Annual National Conference: New Perspectives: Single Parents & Self-Sufficiency, Lexington, KY.

Maass, V. S. (1992, December). *The effects of values on the self-sufficiency of single-parent families*. Paper presented at the Third International Conference on Counseling in the 21st Century, Singapore.

Maass, V. S. (1995). Modern family life and the significance of values. In P. L. Lin & W. Tsai (Eds.), *Marriage and the family: A global perspective* (pp. 19–28). University of Indianapolis Press.

Maass, V. S. (1996, September). *Single parent families*. Paper presented at the III European Conference in Counselling, Athens, Greece.

Maass, V. S., & Featherstonaugh, H. G. (1981, September). *Conflicting motivators in cognitive behavioral therapy*. Paper presented at the First European Meeting on Cognitive-Behavioural Therapies, Lisbon, Portugal.

Maccoby, E., & Martin, J. A. (1983). Socialization in the context of the family: Parent-child interaction. In P. Mussen (Ed.), *Handbook of child psychology: Vol. 4: Socialization, personality, and social development* (pp. 1–101). New York: Wiley.

Maddux, J. E. (1991). Personal efficacy. In V. Derlega, B. Winstead, & W. Jones (Eds.), *Personality* (pp. 231–262). Chicago: Nelson-Hall.

Mahoney, M. J. (1991). *Human change processes*. New York: Basic Books.

Mann, B. J., & MacKenzie, E. P. (1996). Pathways among marital functioning, parental behaviors, and child behavior problems in school-age boys. *Journal of Clinical Child Psychology, 25*, 183–191.

Marks, S. R., & MacDermid, S. M. (1996). Multiple roles and the self: A theory of role balance. *Journal of Marriage and the Family, 58*, 417–432.

Masten, A. S., & Coatsworth, J. D. (1998). The development of competence in favorable and unfavorable environments: Lessons from research on successful children. *The American Psychologist, 53*, 205–220.

Maultsby, M. C., Jr. (1971). Systematic written homework in psychotherapy. *Psychotherapy: Theory, Research and Practice, 8*, 195–198.

Maultsby, M. C., Jr. (1975). *Help yourself to happiness*. Boston: Esplanade Books, Marlborough House.

Maultsby, M. C., Jr. (1984). *Rational behavior therapy*. Englewood Cliffs, NJ: Prentice-Hall.

McCrone, J. (1993). *The myth of irrationality*. New York: Carroll & Graf.

McKeehan, J. C. (1992). *Effects of survival skills workshops on depression and attributional style of urban women in poverty*. Unpublished dissertation, Kansas State University, Manhattan, KS.

McLanahan, S. S., & Booth, K. (1989). Mother-only families: Problems, prospects, and politics. *Journal of Marriage and the Family, 51*, 557–580.

McLanahan, S. S., & Bumpass, L. (1988). Intergenerational consequences of family disruption. *American Journal of Sociology, 94*, 130–152.

McLean, V. (1988). *Modeling influences on athletic performance and attitude*. Unpublished dissertation, Kansas State University, Manhattan, KS.

Meyer, D. R., & Cancian, M. (1998). Economic well-being following an exit from aid to families with dependent children. *Journal of Marriage and the Family, 60,* 479–492.

Meyer, D. R., & Garasky, S. (1993). Custodial fathers: Myths, realities, and child support policy. *Journal of Marriage and the Family, 55,* 73–89.

Minuchin, S. (1974). *Families and family therapy.* Cambridge, MA: Harvard University Press.

Morrison, W., Page, G., Sehl, M., & Smith, H. (1986, Fall). Single mothers in Canada: An analysis. *Canadian Journal of Community Mental Health, 5*(2), 37–46.

My family right or wrong. (1992, September 19). *The Economist, 324,* p. 72.

Needleman, J. (1963). *Being-in-the-world: Selected papers of Ludwig Binswanger.* New York: Harper & Row.

Neely, M. A. (1982). *Counseling and guidance practices with special education students.* Homewood, IL: Dorsey.

Neely, M. A. (1992a, May). *Conflict and single parent family.* Paper presented at Conference on Conflict Resolution: Tools for School Counselors. Emporia, KS.

Neely, M. A. (1992b, December). *Single parents and family dynamics.* Paper presented at the Third International Conference of Counseling in the 21st Century, Singapore.

Newhouse, R., & Neely, M. A. (1993). Conflict resolution: An overview for classroom managers. *The International Journal of Educational Management, 7*(3), 4–8.

Nickerson, R. S. (1998). Confirmation bias: A ubiquitous phenomenon in many guises. *Review of General Psychology, 2,* 175–230.

Norwood, R. (1985). *Women who love too much.* Los Angeles: Jeremy Tarcher.

Orlinsky, D. E., & Howard, K. I. (1986). Process and outcome in psychotherapy. In S. L. Garfield & A. E. Bergin (Eds.), *Handbook of psychotherapy and behavior change* (pp. 311–381). New York: Wiley.

Perosa, L. (1996). Relations between Minuchin's structural family model and Kohut's self-psychology constructs. *Journal of Counseling & Development, 74,* 385–392.

Perosa, L., & Perosa, S. (1990, August). *The revision and validation of the structural family interaction scale.* Paper presented at the annual convention of the American Psychological Association, Boston, MA.

Perry, J. W. (1966). *The lord of the four quarters.* New York: George Braziller.

Pfeiffer, J. W., & Jones, J. E. (1974). *A handbook of structured experiences for human relations training: Vol. II* (Rev. ed.). La Jolla, CA: University Associates.

Prater, L. P. (1991, June). *Adolescent African-American single parents: Barriers to self-sufficiency.* Paper presented at the Third Annual National Conference, New Perspectives: Single Parents & Self-Sufficiency, Lexington, KY.

Prochaska, J. O., DiClemente, C. C., & Norcross, J. C. (1992). In search of how people change: Applications to addictive behaviors. *American Psychologist, 47,* 1102–1114.

Quintana, S. M., & Kerr, J. (1993). Relational needs in late adolescent separation individuation. *Journal of Counseling & Development, 71,* 349–35.

Raimy, V. (1975). *Misunderstandings of the self.* San Francisco: Jossey-Bass.

Raimy, V. (1976). Changing misconceptions as the therapeutic task. In A. Burton (Ed.), *What makes behavior change possible?* (pp. 199–226). New York: Brunner/Mazel.

Rehm, L. P. (1973). Relationships among measures of visual imagery. *Behavior Research and Therapy, 11,* 265–270.

Risman, B. J. (1987). Intimate relationships from a microstructural perspective: Men who mother. *Gender and Society, 1,* 6–32.

Risman, B. J., & Park, K. (1988). Just the two of us: Parent-child relationships in single-parent homes. *Journal of Marriage and the Family, 50,* 1049–1062.

Rogers, C. R. (1961). *On becoming a person.* Boston, MA: Houghton Mifflin.

Rosenbaum, M. (1983). Learned resourcefulness as a behavioral repertoire for the self-regulation of internal events: Issues and speculations. In M. Rosenbaum, C. M. Frank, & Y. Jaffe (Eds.), *Perspectives on behavior therapy in the eighties* (pp. 54–73). New York: Springer Publishing Co.

Rychlak, J. F. (1973). *Introduction to personality and psychotherapy.* Boston: Houghton Mifflin.

Salzman, L. (1976). The will to change. In A. Burton (Ed.), *What makes behavior change possible?* (pp. 13–33). New York: Brunner/Mazel.

Sandfort, J. R., & Hill, M. S. (1996). Assisting young, unmarried mothers to become self-sufficient: The effects of different types of early economic support. *Journal of Marriage and the Family, 58,* 311–326.

Sanford, A. J. (1985). *Cognition and cognitive psychology.* New York: Basic Books.

Schacht, T. E., & Henry, W. P. (1992). Reaction to Lambert, Ogles, and Masters: "Choosing outcome assessment devices." *Journal of Counseling & Development, 70,* 533–534.

Schachter, S., & Singer, J. (1962). Cognitive, social, and physiological determinants of emotional state. *Psychological Review, 69,* 379–399.

Seaburn, D. B. (1990). The ties that bind: Loyalty and widowhood. *The Psychotherapy Patient, 6,* 139–146.

Seccombe, K., James, D., & Battle Walters, K. (1998). "They think you ain't much of nothing": The social construction of the welfare mother. *Journal of Marriage and the Family, 60,* 849–865.

Seligman, M. E. P. (1975). *Helplessness: On depression, development and death.* San Francisco: Freeman.

References

Seligman, M. E. P. (1998). The American way of blame. [President's column]. *APA Monitor* (July). www.apa.org/monitor/jul98/pc.chtml.

Seligman, M. E. P. (1999). Seligman on positive psychology: A session at the National Press Club. *The General Psychologist, 34*, 37–45.

Shapiro, A., & Lambert, J. D. (1999). Longitudinal effects of divorce on the quality of the father-child relationship and on fathers' psychological well-being. *Journal of Marriage and the Family, 61*, 397–408.

Silverstein, L. B., & Auerbach, C. F. (1999). Deconstructing the essential father. *American Psychologist, 54*, 397–407.

Simons, R. L., Beaman, J., Conger, R. D., & Chao, W. (1992). Gender differences in the intergenerational transmission of parenting beliefs. *Journal of Marriage and the Family, 54*, 823–836.

Simons, R. L., Beaman, J., Conger, R. D., & Chao, W. (1993). Childhood experience, conceptions of parenting, and attitudes of spouse as determinants of parental behavior. *Journal of Marriage and the Family, 55*, 91–106.

Skinner, B. F. (1972). *Cumulative record: A selection of papers (3rd ed.)*. New York: Meredith.

Skinner, H. A., Steinhauer, P. D., & Santa-Barbara, J. (1983). The family assessment measure. *Canadian Journal of Community Mental Health, 2*, 91–105.

Smith, H. B., & Robinson, G. P. (1995). Mental health counseling: Past, present, and future. *Journal of Counseling & Development, 74*, 159–162.

Sniezek, J. A., & Buckley, T. (1993). Becoming more or less uncertain. In N. J. Castellan, Jr. (Ed.), *Individual and group decision-making* (pp. 87–108). Hillsdale, NJ: Erlbaum.

Sprenkle, D. H., & Cyrus, C. L. (1983). Abandonment: The stress of sudden divorce. In C. R. Figley & H. J. McCubbin (Eds.), *Stress and the family Vol. 2: Coping with catastrophe*. New York: Brunner/Mazel.

Staub, E. (1999, January). Aggression and self-esteem [Point]. *APA Monitor*, p. 6.

Steenbarger, B. N., & Smith, H. B. (1996). Assessing the quality of counseling services: Developing accountable helping systems. *Journal of Counseling & Development, 75*, 145–150.

Steinberg, L. (1990). Autonomy, conflict, and harmony in family relationships. In S. S. Feldman & G. R. Elliot (Eds.), *At the threshold* (pp. 255–277). Cambridge, MA: Harvard University Press.

Sternberg, R. J. (1998). A balance theory of wisdom. *Review of General Psychology, 2*, 347–365.

Sternberg, R. J., & Grigorenko, E. L. (1997). Are cognitive styles still in style? *American Psychologist, 52*, 700–712.

Strong, S. (1968). Counseling: An interpersonal influence process. *Journal of Counseling Psychology, 15*, 215–224.

Swann, W. B., Jr. (1983). Self-verification: Bringing social reality into harmony with the self. In J. Suls & A. G. Greenwald (Eds.), *Social psychology perspectives* (Vol. 2, pp. 33–66). Hillsdale, NJ: Erlbaum.

Tan, E. (1992, December). *The Singapore family in the 90's: Implications for counseling.* Paper presented at the Third International Conference on Counseling in the 21st Century, Singapore.

Tavris, C. (1982). *Anger: The misunderstood emotion.* New York: Simon and Schuster.

Tavris, C. (1995). Diagnosis and the DSM: The illusion of science in psychiatry. *The General Psychologist, 31,* 72–76.

Thailand Ministry of the Interior. (1988). *Registered divorces.* Bangkok: Author.

Thomas, G., Farrell, M. P., & Barnes, G. M. (1996). The effects of single-mother families and nonresident fathers on delinquency and substance abuse in black and white adolescents. *Journal of Marriage and the Family, 58,* 884–894.

Tschann, J. M., Johnston, J. R., Kline, M., & Wallerstein, J. S. (1989). Family process and children's functioning during divorce. *Journal of Marriage and the Family, 51,* 431–444.

U.S. Bureau of the Census. (1997). *Marital status and living arrangements.* (Current Population Reports, Series P20, No. 506). Washington, DC: U. S. Government Printing Office.

Walker, B. G. (1983). *The woman's encyclopedia of myths and secrets.* San Francisco: Harper and Row.

Wallerstein, J. S., & Blakeslee, S. (1989). *Second chances.* New York: Ticknor & Fields.

Warner, R. E. (1991). Canadian university counsellors: A survey of theoretical orientations and other related descriptors. *Canadian Journal of Counselling/Revue Canadienne de Counseling, 25*(1), 33–37.

Watzlawick, P. (1983). *The situation is hopeless, but not serious.* New York: Norton.

Watzlawick, P. (1990). *Münchhausen's pigtail: Or psychotherapy & "reality": Essays and lectures.* New York: Norton.

Whisnant, P. S., Hammond, R., & Tilmon, R. (1999). Comparing methods of counseling among Arkansas CADCs. *The Counselor, 17,* 33–36.

Wills, T. A., & DePaulo, B. M. (1991). Interpersonal analysis of the help-seeking process. In C. R. Snyder & D. R. Forsyth (Eds.), *Handbook of social and clinical psychology* (pp. 350–375). New York: Pergamon.

Wolpe, J. (1976). Conditioning is the basis of all therapeutic change. In A. Burton (Ed.), *What makes behavior change possible?* (pp. 58–72). New York: Brunner/Mazel.

Women and work survey: At the double. (1998, July 18). *The Economist*, 12–15.
Yalom, I. D. (1980). *Existential psychotherapy*. New York: Basic Books.
Yauman, B. E. (1991). School-based group counseling for children of divorce: A review of the literature. *Elementary School Guidance & Counseling, 26*, 130–138.
Yeung, C. S. (1992, December). *Changes in marriage patterns in Hong Kong: Implications for counseling*. Paper presented at the Third International Conference on Counseling in the 21st Century, Singapore.
Zelnik, M., & Kantner, J. F. (1979). Reasons for nonuse of contraception by sexually active women aged 15–19. *Planning Perspectives, 11*, 289–296.

Name Index

Acock, A. C., 6, 99
Adkins, A. W. H., 102
Adler, A., 248
Allen, K. R., 9
Almeida, D. M., 8
Amato, P. R., 9, 13
American Psychiatric Association, 20, 332
Anderson, E. R., 2, 10
Anderson, S. A., 127, 162
Anderson, W. P., 278
Ashby, J. S., 248
Assagioli, R., 64, 166, 219
Auerbach, C. F., 10
Avison, W. R., 6

Bagarozzi, D. A., 127, 162
Bakan, D., 248, 272, 279
Baldwin, L. M., 149
Bandura, A., 24, 30, 31, 46, 275, 277, 299
Bank, L., 7, 151
Barber, B. K., 149
Barnes, G. M., 6, 150
Barrett-Lennard, G. T., 277
Barrios, B. A., 227
Bart, M., 3
Battle Walters, K., 289
Baumeister, R. F., 275, 280
Beach, S. R., 274
Beal, D., 232, 246
Beaman, J., 147, 151, 162

Beamish, P. M., 217, 218
Beck, A. T., 19, 22, 33, 34, 46, 88, 122, 216, 217, 340
Bender, B. A., 217, 218
Bester, N., 2
Betz, N. E., 277
Binswanger, L., 39, 80, 311, 312
Bishop, D. S., 149
Blakeslee, S., 9
Blascovich, J., 276
Bogolub, E, B., 13, 25
Booth, A., 13
Booth, K., 4, 5, 6
Bridges, M., 3, 9, 14, 100
Brock, T. C., 228
Brown-Azarowicz, M. J., 51
Buckley, T., 164, 165, 199
Buehler, C., 4, 149
Bumpass, L., 4
Burnett, J. W., 278
Burnett, P. C., 280

Call, V., 15
Cancian, M., 15
Cannon-Bowers, J. A., 165
Chandler, A. L., 8
Chao, W., 147, 151, 162
Chase-Lansdale, P. L., 14
Coatsworth, J. D., 13
Coleman, L., 25
Coley, R. L., 14
Collins, W. A., 147

Conger, R. D., 147, 151, 162
Cooksey, E. C., 99, 122
Corsini, R. J., 27
Crosbie-Burnett, M., 13
Crutchfield, R. S., 218
Csikszentmihalyi, M., 305
Cyrus, C. L., 4

Danaher, B. G., 217
Davies, L., 6
Davis, D., 217
Deese, J., 279
Dell, D. M., 143
Demo, D. H., 6
DePaulo, B. M., 143
DiClemente, C. C., 87
Diener, E., 311
DiGiuseppe, R., 232, 246
Downs, J., 167
Driscoll, A. K., 15
Dryden, W., 22

Ellis, A., 17, 19, 20, 26, 28, 36, 37, 47, 164, 198, 217, 225, 247, 249, 272, 291, 299, 325, 326, 328, 331, 336
Emery, G., 19, 22, 33, 34
Emmons, R. A., 311
Epstein, N. B., 149
Evans, V. J., 15

Farrell, M. P., 6, 150
Featherstonaugh, H. G., 89
Fetrow, R. A., 7, 151
Fischoff, B., 167
Fondell, M. M., 99, 122
Forgatch, M. S., 7, 151
Foster, M. E., 14

Ganong, M. H., 25
Garasky, S., 4, 122, 259
Garfinkel, I., 4
Gaylin, W., 124
Gillis, A. R., 151
Gillman, S., 7, 8
Glasser, W., 164, 199
Good, G. E., 143
Goodnow, J. J., 147

Granello, D. H., 217, 218
Granello, P. F., 217, 218, 228, 246
Green, M. C., 228
Greenberg, R. L., 33, 34
Grigorenko, E. L., 54, 86

Hagan, J., 151
Hagan, M. S., 2
Haines, J. M., 11, 26
Hall, L. D., 99
Hammond, R., 17
Harper, R. A., 28, 47
Harshbarger, J., 277
Hattie, J., 280
Hayes, S. C., 334
Hearn, G. K., 15
Heiby, E., 334
Henderson, A. J., 13
Henken, E. R., 127
Henry, W. P., 228
Heppner, P. P., 102, 278
Herlihy, B., 333
Hermon, D. 217, 218
Hetherington, E. M., 2, 3, 9, 10, 14, 100
Highlen, P. S., 20, 279
Hill, C. E., 20, 279
Hill, M. S., 16
Hines, A. M., 3
Hinson, J. A., 142
Hodgkinson, H., 2
Hoffman, S. D., 14
Hogan, M. J., 4
Hohenshil, T. H., 332, 348
Hollon, S. D., 340
Howard, K. I., 21, 334, 338, 340, 345

Insabella, G. M., 3, 9, 14, 100
Ivey, A. E., 20, 38, 333, 348
Ivey, M. B., 20, 38, 333, 348

Jackson, B. J., 12
James, D., 289
Johnston, J. R., 8
Jones, D., 14
Jones, J. E., 33

Name Index

Kantner, J. F., 127
Katz, J., 274
Kelly, G., 292
Kelly, J. B., 14
Kerr, J., 150
Kimble, G. A., 280
Kitson, G. C., 6
Klein, K., 277
Kline, M., 8
Knaus, W. J., 190
Kohut, H., 150
Kopec, A. M., 232, 246
Kottman, T., 248
Krauskopf, C. J., 102
Krech, D., 218

Lambert, J. D., 4
Lambert, M. J., 228
Langs, R., 166
LaRossa, R., 141
Larsen, R. J., 311
Larson, R. W., 7, 8
Lazarus, A. A., 88
Lazarus, B. N., 117, 210, 211, 212, 225
Lazarus, R. S., 117, 210, 211, 212, 225
Lecky, P., 163, 279, 297
Li, E. B. C., 2
Lipson, A., 32
Livson, N., 218
London, P., 217

Maass, V. S., 10, 14, 89, 161 211, 217, 314, 316
Maccoby, E., 151, 152
MacDermid, S. M., 302
MacKenzie, E. P., 8
Maddux, J. E., 31, 276
Mahoney, M. J., 18, 292, 299, 346
Mann, B. J., 8
Marks, S. R., 302
Martin, J. A., 151, 152
Masten, A. S., 13
Masters, K. S., 228
Maultsby, M. C., Jr., 17, 28, 38, 216, 225
McAlpine, D., 6

McCrone, J., 273
McKeehan, J. C., 289
McLanahan, S. S., 4, 5, 6
McLean, V., 64
McLemore, C. W., 217
McSteen, P. B., 217, 218
Meyer, D. R., 4, 15, 122, 259
Mintz, L. M., 143
Minuchin, S., 151
Moore, K. A., 15
Morgan, L. A., 6
Morrison, W., 14, 304

Needleman, J., 312
Neely, M. A., 11, 14, 26, 29
Newhouse, R., 14
Nickerson, R. S., 275
Norcross, J. C., 87
Norwood, R., 139

Ogles, B. M., 228
Orlinsky, D. E., 20, 334, 338, 340, 345

Page, G., 14, 304
Park, K., 100
Patterson, G. R., 7, 151
Perkins, D. N., 32
Perosa, L., 149
Perosa, S., 149
Perry, J. W., 127
Pfeiffer, J. W., 33
Prater, L. P., 14
Prochaska, J. O., 87
Pruitt, J. S., 165
Pulvino, C. J., 13

Quintana, S. M., 150

Raimy, V., 337
Rehm, L. P., 217
Reich, D. A., 228
Reitzes, D. C., 141
Remley, T. P., Jr., 333
Rice, K. G., 248
Risman, B. J., 99, 100
Robinson, B., 4
Robinson, G. P., 333

Rogers, C. R., 277, 300
Rosenbaum, M., 73
Rush, A. J., 22
Rychlak, J. F., 216, 312, 328, 330, 331

Salas, E., 165
Salzman, L., 60
Sandfort, J. R., 16
Sanford, A. J., 60, 64, 85, 125
Santa-Barbara, J., 149
Schacht, T. E., 228
Schachter, S., 217
Seaburn, D. B., 102
Seccombe, K., 289
Sehl, M., 14, 304
Seligman, M. E. P., 13, 167, 280
Serling, D., 277
Shapiro, A., 4
Shaw, B. F., 22
Silverstein, L. B., 10
Simons, R. L., 147, 151, 162
Simpson, J., 151
Singer, J., 217
Skinner, B. F., 28
Skinner, H. A., 149
Smith, H., 14, 304
Smith, H. B., 228, 333
Sniezek, J. A., 164, 165, 199
Sprenkle, D. H., 4
Staub, E., 280
Steenbarger, B. N., 228
Steinberg, L., 149
Steinhauer, P. D., 149
Sternberg, R. J., 54, 86, 311, 328
Strong, S., 338

Sugland, B. W., 15
Swann, W. B., Jr., 274
Swanson, J. L., 142

Tan, E., 2
Tavris, C., 42, 332, 333, 349
Thailand Ministry of the Interior, 1998, 2
Thomas, G., 6, 150
Thoresen, C. E., 217
Tilmon, R., 17
Tomaka, J., 276
Tschann, J. M., 8

U.S. Bureau of the Census, 1997, 3

Walker, A. J., 99
Walker, B. G., 126
Wallerstein, J. S., 8, 9
Warner, R. E., 17
Watzlawick, P., 45, 141
Wedding, D., 27
Wethington, E., 8
Whatley, M. H., 127
Whisnant, P. S., 17
Wills, T. A., 143
Witmer, J. M., 228, 246
Wohlgemuth, E., 277
Wolpe, J., 30
Women and work survey, 1998, 2

Yalom, I. D., 166
Yauman, B. E., 13
Yeung, C. S., 2

Zelnik, M., 127

Subject Index

Index note: page references in italics indicate a figure or table

activities list in therapy, case study of, 180, *180*, 181, *181*, 182–186
advice, types of
    lay *vs.* professional advice, 141–147
    syndicated newspaper columns and TV talk shows, 141
AFDC mothers, 13–16, 289
Aid to Families with Dependent Children (AFDC), 13–16, 289
anger and the addiction cycle, 41–42
"as-if," concept of, 40
autobiographies
    in therapy, case study of, 170–180
    use in counseling, 339

balancing of three worlds, 24, 301–328
    case study of perceived lack of personal competence, 305–311
    change in role, case study of, 316, *317*
    environment and larger world, 311–316, *317*, 318, 327
    interconnectedness and influences of, 314–316, *317*, 318, 327
    interpersonal world, 311–316, *317*, 318, 327
    personal world, 311–316, *317*, 318, 327
    role balance and role ease, 302–305
    sudden widowhood, case study of, *317*, 318
    temporary single parenthood, case study of, 319–325

three worlds, the, 311–316, *317*, 318, 327
welfare mother, case study of, 318–319
Barrett-Lennard Relationship Inventory (BLRI), 277
Beck Depression Inventory (BDI), 274
behavior modification theory and case study of, 28–30
behavior rehearsals, 63–64, 202–224
Behavior Therapy, 17
behavior *vs.* conduct, 248–249
Behavioral Indicators of Self-Esteem Scale (BIOS), 280
beliefs
    case study of, 39
    challenging/disputing of, 38, *38*, 39, 341–342
    effects on decision making and case study of, 191–197, 240–245
    and faulty perceptions, 18–19
    myths and mystery of, 43–44
    of single parents, 35, *35*, 36
body language, in therapy, 44–45

case studies
    activities list in therapy, 180, *180*, *181*, 182–186
    autobiographies in therapy, 170–180
    behavior modification, 29
    beliefs system, 39, 191–197, 240–245
    change in role, 316, *317*

369

changed outlook, 293–297
conflicting values, 191–197, 240–245
conjoint therapy, 16, 167–186, 202–210, 229–232
coping skills, 70–72
designating the problem areas, 51–54
exploring affect in attempted strategies, 55–59
focus on the future, 133–140
forced choices, 186–190
generalizing learning onto other situations, 73–77
guiding reality check, 64–69
idea of choices, 61–63
identifying what does not work, 55–59
journals, starting and using, 131–140
lay advice, 143–147, 156–160
long-range planning, 260–264
myths and folk sayings, 128–140
perceived lack of self competence, 305–311
reconceptualizing the Self, 78–80
reevaluating progress, 70–72, 229–245
reinforcing initiative, 73–77
relief and behavior change, 212–224
Self as single, 281–284
self-image changes, 78–80
Social Learning Theory, 30–32, 45
sudden widowhood, 103–117, 121, 317, 318
taking control, 284–288
temporary single parenthood, 264–272, 319–325
too many problems, 249–260
unexpected options, 112–117, 121
unrequited love, 117–121
unresolved emotions, 202–224
unresolved requests and feelings of guilt, 107–111, 121
unwanted divorce, 92–99, 233–239
validating interconnectedness, 81–85
values and decision making, 191–197, 240–245

welfare mother, 290–292, 318–319
what does not work, 55–59
worlds of human existence, 81–85
change
  attributes and therapy, 42
  and client satisfaction, 228
  personality system resistance of, 279–280
  in self-image, case study of, 78–80
characteristics of single-parent households, 3–4
Chelune Self-Disclosure Situations Survey (SDSS), 142
children
  effects of mother-only households, 6–10
  race and single-parent households, 6–7
Choice Theory, 155, 189
choices, idea of, 23
chosen path, starting and proceeding, 23, 63–69
clients
  role and involvement of, 338–345
  satisfaction and change, 228
cognitive-behavioral theory, counseling, therapy, 7, 22–23, 34
cognitive therapies, 17–18, 21–24
Cognitive Therapy, 33–34
communication, in therapy, 44–45
Community psychiatry, concept of, 331–332
compatibility of client and therapist, 334–336
conduct vs. behavior, 248–249
conflicting values, case study of, 191–197, 240–245
conjoint therapy, case study of, 16, 167–186, 202–210, 229–232
Constructivist vs Rationalist views, 292–293
Contextualism and self-consistency, 279–280
Coopersmith Self-Esteem Inventory (SEI), 278
coping

emphasizing skills, case study of, 70–72
with multiple worlds, 39–40
counter-anxiety responses, 30
cultural awareness in therapy, 20

Dasein, 312–313
Daseinsanalyse, 313
decision-maker, characteristics of, 165–166
designating the problem
   developing priorities, case study of, 51–54
   horizontal and vertical loyalties, 102
   identifying and prioritizing, 88–89
   Interpersonal/Intrapersonal Growth Scales, 89–101
   subjective perceptions of problems, 102
   sudden widowhood, case study of, 103–105, *106*, 107–117, 121
   unrequited love, case study of, 117–121
   unwanted divorce, case study of, 92–96, *96*, 97–99
Developmental Counseling and Therapy (DCT), 38
Diagnostic and Statistical Manual of Mental Disorders (DSM-IV), 20, 40, 332
discipline, parental differences in, 10–11
Discipline Beliefs Scale, 148
disclosure and trust, 264
disorders, classification of, 332
divorce
   impact on single-parent households, 5–6
   incidence in the world, 2–3
Driving Forces of Force Theory, 33

Eigenwelt, 40, 80–84, *84*, 85, 311–316, *317*, 318, 327
emotions
   arousal of self-efficacy, 276
   investment in counseling, 77–80
   unresolved and unexpected, 202–224

enmeshed parent-child relations, 149–156
ethical structure for therapists, 19–20, 342–343
existence in the three worlds, 312–314
exploring affect and attempted strategies
   case study of, 55–59

faulty thinking in Cognitive Therapy, 33–34
fear
   and anxiety, causes of, 217–219
   attributes in therapy, 42
female gender and self-esteem, 278–279
Force-Field Analysis, 33
Force Theory, 32–33
forced choices, case study of, 186–190

Gamblers Anonymous, 18
Game Without an End, The, 45
gender role and self-esteem studies, 278–279
generalizing learning onto other situations, 23–24, 247–272
   effects on personality, 248–249
   long-range planning, case study of, 260–264
   reinforcing initiative, case study of, 73–77
   temporary single parenthood, case study of, 264–271
   too many problems, case study of, 249–255, *255*, 256–260
Giving and Getting in Love Relations, *140*
growth, opportunities for, 11–13
guiding reality check, case study of, 64–69
guilt feelings from unresolved requests, case study of, 107–111, 121

historical perspective of psychotherapy, 329–337, 347–348
homework and client responsibility, 339–340

hope and determination in pursuit of goals, 117
human worth and self-rating, 291–292

identifying what does not work
case study of, 55–59
focus on the future, case study of, 133–140
intergenerational transmission of parenting styles, 147–149
lay advice, case study of, 143–147, 156–160
myths and folk sayings and case study of, 126–140
problem-solving goals, 124–126
readily available types of advice, 140, *140*, 141–160
Impact of Parenting Scale, 148
Implosion Therapy, 216
inclusionary communication style, 45
Individual Psychology Clinics, 330–332
Individualist *vs.* Microstructural theories and sex differences in parenting, 100–101
intergenerational transmission of parenting styles, 147–149
intervention targets, 23
Interpersonal/Intrapersonal Growth Scales, 89–90, *90*, 91, *91*, 92, 93–96, *96*, 97–101, 339
introducing the idea of choices, 59–63, 163–199
activities lists, 180–186
case study of, 61–63
effects of values and beliefs, 190–198
factors involved in decision making, 164–167
forced choices, 186–190

Jourard Self-Disclosure Questionnaire (SDQ), 142
journals, use in counseling, 131–140, 339

Kennedy Bill, 332

learning curve in cognitive therapies, 22–24

marital tension, effects on children, 8–10
medical *vs.* developmental model of disorder classification, 332
mental imagery
preparation for new behaviors, 202–224
in problem solving, 63–64
Mental Retardation Facilities and Community Mental Health Centers Construction Act of 1963, 332
Mitwelt, 40, 80–84, *84*, 85, 311–316, *317*, 318, 327
motivational forces in Force Theory, 32–33
multiple worlds, interacting with, 39–40
myths and folklore in problem solving case study of, 128–140

National Longitudinal Survey of Youth (NLSY), 15
National Survey of Families and Households (NSFH), 4, 15
never-married parents, incidence of, 5
new behaviors, preparation for, 63–64, 202–224
nonjudgmental approaches to problem solving, 59–63

options, choices of, 163–199

pacing of therapy, 341
Panel Study of Income Dynamics (PSID), 14
parent-child relationships, effects of divorce, 6–13
parents/parents-in-law of single-parent-households, 12–13
Partner-Specific Support Scale, 274
perception
by others, 274–275
response to, 40, 41
person-centered therapy, 17
Personal Attributes Questionnaire-Environmental form (PAQ-env), 278

Subject Index

Personal Attributes Questionnaire (PAQ), 278
phases of learning in cognitive therapies, 22–24
phases of the counseling process, 281
   coordinating and balancing the worlds, 80–84, *84*, 85, 301–328
   designating the problem areas, 50–54, 87–122
   generalizing learning onto other life situations, 72–77, 247–272
   identifying what does not work, 54–59, 123–162
   introducing the idea of choices, 59–63, 163–199
   nonjudgmental approaches to problem solving, 59–63
   reevaluating progress, 69–72, 227–246
   reconceptualizing the Self, 77–80, 273–300
   starting and proceeding along the chosen path, 63–69, 201–225
   unresolved affect, 63–69
posttraumatic stress disorder (PTSD), 36, 38
Premack's principle, 29–30
priorities, development of, 51–54
problem areas, designation of, 23, 50–54, 87–122
problem-solving goals and process, 59–63, 124–126
problems in single-parent households, 4–10
progress, reevaluating, 69–72
psychoanalytic therapy, 17
psychological study, categories for, 280–281
psychotherapy
   client's role in, 338–340
   historical perspective of, 329–337, 347–348
   involvement of the client, 338
   process variables, 21
   themes in counseling, 337–338
   theories, types of, 28–35
   therapist, role and as a person, 334–337, 340–347
   variables of, 21

quality-of-care issues in counseling, 228
Quality of Marriage Index (QMI), 274

rapport, as element of therapeutic relationships, 19
Rational Emotive Behavior Therapy (REBT), 17, 22, 36–37, 45, 247–249, 325–326
rationalist therapies, 292–293
reality, consideration during problem solving, 64–69
Reality Therapy, 17
reconceptualizing the Self, 23, 273–300
   changed outlook, case study of, 293–297
   emphasizing coping skills, case study of, 78–80
   Self as single, case study of, 281–284
   taking control, case study of, 284–288
   therapist's task and timing of, 297–298
   welfare mothers, concepts of, case study of, 290–292
reevaluating of behaviors, 23
reevaluating progress, 227–246
   conjoint therapy, case study of, 229–232
   emphasizing coping skills, case study of, 70–72
   procedures for, 232
   treatment outcome criteria, 228
reinforcing initiative, case study of, 73–77
relief and behavior change, case studies of, 212–224
responsibility of client in counseling, 338–340
Restraining Forces of Force Theory, 33
returning clients, evaluation of, 239–240

Rogerian therapy approach, 17
"role constructs" of self-identity, 292
Rosenberg Self-Esteem Scale (RSE), 274

self-acceptance, 276–279
self-concept
   opportunities for growth, 11–13
   and self-esteem, 276–279
self-consistency, 279–280
self-defeating/self-destructive behavior, 275
self-efficacy, 275–277
self-image, changes in, case study of, 78–80
self-imposed helplessness, learned helplessness, 166–167
Self in World, 80–84, *84*, 85, 311–314
self-perceptions in counseling, 77–80
self-regard, 276–279
self-regulation, failure of, 275, 280
self-sufficiency, finding solutions for, 16
Self-Verification Theory, 274–275
single-father households
   fathers as primary parents, 99–101
   incidence of, 3–5
single-mother households
   incidence of, 3–4, 5–6
   mental-health, studies of, 6
single-parent households
   attitudes and perceptions about, 13–16
   beliefs of single parents, 35, *35*, 36
   incidence of, 2–3
   temporary single parenthood, case study of, 264–272
skillful will in problem solving, 63–64, 209–210
Social Learning Theory and case study of, 30–32, 45
socioeconomic disadvantage, in single-mother households, 6–7
standards of practice, 228
starting along the chosen path, 63–69, 201–225

relief and behavior change, case studies of, 212–224
unresolved emotions, case studies of, 202–224
strengths and potential strengths in single-parent households, 10–13
subjective uncertainty *vs.* environmental uncertainty, 164–165
subjective well-being, 311
sudden widowhood, case study of, 103–105, *106*, 107–117, 121
suddenly-single parents, causes of, 3, 12–13
Supportive Parenting Index, 148
Supportive Parenting Scale, 148

teachable moments in therapy, 343–344
Temporary Assistance to Needy Families (TANF), 289
temporary single parenthood, case study of, 264–272, 319–325
tension, transmission of, 7–8
termination part of counseling process, 80–84, *84*, 85
themes in counseling, 337–338
therapeutic alliance in counseling, 20–21, 244–245, 344–345
therapeutic approaches, 16–18
therapists
   ethical structure of, 19–20, 342–343
   as a person, 345–347
   role in counseling, 340–345
therapy, conceptual elements of, 21
transmissions of emotions, in single-mother households, 7–10
treatment
   categories and specialties, 333–334
   outcome criteria, 228

Umwelt, 40, 80–84, *84*, 85, 312–316, *317*, 318, 327
Unconditional Self-Regard Scale (USRS), 277–278
unexpected options, case study of, 112–117, 121

Subject Index

United States Bureau of the Census, 3–4
unrequited love, case study of, 117–121
unresolved affect, 63
unresolved emotions in problem solving, 202–224
unwanted divorce, case study of, 92–96, *96*, 97–99, 233–239

validating interconnectedness, case study of, 81–84, *84*, 85
values
  effects on decision-making and case study of, 190–198, 240–245
  systems in different cultures, 20

verbal persuasion of self-efficacy, 276
vicarious experiences of self-efficacy, 276
victimology, attitudes of, 13

"welfare" mothers
  perceptions of, 14–16
  self-concepts and concepts of others, 288–292
widowhood and forced choices, 186–190
wisdom, balance theory of, 311
worlds of human existence and case study of, 80–84, *84*, 85
Worry-Relief cycle, 43

Springer Publishing Company

Evidence-Based Social Work Practice with Families
A Lifespan Approach
Jacqueline Corcoran, PhD

"This book is a practice overview of family social work. One of the goals is to help the reader—practitioner and student alike—to actually "do" family therapy, and Professor Corcoran reaches that goal. She also hopes to further span the gap between theory, practice, and research. Dr. Corcoran does so very nicely in this useful volume."

—**Kevin Corcoran**, PhD, JD
Professor, Graduate School of Social Work
Portland, OR

In this comprehensive text Dr. Corcoran makes implementing evidence-based clinical practice easy. She reviews the most common problem areas social workers encounter. Each chapter reviews the family treatment outcome literature, addresses different theoretical orientations, summarizes the most current clinical research studies, and provides information on standardized, self-report instruments and their validity. Topics include: child physical abuse and neglect, ADHD, sexual abuse, eating disorders, schizophrenia, caregiving of the elderly, and more.

Contents:
• Family Preservation Approaches
• Child Physical Abuse and Neglect
• Conduct Disorder
• Attention Deficit and Hyperactivity Disorder
• Sexual Abuse
• Eating Disorders
• Juvenile Offending
• Adolescent Substance Abuse
• Adult Substance Abuse
• Family Violence
• Schizophrenia
• Caregivers of the Elderly

Springer Series on Social Work
2000   600pp.   0-8261-1303-6   hardcover   www.springerpub.com

536 Broadway, New York, NY 10012-3955 • (212) 431-4370 • Fax (212) 941-7842

S *Springer Publishing Company*

Counseling Adults in Transition, 2nd Edition
Linking Practice with Theory
Nancy K. Schlossberg, EdD, **Elinor B. Waters**, EdD, and **Jane Goodman**, PhD

"A creative piece of work...It should be in every counselor's library."
—**G.M. Gazda**, EdD

"...one of the most well written and informative books I have read for some time." —**Kay Gavan**, Behaviour Research Therapy

In this updated edition of the highly successful text, the authors expand on their transition model, which offers effective adult counseling through an integration of empirical knowledge and theory with practice. The authors combine an understanding of adult development with strategies for counseling clients in personal and professional transition. A framework is provided for individual, group, and work settings. The final chapter goes beyond intervention to discuss issues such as consulting and advocacy.

Counselors, counselor educators, counselors-in-training, and other mental health professionals will find this volume an essential addition to their library of resources.

Contents:
• What Do We Need To Know?
• Adult Development Theories
• The Transition Framework
• Factors That Influence Transitions
• What Are We Likely to Hear?
• Individual Transitions
• Relationship Transitions
• Work Transitions
• What Can We Do With What We Know And Hear?
• Individual Counseling
• Group Counseling
• Consultation, Program Development, and Advocacy

First Edition: *Beahvioral Science Book Service Selection*
1995   320pp.   0-8261-4231-1   hardcover   www.springerpub.com

536 Broadway, New York, NY 10012-3955 • (212) 431-4370 • Fax (212) 941-7842